D0984251

CLINICAL LECTURES
OF SENILE
AND CHRONIC DISEASES

AGING AND OLD AGE

Advisory Editor

Robert Kastenbaum

Editorial Board

See last page of this volume
for a complete list of titles.

CLINICAL LECTURES
OF SENILE
AND CHRONIC DISEASES

J(éan) M(artin) Charcot

ARNO PRESS
A New York Times Company
New York • 1979

Editorial Supervision: Joseph Cellini

———

Reprint Edition 1979 by Arno Press Inc.

Reprinted from a copy in the Duke University Medical Library

AGING AND OLD AGE
ISBN for complete set: 0-405-11800-7
See last pages of this volume for titles.

Publisher's Note: Plates III and IV, originally in color, have been
reproduced in black and white in this edition.

Manufactured in the United States of America

———

Library of Congress Cataloging in Publication Data

Charcot, Jean Martin, 1825-1893.
    Clinical lectures on senile and chronic diseases.

    (Aging and old age)
    Translation of Leçons cliniques sur les maladies des
vieillards et les maladies chroniques.
    Reprint of the 1881 ed. published by the New Sydenham
Society, London, and issued as v. 95 of its Publications.
    1. Geriatrics. 2. Chronic diseases. I. Title.
II. Series. III. Series: New Sydenham Society,
London. Publications ; v. 95.
RC952.C4613   618.9'7   78-22189
ISBN 0-405-11807-4

A Note About This Book

J.-M. Charcot (1825-1893) was an austere, dignified and distinguished French clinician who married a wealthy woman, which made it possible for him to dedicate his life to clinical medicine, the study of Shakespeare, music, the study of diseases revealed in the art of famous painters, and other interests. His chief fame was in the field of neurology — indeed, he has been called the Father of Neurology. With a great sense of the dramatic, Charcot presented his unusual neurological cases on a small stage with candlelights. In 1867 he gave a series of lectures on old age to his students. The first lecture was a remarkable single contribution to the subject which marked the beginning of a new era in clinical medicine. He said that the need for the teaching of the clinical aspects of aging could not be disputed. His own book contains a number of valuable descriptions of pathological conditions in the aging.

THE NEW SYDENHAM SOCIETY.

Instituted MDCCCLVIII.

VOLUME XCV.

CLINICAL LECTURES

ON

SENILE AND CHRONIC DISEASES.

BY

J. M. CHARCOT,

Professeur à la Faculté de médecine de Paris, Médecin de la Salpêtrière ; Membre de l'Académie de médecine, des Sociétés " Harveian," Clinique, Pathologique, Medico-Psychologique, Medicale de Londres ; de la Société Medico Chirurgicale d'Edimbourg, &c.

TRANSLATED

BY

WILLIAM S. TUKE, M.R.C.S.

WITH PLATES AND WOODCUTS.

London :

THE NEW SYDENHAM SOCIETY.

MDCCCLXXXI.

PREFATORY NOTE BY THE AUTHOR.

LES LEÇONS "*Sur les Maladies des Vieillards et les Maladies Chroniques*," commencées à une époque de la vie où l'horizon ne parait pas encore limité, avaient été conçues sur un plan très vaste ; il ne s'agissait, en effet, de rien moins que de remanier, à la lumière d'observations personnelles, l'histoire de ces affections nombreuses et variées qui ne se rencontrent et ne s'étudient guères que d'une façon incidente, dans les hôpitaux ordinaires, tandis qu'elles se montrent, au contraire, à profusion dans les hospices, en particulier dans ce grand asile qu'on appelle la Salpêtrière. Mais des difficultés très sérieuses et qui n'avaient pas été suffisamment prévues, devaient naturellement surgir bientôt. Le champ neuropathologique n'était pas en ce temps là, ouvert à tous comme il l'est aujourd hui, et sillonné sur presque tous les points de larges voies qui en rendent le parcours relativement facile. Pour pénétrer dans ce domaine et apprendre à s'y orienter il fallut se livrer alors à une serie d'études qui exigèrent beaucoup de temps. Cependant les matériaux recueillis, chemin faisant, pendant cette période de recherches, s'etaient accumulés en grand nombre, si bien qu'il parut indispensable, à un moment donné, de les coordonner dans un ouvrage à part.*

Ceci expliquera pourquoi le présent volume est resté, et restera sans doute toujours inachevé. Je tiens à déclarer qu'en l'admettant à figurer tel qu'il est, et malgré tout ce qui lui manque, dans sa collection, la *Société de Sydenham* lui a fait, à mon avis, un très grand honneur. Je tiens également à remercier sincèrement Mr. W. S. TUKE, d'avoir bien voulu, sous la forme d'une traduction à la fois élégante et fidèle, le presenter à l'appréciation de mes confrères anglais auxquels, depuis longtemps déjà, tant de liens de sympathie m'attachent et dont je viens, une fois de plus, invoquer l'acceuil bienveillant.

J. M. CHARCOT.

PARIS, 1*er Octobre*, 1881.

---

* Les " Leçons sur les Maladies du Systême nerveux."

CONTENTS.

---◆---

INTRODUCTION.

LECTURE I.

GENERAL CHARACTERS OF SENILE PATHOLOGY.

LECTURE II.

THE FEBRILE STATE IN OLD AGE.

LECTURE III.

NODULAR RHEUMATISM AND GOUT—STATE OF THE BLOOD IN GOUT.

LECTURE IV.

MORBID ANATOMY OF GOUT.

LECTURE V.

MORBID ANATOMY OF VISCERAL GOUT.

LECTURE VI.

THE SYMPTOMS OF GOUT—THE URIC DIATHESIS—ACUTE AND CHRONIC GOUT.

LECTURE VII.

SYMPTOMS OF VISCERAL GOUT.

LECTURE XIV.

VISCERAL AFFECTIONS IN ACUTE AND CHRONIC ARTICULAR RHEUMATISM.

LECTURE XV.

SYMPTOMATOLOGY OF PROGRESSIVE CHRONIC ARTICULAR RHEUMATISM.

LECTURE XVI.

LECTURE XVII.

LECTURE XVIII.

PAGE

LECTURE XIX.

LECTURE XX.

LECTURE XXI.

LECTURE XXII.

CEREBRAL HEMORRHAGE AND SOFTENING OF THE BRAIN—MORBID ANATOMY OF
CEREBRAL HEMORRHAGE.

LECTURE XXIII.

MORBID ANATOMY OF CEREBRAL HEMORRHAGE.

LECTURE XXIV.

DIFFUSE PERIARTERITIS AND MILIARY ANEURISMS.

DESCRIPTION OF THE PLATES.

―――◆―――

PLATE I.

FIG. 1.—The right hand of a man aged 69, suffering from gout since the age of 32. A large tophus is seen at the base of the index finger, close to the metacarpo-phalangeal articulation. Another tophus, less bulky than the former, is situated at the base of the middle finger. This patient has numerous concretions of urate of sodium on the external ear.

FIG. 2.—The left hand of a woman aged 84, the subject of gout, who died at the Salpêtrière in 1863. Both hands were symmetrically affected and to the same degree. There was no appearance of tophaceous swellings in the neighbourhood of the joints. We see here the exact reproduction of one of the types of deformity of the upper extremities observed most frequently in progressive chronic articular rheumatism. The metacarpo-phalangeal articular cartilages were encrusted with urate of sodium. There were, besides, tophaceous deposits upon the dorsal aspect of the heads of the metacarpal bones, which, situated immediately under the skin and pressed against the extremities of the bones, were flattened and did not form any appreciable elevation upon the back of the hand ; so that before dissection their existence could not be recognised.

FIGS. 3, 4, 5, 6.—These figures refer to the anatomy of Heberden's nodosities. In Fig. 3 is seen the second phalangeal articulation deformed, and still covered with the soft parts. The pisiform prominences described by Heberden are well marked. Fig. 4 shows the bone exposed by dissection ; the articular extremities are enlarged in all directions in consequence of the formation of osteophytes. Fig. 5 shows the same preparation, sideways. The 4th figure should be compared with Fig. 6, which is healthy.

PLATE II.

FIGS. 1 and 2.—Deformities of the hands in general chronic articular rheumatism. The characters of the first type are well marked in Fig. 2. Fig. 1 gives a good idea of the deformities of the second type.

FIG. 3.—Alterations in the mitral valve in a case of general primarily chronic articular rheumatism.

PLATE III.

FIG. 1.—*Gouty nephritis.* Section of kidney magnified 10 diameters ; the white lines resembling chalk, *a*, are deposits of urate of sodium occupying the tubular substance, which are represented in Fig. 3 magnified 150 diameters.

FIG. 2.—Distorted uriniferous tube from the cortical substance, of which the epithelial cells *b*, large and opaque, are also filled with fatty granules (magnified 300 diameters).

FIG. 3.—Crystals of urate of sodium, *d*, forming the deposit represented in *a*, Fig. 1, as visible to the naked eye (section of tubular substance magnified 150 times).

FIG. 4.—This figure illustrates the solution of these deposits under the influence of acetic acid. The free crystals are dissolved and there only remains an amorphous deposit *e*, whose solution is proceeding slowly. It is clearly seen that a part of this deposit is situated in the interior of the uriniferous tubes *g* (section of kidney magnified 200 diameters).

FIG. 5.—Synovial fringes of the knee-joint, covered with epithelium, and presenting at *m* a deposit of urate of sodium chiefly amorphous.

N.B.—These preparations are taken from a woman with gout, aged 84, who died at the Salpêtrière in 1863, and whose left hand is represented in Pl. I., Fig. 2.

FIG. 6.—Left ear of I. M., formerly a coachman, born in Poland in 1807, and in whom the first attack of gout appeared at 25. (Hôpital Rothschild, under M. Worms.)

h. h. h. Large concretions of urate of sodium. These tophi, according to the patient, made their first appearance three years after the first attack of articular gout.

PLATE IV.

FIG. 1.—Lesions of diffuse periarteritis. *a.* Lymphatic sheath loaded with nuclei. *b.* Nuclei of this sheath notably multiplied. *c.* Artery whose muscular fibres are thinned without fatty substitution. *d.* One of the branches of the same artery whose adventitia has assumed a fibrous appearance.

FIG. 2.—Appearance presented by miliary aneurisms, *a a a,* in the cerebral convolutions.

FIG. 3.—Miliary aneurisms, *a a,* in the pons and cerebellum. *b.* Ochre-coloured focus of cerebellar hemorrhage at a point symmetrical with one where some aneurisms are intact.

PLATE V.

FIG. 1.—Periarteritis where the muscular fibres have disappeared at the same time that the nuclei of the adventitia are multiplied and the vessel is dilated.

FIG. 2.—*a.* Middle cerebral artery. *b.* Artery of the optic thalamus. *c.* Aneurism in the optic thalamus.

FIG. 3.—Arterioles affected with periarteritis and presenting moniliform dilatations.

PLATE VI.

FIG. 1.—Vessel broken and surrounded by a fragment of clot, which to the naked eye simulated a miliary aneurism.

FIG. 2.—Arteriole from the wall of a recent focus. *a.* Miliary aneurism broken. *b.* Clot formed by the extravasated blood which has distended, then burst the sheath. *c.* Lymphatic sheath burst. *d.* Another aneurism also burst.

FIG. 3 —Miliary aneurism which has been burst by pressure, showing its coagulated contents.

FIG. 4.—Arteriole with three aneurismal dilatations, one of which has burst under pressure.

INTRODUCTION.

---◆---

EMPIRICAL AND SCIENTIFIC MEDICINE—COMPARISON BETWEEN
THE ANCIENTS AND MODERNS.

GENTLEMEN,—The course which we commence to-day is
intended to make you acquainted with the general characters
which distinguish the pathology of old age from that of adult
life, and to fix your attention upon certain of the diseases which
are more especially met with in hospitals for the aged.

I shall restrict myself as much as possible to giving that
methodic character to my lectures which is adapted to all
theoretic teaching. I shall never lose sight of the clinical
aspect, and quite hope to show you at the bedside examples
of the types which will serve as the starting-point of my
descriptions.

You now know the object of these studies; we might plunge
directly into the subject, for I am of Condillac's opinion, and
think that general considerations are better placed at the end,
than at the beginning, of a course. But there exists a kind of
classical tradition which obliges the professor first of all to
explain himself, more or less categorically, on certain fundamental questions, and to declare, so to speak, his profession of
scientific faith.

I do not think it right to disregard this obligation, and I
shall enter boldly upon the accomplishment of this often
thankless and always difficult task, reckoning upon your
indulgence and the kindness you have so often shown me.

There is a simple and, so to speak, natural means of approaching these larger questions : it is to examine how, in the
course of the progressive development of scientific culture, such
questions have arisen, and how they have been solved; history
thus becomes a means of criticism. Now, in following this
method one soon perceives that at no period has pure observation succeeded in dominating the spirit of speculation without

B

supreme efforts.   As for Medicine, which is alone to occupy us
here, even the most stoical intellects have never been found to
limit themselves to establishing facts without trying to connect
them by some sort of theory ; from the beginning we see minds
occupied as much (or even more) with the subjective relations of
things as with their actual reality; newly acquired empirical
observations are compared and tested with one another, in order
to make theories or systems issue from them.*   There, let us
remember, lies a necessity of the human mind, and it seems, to
use a celebrated expression of Kant's, that our thoughts are
necessarily formed in this uniform mould.   This was clearly
recognised by the founder of the Positive Philosophy himself,
and no one will reproach him with opening the door to
hypotheses when he declared that, though a theory should be
exclusively based on observations, it is absolutely necessary to
be guided by a theory in order to devote oneself to observation
fruitfully.

But with reference to this, we can always distinguish the real
needs of our intellect from the exaggerations of every kind into
which the lovers of systems allow themselves to be drawn.   We
recognise in fact the existence of a speculative method based
rigorously upon facts, as well as the existence of a method of
observation which keeps itself as far as possible from premature
speculations ; and consequently we have now only to find out on
what ground these two methods can unite.

Gentlemen, from our point of view I think I recognise an
essential difference between ancient and modern medicine.   The
former has always wanted the elements necessary to build up a
positive theory, and that is why the numerous attempts it has
made in that direction have always come to grief.   The moderns
on the contrary possess some of the materials which can be used
in this work of construction ; but above all, they know, profiting
by the errors of their predecessors, which roads ought to remain
closed to speculation, and which, on the contrary, they may
traverse without fear of losing themselves.

It is to develop this position that I shall devote this lecture ;
but first I must indicate at what point in history the old
medicine came to an end in order to give place to the new.

* Dechambre, Introduction to the *Dictionnaire encyclopédique des sciences médicales*,
p. xix.

I.

In our days Medicine has seen a profound and radical revolution taking place.

We should no doubt have to go back to very distant times to discover the first origin and starting-point of this great change, the influence of which we feel to this day. But it was only towards the close of last century, and at the beginning of our own, that the direction of this movement became clearly marked, and the end whither it is tending became revealed in vivid colours. To say that an impassable gulf opened between the old and the new medicine, would evidently be going much too far. No, the links of tradition are not broken. The labour of past times has not been lost, and we carefully preserve the immense heritage which our predecessors have accumulated as the centuries rolled on, but it must be admitted that new horizons have opened for us, and that the point of view of modern science has been elevated by the change.

The pioneers in this reform were Vesalius, Harvey, Morgagni, and Bichat, the creator of general anatomy. Corvisart, Laennec, Broussais were powerful aiders of the movement. Then came our immediate teachers, Andral, Rostan, Bouillaud, Cruveilhier, Magendie, Rayer, and I am glad to point out to you that all these names are French. It seems that the marvellous progress lately attained by experimental physiology under the influence of Müller, Claude Bernard, Longet, Brown-Séquard, has at last carried away the halting and the timid, and decided the situation.

The essential character of this revolution consists in the direct, immediate—and let us add, legitimate—intervention of anatomy and physiology in the domain of pathology.

Before this period Medicine was almost entirely occupied in the study of symptoms ; afterwards it became first anatomical, then physiological, and acquired really scientific tendencies.

I believe it is possible to reduce to two characteristic features the fundamental principles adopted by modern Medicine :—

1. Firstly, while symptoms were formerly considered in an abstract manner, and to a certain extent as outside the organism, to-day they are closely bound up with it. We have to search for the seat of the mischief, according to the doctrine of Bichat.

B 2

Carried along by his inflexible logic, Broussais proclaims that there can be no derangement of functions without a corresponding lesion of organs (to-day we should say, of tissues) : in short, symptoms are henceforth only the cry of the suffering organs.

2. Secondly, while the disease was formerly considered as a being independent of the organism, a kind of parasite attached to the economy ; to-day—and it is again to Broussais that we owe the clear enunciation of this principle—it is nothing but a disturbance of the inherent properties of our organs. We have to do not with the appearance of fresh laws, but with the perversion and derangement of pre-existing laws.

The enormous part which must be taken in future by the facts of anatomy and physiology in the interpretation of morbid phenomena is now understood ; may we say that these two sciences will absorb pathology and rule it absolutely ?

Gentlemen, here a serious difficulty occurs, which calls for discussion ; I ask your permission to enter for this purpose on certain digressions.

No doubt pathology may be vividly illumined by physiology, but certainly it could not have been deduced from it.

Allow me therefore to recall to you a profound thought which we find in Hippocrates : " Who could have foreseen from the structure of the brain that wine can derange its functions ? " Who would have learnt from his knowledge of the human body, adds Littré, who cites this passage, that emanations from marshes produce intermittent fever ? The problem, you see, is complex. In short, beyond the physiological condition supposed to be known, the kind of effect produced by a morbific agent has still to be sought for. In other terms, in order to know what will be the effects upon a healthy organism, of a morbific agent, it is absolutely necessary that the experiment should be made.

One sees in this way that pathology rightly maintains a certain autonomy and independence of anatomy and physiology. The mere establishment of pathological facts evidently furnishes us with data of much importance and independent value, and here we have what may be called the material of Medicine. The intervention of the biological sciences, including the physico-chemical knowledge belonging to them, is here, doubtless, indispensable ; our researches without their point of support,

would most often be made at random and in the dark;* but
their *rôle*, in so far as we have to do with pathological observation, is in some degree subordinate; they are the means, not
the end. The observer limits himself, as he wishes to do, to
recording facts and contemplating them in their natural con-
nections. This we take to be the true character of empirical
medicine, using the word in all the dignity of its etymological
meaning. In short, by this expression is meant science in a
still imperfect state and at a time when facts are not united
together by a physiological theory.†

"The day when science," said Requin, "has attained to a
complete knowledge of normal man to the utmost depths of his
organisation and the most hidden mysteries of his life; the day
on which she has unveiled all the secrets of the pathological
state, and comprehended all the modifications which external
agents produce upon the economy, on that day science will be
complete."‡ But to-day the reality is very far from reaching
this ideal; pathology, physiology, anatomy itself, are in process
of evolution.

I believe it also to be a wise method to keep systematically
separate, though only provisionally, the two points of view which
I have indicated, while I should favour as much as possible
their legitimate meeting. In one word, we must, as Bordeu
would have said, avoid marrying doctrine and practice by force
and against the grain.

Having made these reservations, I am foremost in recognising
the immense services rendered to pathology by the well-directed
application of modern physiology, and to proclaim loudly that
in this direction lies the future of medicine.

For the rest, what was wanting in our predecessors was not a
feeling of the importance to be accorded to physiology in medical
studies, but more exact and extended notions about the difficult
problems which they sometimes tried to solve without having

* "The clinical observations collected now-a-days are not superior to those of former
centuries, except by reason of the advance of the moderns beyond the ancients in the
matter of anatomical and physiological knowledge."—C. Robin, *Journal de l'Anatomie,*
etc., 1867, p. 297.

† Littré, *Dictionnaire de la langue française,* article, "Empirisme."

‡ Boerhaave had said: "Qui itaque haberet perfecte intellectas omnes conditiones
requisitas ad actiones, ille perspiceret clare defectum conditionis ex cognito morbo, et
rursus bene caperet ex cognito defectu naturam morbi inde necessario sequentis."

measured their depth. It may indeed be said that at all times people have been obliged to interpret pathological facts from the point of view of the then reigning physiology.

Let me quote to you the appropriate words of Daremberg, who speaks on this point with all the authority given by a thorough knowledge of history : " Nothing is better than a wise physiology, or at least, a physiology which, resting on experiment, bears within itself the inexhaustible germs of perfectibility. Such a physiology transforms medicine and reforms therapeutics ; but there is nothing more disastrous, more contrary to the progress of pathology, than a bad physiology, a physiology *a priori*, which, each day, finds in itself the best reasons for sinking deeper and deeper into darkness and of restraining the free play of science. In vain the most delicate and difficult observations became multiplied in the Hippocratic school at Alexandria; ideas were more obstinate than facts. Physiology resisted so well that it distorted the discoveries of anatomy and the conquests of pathology, in order to range them under its laws. When on the contrary, in the hands of Galen, the experimental method, already attempted in the school of Alexandria, had transformed the physiology of the nervous system, then medicine changed its front." *

Now, gentlemen, this physiology *a priori* is alone responsible for those too famous systems, which on divers occasions have exercised so fatal an influence on the development of science. Naturalism, Stahlianism, and all the forms of ancient and modern Vitalism, without excepting that of Bichat, are bound to it on one side ; Iatro-mechanicism, Iatro-chemism are bound to it on the other. The former detach from the organism the principles of life, in order to make them rule over it as capricious tyrants; the latter rashly endeavour to give a physical or chemical interpretation of life, and that at a time when no one even suspected the true relationships between biology and the physical sciences. Such errors are happily impossible in our days. Standing on positive foundations, physiology can no longer be a danger to Medicine : it has become on the contrary Medicine's most solid support. It envelopes it on every side, and, if I may so speak, in a close-netted armour, which no longer gives passage to rash speculations ; and if in our days errors are still sometimes com-

* " Résumé de l'histoire de la médecine," etc., *Union médicale*, 1865.

mitted, they point only to a vice in the application of the method, and not to an error in its principles.

Against the usurpation of a mistaken physiology, wise and well-poised minds have always protested with energy; and it is especially this point which is so admirable in those physicians, who have been devoted by principle to the culture of pure observation, and in whose foremost rank stands out the grand figure of Hippocrates.

Gentlemen, what have been the results of this Medicine, carefully isolated from all outside contact, reduced in consequence to its own powers, and founded on pure observation? What has been its character, to what does it aspire, where does its dominion cease? These are questions which well deserve examination. History offers us on this subject an experiment ready-made, which has been prolonged for many centuries, and the results of which are to-day offered for our judgment.

II.

But this conducts us deep into antiquity, to the grandest days of Greece, the age of Pericles.*

At that period anatomy only existed in the most rudimentary state; the nervous system was not yet distinguished from tendinous structures. The brain was regarded as a gland. The arteries were supposed to be full of air, and the real arrangement of the venous system was entirely unknown.

Physiology was at an even lower point; it rested only on fanciful notions; it had not even disengaged itself from the speculative philosophy of the time, which in its audacious aspirations for an immediate comprehension of the universe, neglected the patient modest search for facts, and considered that almost unworthy of a sage. For the radical error of Greek philosophy, as Herschel† has well said, was in imagining that the method which had been so splendidly successful in mathematics, could also be applied to objective reality, and that by starting with the most elementary notions or the most evident axioms, everything could be argued out.

* In this section the influence of Littré's fine interpretation of the work of Hippocrates will be readily recognised.
† Discourse on *The Study of Natural Philosophy.*

In the midst of such apparently unfavourable circumstances, we see the school of Cos make its appearance. It appears before us directing all its criticism against the Cnidian physicians, who had not been able, like it, to resist the invasion of the philosophy of the period. It affirmed that Medicine must proceed in its own paths, supporting itself on facts, not on hypotheses ; in this way it built up that edifice, which has been the admiration of every age.

It might be compared to those *chefs-d'œuvre* of Greek sculpture, executed by artists who had only observed external forms, and the beauty of which all our anatomical knowledge has not enabled us to surpass.

Hippocrates regarded the body in its entirety, and, so to speak, in its broad outlines, without pretending to penetrate its internal mechanism.

He considered it too in its relation with the external world, so as to establish the modifications which it receives therefrom.

This latter point of view led him to a broad and comprehensive etiology, in which the influence of season and climate, and among individual causes, that of age, appeared in especial relief.

Just as the year passes through successive stages of heat and cold, dryness and humidity, the human body experiences changes, from which diseases derive their character. On this foundation is established the doctrine of medical constitutions corresponding to particular states of the atmosphere, which doctrine has lasted to our day in spite of the exaggerations it has often been subjected to, because it contains a nucleus of truth.

As to climate, it is only a kind of permanent season, the effect of which is more marked because its influence is always in operation. If the Greeks are brave and free, while the Asiatics are emasculate and enslaved, that has to do with the climate in which these races dwell. This idea, you see, contains in germ, the geographical fatalism developed in modern times by Herder, whose doctrine has lately been so cleverly worked out by a philosophic writer, M. Taine, under the name of Theory of Surrounding Conditions [*milieux*]. Their exaggeration was flagrant ; yet who would contest the influence of climates on the habitual temper both of body and mind, and above all, on the diseases with which we may be affected ?

Following this analogy, Hippocrates considered different ages as the seasons of life, and consequently attributed to them special maladies. Without accepting this interpretation, modern science has fully confirmed the reality of the fact ; and we know that there exist diseases which are in close relation with people's ages.

What strikes us at once, and impresses us most vividly in the Hippocratic pathology, is the importance he attributes to the general, and his indifference to the local, state. This point of view would seem curiously exclusive if one forgot the conditions under which Hippocrates was observing. For he had specially concentrated his attention upon acute febrile diseases, and especially no doubt, as Littré's remark implies, upon the remittent or pseudo-continued fevers, which are still prevalent in Greece as they were in the days of Hippocrates. Now it must be admitted that the febrile state is always an almost identical process, independent of the causes which produce it, and of the varied forms which it assumes. What Hippocrates regarded as most important was to look for certain signs which would enable him to foresee the crises, incidents, and issue of the malady, and furnish him with indications in the employment of remedies.

To arrive at this result, he examined attentively the expression of the features, the colour of the face, the attitude of the patient, the heat of the body, the respiratory movements, the urine, the sweat, the various evacuations. Is it not with the same end in view that we try to estimate the patient's strength, the degree of tension of his arterial system, the oscillations of his general temperature, when the local condition furnishes no useful indications ? It was not merely for the sake of the theory of crises, which, submitted to the rude test of modern criticism, has not survived, deprived as it has been of the practical character which the ancients gave it.

You see, gentlemen, by this rapid sketch of the Hippocratic pathology to what results the method of observation may lead; the facts which it collects, the points of view which it allows, can resist the action of time. They have come down to us without losing anything of their striking truth. We see also how, without leaving its legitimate sphere, this method may suggest generalisations, as well as furnish data of a superior order.

If there exists a method of observation which is specially analytical and limited to matters of detail, in which method the moderns have particularly excelled, there exists also a general kind of observation, more familiar perhaps to the ancients, which does not limit itself to an examination of isolated phenomena, but which regards them on the contrary in their mutual bearings, in their order of succession ; in short, as Nature presents them to him who can get a bird's-eye view of things.

Thus it has come to be recognised that each disease has an evolution of its own, a special mode of development, a particular grouping of symptoms, which allow us to describe it according to a common type, in spite of the variability of accessory circumstances. Thence arose the notion of morbid unities or species, a notion perfectly exact, since it corresponds to a fact of experience, but the meaning of which became singularly altered when people went so far as to consider diseases as concrete beings like individuals, and on the same footing as animals or plants.

It is now seen that sometimes the disease goes rapidly through its successive periods to reach its natural termination ; while sometimes, on the contrary, it requires a long space of time to pass through the different phases of its evolution. Thence comes the distinction established between acute maladies and chronic affections, which evidently corresponds to the facts of clinical observation, but which must not be regarded as an absolute line of demarcation, since the acute and the chronic form of one and the same pathological state merge into one another by insensible transitions.

Again, it has been determined by multiplied observations that different morbid states may coexist or succeed one another in the same individual or family according to a determined order and certain laws; and it has been concluded by very simple reasoning, or rather by a direct intuition, that these affections are not isolated, but are dependent on a common cause which serves as a link between them. Thus was produced the great conception of constitutional and diathetic diseases. This idea arose, then, from pure observation. Hypothesis only commences at the moment, when, to give a body to this unknown cause, the mind has imagined, according to the taste of the period, sometimes an influence of the nervous system, sometimes a modification of the crasis of the humours, or the presence of morbific matter in the blood.

In the course of time, analytic succeeded synthetic observation, though the latter was not altogether neglected. And thus as the world grew older, science was constantly enriched by general or partial facts, and these constitute indeed the only traditional medicine that commands our respect. We may close here this rapid review. The examples which we have given are sufficient to enable us to understand the resources of the method of observation as applied to medicine, even when it voluntarily limits itself to the sphere of the external phenomena of the disease, that is to say, of the symptoms.

But at the same time it is easy to see that a pathology thus deprived of its natural supports could, even in the cleverest hands, only end in a more or less elevated empiricism. That, no doubt, is what constitutes at the beginning the basis of every scientific structure, and on such foundations it has even been possible to establish a practical system of medicine, which nothing could hinder from reaching a certain degree of perfection. But the work remains incomplete, and the human mind, pushed on by an irresistible force, cannot stop on the way.

The efforts which it made to complete its task necessarily remained sterile so long as anatomy and physiology remained undeveloped. It is this which should make us indulgent to the successive systems which have been constructed from antiquity to our own times. But at last the hour has come, the reform has been accomplished, and we can perceive to-day the fruits which it has borne, as well as foresee those which it will bear in the future.

III.

Passing at a single bound over a space of 2,000 years, we will now place the results of pure observation in comparison with the labours of the modern mind, armed with all the means of investigation which it possesses to-day. And to make the contrast more striking, we will pass silently over the periods of transition so as to occupy ourselves only with the scientific movement which actually belongs to our own century.

No doubt, gentlemen, you have often heard of a new as opposed to an ancient pathological anatomy. It will be convenient to determine, first of all, what these expressions mean.

Here we come upon a historical point to which I must draw your attention for a moment ; it belongs to quite modern history, for it is not long since pathological anatomy first asserted itself as a special branch of learning. One of the first attempts at systematisation, which was made in France, dates from 1812. The enunciation of the doctrine, its code, if one may say so, is found recorded in one of the first articles of the great "Dictionnaire des sciences médicales." This document, precious in so many ways, is signed by two illustrious names, Bayle and Laennec.

I should like, gentlemen, to describe in few words this first pathological anatomy, which for nearly half a century reigned without opposition.

Its means of investigation are very simple : it takes the word anatomy in its strictly etymological sense, and is as yet only acquainted with the scalpel.

In its view the alterations in organs are to be described only according to their relation to neighbouring parts, their volume, consistence, density, colour, and general aspect.

It is not possible for it as a rule to look for characters in modifications of texture, this being nearly always almost ignored.

What efforts are not necessary to establish, by help of such methods, the identity of an anatomical type ! But the masters of this subject surpassed themselves and produced more than one inimitable model. After all, every one understands how difficult it is to fix in the mind characters so fugitive as those drawn for example from *aspect* and *colour*. Shades and contrasts can only be pourtrayed with difficulty by the most imaginative language. Moreover, the morbid anatomist has often felt the need of being an artist himself, or of invoking aid from an outsider's brush. It was natural that Art should intervene where the external appearance is so important. We owe to its aid more than one precious collection, and, above all, the imperishable monument raised by Prof. Cruveilhier, the "Atlas d'Anatomie pathologique du corps humain."

It was foreseen from the beginning that a day would come when all the lesions which the naked eye can recognise would be definitely described, classed, and catalogued. The work, they thought, would then be completed ; for they did not see from what side perfection would come. That is why, no doubt, the

masters of the school only ascribed to their science a very modest *rôle* in the sum of pathological knowledge. They always obliged themselves to circumscribe it within narrow limits, as though they wished in this way to preserve it from all the temptations which might have compromised it.

In the first place, they are quick to declare that their anatomy has no applications except in a restricted number of diseases, since in many of them there are no lesions appreciable to its modes of investigation.

Again, even in the domain of structural diseases where it seemed right for it to enter, its *rôle* is still by no means ambitious. Its object is mainly that of enriching nosography by new light, permitting the distinction of diseases whose symptomatic resemblance might have caused them to be confounded. The distinction once made, the object is attained, for morbid anatomy voluntarily limits itself to contemplating the lesion itself independently of the symptoms which accompany it. No explanation is to be sought in this direction of the immediate cause of diseases or their mode of production.

Such, gentlemen, if I mistake not, are the most essential characters of that morbid anatomy which has sometimes been ironically called *dead anatomy*. I have exaggerated nothing; I think I have faithfully expressed what were the tendencies of its first exponents.

It is true that their successors or rivals have often overstept the limits which they had imposed, and it is easy still to trace their brilliant incursions into more than one region which had been considered closed to morbid anatomy.

But the method remained in use, at least as a whole, though the moment was near when it was to undergo a radical reform.

You know, gentlemen, the profound changes introduced into Medicine by the Anatomical School, as it is called, although it had imposed on itself such limited and circumscribed functions. It is a point on which I need not insist. I wish to make it especially clear, that even to-day, in spite of so much progress accomplished in all directions, its teachings have preserved in great measure all their authority and reality. Thus, naked-eye studies, such as it instituted, the autopsy, as conducted by it, will ever form the first operation through which every regular investigation must necessarily pass.

These considerations make it easy to foresee that the new anatomy may be called in to complete the old, in order to extend and develop it, but the former will never be substituted for the latter. Gentlemen, if I were to describe in a single word the services rendered to us by this first pathological anatomy, the creation of which must be reckoned among the glories of our country, I should say that it has taught the physician to *think anatomically.*

When circumstances, long in preparation, had made development and reform possible, this commenced through the influence of physiology, which had been entirely renovated, and had entered decidedly on the path of experiment—the physiology of Magendie and Legallois. It was ultimately accomplished by the intervention of histology armed with the microscope.

It became recognised then, that the physician has not merely to know about the dead organ as it is seen at the autopsy, but that he must be able to image in the light of physiological notions the living active organ, exercising its proper functions and modified by the morbid state. The lesion which he has before his eyes represents only one of the phases, and often the last, of a morbid process, the course of which he must trace back to the primitive effects of the morbific agent.

There I have traced the physiological programme, but as you will see for yourselves, it would long have remained an unknown region had it not been for the aid of histology.

As we have seen, the anatomist's principle was to stop abruptly at the surface of the organ. If now and then the microscope was used in studying the lesions, its employment was directed in this kind of research by no systematic idea. But, gentlemen, in histology the microscope is not the only thing to be thought of ; there is, besides, a system, a doctrine. Herein especially does this doctrine consist : *The analysis must penetrate the depths of the organ even to its elements or indecomposable anatomical parts.*

It is in these elements that the real conditions of local life exist ; the organ is but an aggregate, a total, a resultant. We must then penetrate as far as the elements by the help of microscope and reagents, in order to grasp the modifications which they undergo under the influence of morbific causes, and in order

to deduce from these modifications the *rationale* of the disturbance experienced by the whole.

Thus, gentlemen, morbid histology, from which histo-chemistry cannot be separated, does not merely aim at a diminution of the number of non-structural diseases, by showing that lesions may exist where the naked eye cannot perceive them, not only at the furnishing of new means of diagnosis and nosographic characters ; neither is its *rôle* limited to unveiling the hidden reason of the morbid appearances recorded and arranged by means of the microscope, and in impressing upon them a more definite and scientific character by associating each of them with a corresponding modification of the texture of the organs : its aims are far wider—a kind of intimate morbid physiology, which, so to speak, follows step by step in each elementary part, the varied phases of the morbid process, seizing upon the least transitions which connect the morbid with the normal state.

In this direction, you see, *histological morbid anatomy* comes in contact with pathogenesis, or rather merges in it. At the same time it is allied to physiology, which in this special direction assumes the name of pathological physiology.

But observe, gentlemen, for this is an essential point, the aim which morbid anatomy proposes to itself cannot be attained without establishing a constant association between the lesion, studied even in the finest details of its development, and those morbid occurrences which have been carefully observed at the bedside of the patient. In this way, by an inevitable consequence and a logical necessity, morbid anatomy, as it penetrates more deeply into the real nature of the tissues, becomes at the same time more animated, more living, and tends to mould itself more accurately with clinical teaching.

Nevertheless, gentlemen, before a manifest functional disturbance, the seat of which is indicated by physiology, histological analysis is still often powerless to demonstrate a structural abnormality, corresponding to the disturbance of function. Are we obliged to recognise, contrary to all analogy, that a functional lesion, a disturbance of the properties of an organ, can exist without any corresponding structural modification ? For myself, pressed on this question, I should not hesitate immediately to place myself on the side of Reil, Broussais, Georget, and so

many other eminent minds; I should recollect that even in
normal vital processes the action of our organs is not accomplished without material change, without destruction and cor-
relative repair. All functioning tends to destroy the machinery
by means of which it is effected. Muscle in repose has an
alkaline reaction, but becomes acid when fatigued. A similar
modification has been observed in nerve and spinal marrow,
and, according to Heynsius and Funke, the cerebral substance
itself is acid while we are awake, alkaline during sleep. Such
examples make us see well enough that the maintenance of life
is bound up with a ceaseless molecular activity in the anatomical
elements, which expresses itself by appreciable chemical phenomena. Is it not easy to conceive that there may exist lesions
of elements, which, without altering their form, interfere with
this organic motion without which the functions could not be
accomplished? Without altering their shape, carbonic oxide
takes from the red disks their power of absorbing oxygen.
Thenceforth they roll like an inert dust in the torrent of the
circulation; and without the change of colour which they present, nothing would indicate the profound alteration they have
undergone. May not an analogous alteration of the blood
corpuscles be at least suspected in those grave states of the
organism which are shown by intense dyspnœa without there
being any lesion of the lungs or heart? In those who have
succumbed rapidly in the course of acute articular rheumatism,
the blood, and the serosity contained in the pericardium and
synovial cavities often give an acid reaction. In those struck
by lightning, anatomy often reveals no appreciable lesion, and
yet cadaveric rigidity comes on almost directly after death,
scarcely persists at all, and almost immediately gives place to
rapid putrefaction. The same thing happens in over-driven
animals, and also, as Brown-Séquard has shown, in a limb whose
vital properties have been exhausted by the prolonged action of
an electric current. Is it not nearly certain that almost all
these changes, which only death enables us to demonstrate, correspond to structural changes which already existed during life,
but which have remained till now inaccessible to our means of
investigation? But let us not insist on this point; let it
suffice to have led you into a region but little explored, yet which
promises abundant harvests for the future.

IV.

Gentlemen, we have still to determine the relations which now exist between pathology and physiology.

It is no longer a question of the speculative or contemplative physiology of past times, but of the science which the modern masters, the successors of Haller, Legallois, and Magendie, have made for us.

Always remembering that living beings present phenomena which are not found in dead nature, and which consequently are their especial property, the new physiology absolutely refuses to consider life as a mysterious and supernatural influence, which acts at the instigation of caprice and is free from every law.

It goes so far as to believe that vital properties will one day be combined with properties of a physical order; at least, it insists for the future that a correspondence, not an antagonism, must be established between these two forms of energy.

It sets itself to reduce all the vital manifestations of a complex organism to the action of certain organs, and this again to the properties of certain tissues, of certain well-defined elements.

It does not seek the ultimate nature, or the *wherefore* of things, for experience has shown it that the human mind cannot go beyond the *how*, that is, beyond the immediate causes or the conditions of existence of phenomena.

It recognises that in this relation the limits of our knowledge are the same in biology as in physics and chemistry. It remembers that beyond a certain point, as Bacon said, Nature becomes deaf to our questions and replies to them no longer.

It has no wish to lord it over medicine, but only to illumine it and furnish a solid basis for its speculations.

It brings to medicine, lastly, a long-tried method, the experimental method, that admirable instrument, which in its hands has already unveiled so many mysteries.

A master of physiology, Claude Bernard, expresses himself as follows in several passages of the remarkable book which you all know, in which he discusses so profoundly the question which here occupies us.*

* *Introduction à l'étude de la médecine expérimentale.* Paris, 1865. See especially pp. 117, 119, 125, 127, 140, 336, 343, 347, 348, 358, 369.

C

I will limit myself to making clear the express condition which he himself imposes upon all allowable intervention of physiology in the domain of medicine. Pathological observation first, physiological interpretation last—such, says he, is the universal rule; establish first the morbid phenomena, seek then to explain them from the physiological point of view, whenever the actual state of science permits it. The inverse method, which consists in starting from anatomy and physiology in order to deduce from them the conditions of the disease, is full of dangers and beset with risks. Let us not be seduced by elegant notions and ingenious views which this method may suggest, for experience shows that too often it has led to a fanciful conventional physiology, which corresponds to nothing in the reality of things.

It seems to me unnecessary, gentlemen, to insist long on the innumerable services already rendered to medicine by a judicious intervention of the data of modern physiology;* but I must stop a moment over what it has been agreed to call experimental pathology.

The mutilations which the physiologist produces in animals, with the aim of penetrating the mechanism of normal action, are almost always accompanied by various morbid disturbances, which may then become a subject of meditation for the physician. But experiment may be applied even more directly to the problems which pathology offers him. We have the power, in short, of creating in animals different morbid states, either by making them undergo certain mutilations, or by submitting them to the action of poisons, viruses, venoms, putrid substances, etc. The idea of thus producing artificial diseases is far from being new, and we must go back to Lower, Baglivi, Van Swieten, Autenrieth, in order to find the first traces of it. But it is especially in these last years, after the impulse given by Magendie, that experimental pathology has been really established and has had full scope. The works of C. Bernard, Longet, B. Séquard, Virchow, Traube, Vulpian, and so many others are evidences of what may be expected from this method. The brilliant results which it has already given in its short career must not make us

* Consult on this subject the remarkable discourse of my ·friend Brown-Séquard before the College of Physicians of Ireland, 3rd Feb., 1865, "On the Importance of the Application of Physiology to the Practice of Medicine and Surgery," in *Dublin Quarterly Review of Med. Sci.*, May, 1865.

forget that certain limits seem imposed upon it. Experiment succeeds in producing a transient glycosuria by means of a traumatic lesion. It reproduces wonderfully the various events of thrombosis and embolism. It accelerates or paralyses at will the movements of the heart. It determines at will the accidents of uræmia. By means of certain lesions of the nervous system it can cause pleurisy, pneumonia, acute pericarditis, more or less like those observed in man. It has recently succeeded in developing in an animal the phenomena of traumatic fever, by injecting into the blood the liquid taken from the surface of a recent wound in another animal; and thus is found confirmed a view long since advanced by a French surgeon. But it may be said that slowly-developed affections usually escape it. Constitutional and diathetic maladies especially seem inaccessible to it;* and how could it be otherwise when the conditions of development of these diseases are generally unknown to the physician himself? But let us not fail to remark the analogies which exist in some respects between so-called spontaneous diathetic diseases and certain slow poisonings, such as plumbism and chronic alcoholism, which have been successfully reproduced in animals, in imitation of the corresponding affections in man. Recall, too, the remarkable experiments by means of which my illustrious friend Brown-Séquard produced in the guinea-pig a sort of epilepsy, which was hereditarily transmissible.

Even if experimental pathology is impotent to produce certain general maladies, it can often imitate their symptoms and make them appear one by one, though not always in the regular order of their natural succession. It can also facilitate the study of certain general questions, such as local susceptibility and predisposition, and throw light on the mechanism of the generalisation of morbid states. We owe to it lastly that splendid analytical study of poisons, the results of which already presage the approaching formation of a really rational system of therapeutics.

And now, gentlemen, it would be easy to me to prove to you that by combining clinical data with those furnished by morbid anatomy and histology and by physiological experiment, we sometimes succeed in reaching a conception of certain morbid states, which is really rational and almost complete. But time presses and I must conclude.

* See G. Sée, *Leçons de pathologie expérimentale*, p. 11. Paris, 1866.

c 2

V.

We must now take note of the conclusions to which the comparison, which we have tried to trace between the pure observation of the ancients and the modern method, ought to lead.

1. I think I have shown that the empirical method is the necessary vestibule of science. We could never abandon this method, tested by the experience of ages. It will always be of use to control and counterbalance scientific speculations.

2. But there is a side on which theoretical views may and must be rightly introduced into pathology. Perfected by the employment of new methods, clinical observation will ally itself with the general sciences, and approach nearer and nearer to physiology, so as to give birth to a really rational system of medicine.

Such is the end towards which we have to advance ; but our progress in this direction must be with prudence, and we must avoid giving way to hasty generalisations. That would be to compromise the future of this great movement of renovation in which we are taking part to-day.

But, some will say, what use are these big words and grand ideas ? Have the scientific tendencies about which you make so much fuss had a beneficial influence on the practice of the art ? Do you cure more patients than they cured of old ? These, gentlemen, are very indiscreet questions, and might easily be thrown back at our adversaries. Let it suffice to reply with an honoured teacher, that art without science is not slow to degenerate into routine.* That hackneyed scepticism, which people so willingly oppose to all progress of the human mind, is a comfortable pillow for lazy heads ; but the period in which we live allows no time for falling asleep.

To put in its true light the happy influence which scientific tendencies may have on the advance of medicine, I need only recall to you the remarkable transformation which in the course of the last twenty years this science has undergone in a neighbouring country to ours, in Germany. Let us transport our-

---

* "Be sure that practice, without incessant scientific renewal, would very soon become a belated and stereotyped routine."—Béhier, *Leçon d'ouverture du cours de clinique médicale*, p. 19. Paris, 1867.

selves a moment across the frontier, and go back in thought towards the year 1830. At that time Schelling and his audacious " Philosophy of Nature " reigned absolute masters over German minds. The fashion was for poetic points of view and transcendental conceptions, while a physician allowed himself in a treatise on mucous fever seriously to compare a blood corpuscle to the terrestrial globe, because both are round, flattened at the poles, and possess a central nucleus surrounded by an atmosphere.*

During this time medicine was thus reduced to a deplorable condition. Although they possessed translations of the chief pathological works recently published in France and England, yet the progress long accomplished in these two countries remained as though it had never taken place, for none of them understood its importance. An accurate local diagnosis was never made either in hospital or in private practice. In more than one German university the stethoscope was almost unknown ; if anybody happened to come across one of these instruments he examined it with a sort of infantile curiosity, or received with unfavourable jokes those few eccentric individuals, who, by means of this bit of wood, professed to hear *unheard of* things. Besides, most chest and heart diseases, as well as chronic skin affections, formed an almost unexplored territory. And when they began to talk of the French it was only to ridicule, this time with more show of justice, the curious mania which made them look upon all diseases as inflammations.†

Things remained thus till near 1840. Then began the work of regeneration (chiefly through Schönlein's influence) by the introduction of the French methods into clinical work. Then it was the turn of morbid anatomy, brilliantly represented at Vienna by Rokitansky. But already Müller had appeared in physiology, and soon created morbid histology, which was long to remain an almost exclusively German science.

Gentlemen, you know the rest. The German universities presented the spectacle, new to them, of an unheard of, almost feverish, activity ; and you are not ignorant that this fever for work, which does not yet seem near extinction, has already produced more than one work of fundamental importance.

* H. Horn, *Darstellung des Schleimfiebers*, 2 aufl.
† C. A. Wunderlich, *Geschichte der Medicin*, p. 332. Stuttgart, 1859.

For more than ten years this great intellectual movement remained almost unnoticed in France. From time to time some foreseeing observer tried to draw public attention to it; but there was general indifference to struggle against, and, whilst everything was astir in Germany, we in France were occupied with other matters. At last the day is come, and it is understood that a great power has arisen in our vicinity, so that we shall have in future to reckon with the science from beyond the Rhine.*

By a very natural reaction people soon got to think extravagantly of the tendencies they had at first opposed; and whilst in France we are perhaps too much inclined now-a-days to think nothing of other than German work, our neighbours, drunk with success, seem persuaded that for the future the empire of Science belongs to them. Gentlemen, we must know how to allow something to the inebriation of such a triumph. Yet it is not without regret that we have recently seen an eminent man confound the rights conferred upon him by his high position as a *savant* with the political mandate entrusted to his charge by the electors of Berlin, and abuse the word *science* in order to excite German minds for the sake of a narrow patriotism.† Nobody should forget that science owns no country and is the property of no race. With the exclusive and illiberal ideas of the Prussian *savant*, we will contrast the grand words of one of England's greatest physicians.

"The empire of reason, extending from the old to the new world, from Europe to the Antipodes, has encircled the earth, the sun never sets upon her dominions—individuals must rest, but the collective intelligence of the species never sleeps." ‡

* This lecture was given in 1867.

† In allusion to a discourse of Prof. Virchow's at Hanover at the Congress of German Naturalists, 20th Sept., 1865. See the *Revue des cours scientifiques*, 1865—1866.

‡ *Clinical Lectures on the Practice of Medicine.* By Rob. J. Graves, M.D. Edited by Dr. Neligan. 2 vols., 1848, p. 43.

LECTURE I.

GENERAL CHARACTERS OF SENILE PATHOLOGY.

SUMMARY.—Object of these meetings.—Organisation of the Salpêtrière from the medical point of view.—Chronic diseases; diseases of old people.—Historical on senile pathology.—Physiology of old age.—Anatomical changes of organs and tissues.—They can all be summed up in a single word, *atrophy*.—Exception in case of heart and kidneys.—Various troubles resulting from these modifications of structure. —Certain functions are curtailed in the aged; others are maintained.—Pathological immunities of old age: special stamp impressed by old age on most diseases.

GENTLEMEN,— The meetings to which you are coming are intended to bring before you the most interesting clinical facts which the Hospital of la Salpêtrière presents for our observation. Those of you, gentlemen, who till now have only frequented the ordinary hospitals, may expect here to see the cases of disease with a very marked local colouring.

You are acquainted no doubt with the internal organisation of this vast establishment.* If we put the employés on one side, and if we abstract the insane, the idiots, the epileptics, who form a class apart, and with whom we shall not concern ourselves, the population of this asylum is composed of about 2,500 women, who, for the most part, belong to the least favoured classes of society, but some of whom have known better days.

From the point of view of clinical medicine, which alone is to receive our attention, they form two very distinct categories.

The first is composed of old women, generally more than 70 years of age (for thus the administration has decided), but who otherwise enjoy habitual good health, and whom misfortune or desertion has placed under the protection of public charity. It is among these, gentlemen, that we shall find the material with which to construct the clinical history of senile affections.

The second category comprises women of every age, affected for the most part with chronic maladies supposed to be incurable, and who have been thus reduced to a state of lasting infirmity.

* Those of our readers who would like fuller details about the internal arrangements of the Salpêtrière, as well as about the history of this establishment, will do well to consult the interesting chapter devoted to the Hospital for old women by M. Husson, former director-general of the "Assistance publique," in his *Etude sur les hôpitaux*. Paris, 1862.

In this way we possess advantages here, of which one is in great measure deprived in the ordinary hospitals, and we are placed in the most favourable conditions for studying diseases of slow development.

For the numerous population of our wards enables us to watch, under the most varied aspects, the chief types of one and the same kind of disease ; but, what is still more important, we are able here to follow the patients for a long period of their existence, instead of being present at a mere episode in their history ; moreover we see unfolding to its utmost limits the pathological process, of which in general we only know the initial phase ; lastly, we are called to determine the structural lesions which characterise the disease, when it ends fatally.

In other cases, unfortunately very rare, we see recovery taking place, sometimes spontaneously, sometimes brought about by the happy intervention of art.   But what we learn here better than anywhere else, is the importance to be attached to measures of alleviation when it is impossible to cure.

To-day I propose calling your attention more especially to the most general characters of the diseases which supervene during the last period of life.

I. The importance of a special study of the diseases of old age would not be contested at the present day.   It is agreed, in fact, that if the pathology of childhood requires clinical consideration of a special kind, and which it is indispensable to be practically acquainted with, senile pathology too has its difficulties, which can only be surmounted by long experience and a profound knowledge of its peculiar characters.

And yet, gentlemen, this very interesting part of medicine has been long neglected, and hardly in our own days has it succeeded in gaining its independence.

It was at a time very near our own, in France, and in this very hospital, that the pathology of old age was constituted and taught in all its peculiarity, so to speak.   One can hardly cite any works before that time in which the peculiar physiognomy of senile diseases had been noticed.   If we except the little treatise of Floyer; the more recent work of Welsted; and lastly, that of Fischer, which goes back to 1766,* most of the medical works of the last century, which refer especially to old age, have a

* Floyer, *Medicina Gerocomica*.   Londini, 1724.—Fischer, *Tractatus de senis*, 1766.

particularly literary or philosophic turn; they are more or less ingenious paraphrases of the famous treatise *De Senectute* of the Roman orator.

It was reserved for Pinel to point out, if not to supply, this want; yet, at the time when he wrote his " Traité de médecine clinique," the Salpêtrière hospital had already been organised as it is to-day; the penitentiary, which at one time formed a part of it, had been abolished, the infirmary had been founded, and they no longer transported the women who were ill to the Hôtel-Dieu, at the risk of seeing them expire on the way.* But Pinel could not think of restricting his studies to a limited portion of our science. Much more ambitious views had taken hold upon his mind; he was desirous of including pathology in its whole extent, and of creating a philosophical nosography, by applying to medicine the analytical method, to adopt the rather emphatic language of the eighteenth century. Moreover, the differences which distinguish senile from ordinary pathology are very rarely pointed out in his works, although he had passed the greater part of his medical existence in hospitals devoted to the aged.

We owe to Landré-Beauvais, one of the pupils and successors of Pinel at the Salpêtrière, the first special description ever traced of an affection which we encounter at every step in our wards, although it does not belong exclusively to old age.† I mean nodular rheumatism, *arthritis pauperum*, a very common disease among the indigent. Landré-Beauvais spoke of it as " primary asthenic gout," though fully recognising that it differs from ordinary gout. That, gentlemen, is a formidable affection, on account of the infirmities which it involves; it deserves, from all points of view, to be placed in the first rank of the chronic diseases collected in this hospital, and to which you will have to give your attention before long.

The clinical lectures given at the Salpêtrière by Rostan towards 1830 made a great stir at that time. Many questions relating to senile pathology were subjected to a searching study by the eminent professor.‡ Two of his works in particular have remained justly celebrated. The first aims at proving that the

---

* Pinel, *Traité de médecine clinique.* Paris, 1815. Introduction, p. xiii.

† Landré-Beauvais, Thèse de doctorat, An viii.

‡ *Mémoire sur cette question: l'Asthme des vieillards est-il une affection nerveuse?* (1817.)—*Recherches sur une maladie encore peu connue, qui a reçu le nom de Ramollisement du cerveau.* By L. Rostan, Physician to the Salpêtrière. (1820.)

asthma of old people is not a nervous affection, but one of the symptoms of an organic lesion : and we now know that, if this proposition, taken in its general sense, is too absolute, it is not less true in the great majority of cases. The second is a remarkable study on cerebral softening, which has completely transformed our ideas on the subject. We know that, as Rostan said, this change, so frequent at an advanced period of life, far from being the result of an inflammatory process, is a senile degeneration, very much like senile gangrene. The researches of observers who have been armed with all the new means of investigation which science to-day possesses, have fully confirmed this idea.

The mass of material laboriously collected by Prof. Cruveilhier during his period at the Salpêtrière, has largely contributed to the construction of that imperishable monument the "Atlas d'anatomie pathologique." Innumerable observations, which have opened a new era, not only for senile pathology, but also for the history of many chronic maladies, are found collected in this vast store-house.

From the more or less direct stimulus of the authorities whom we have mentioned, many important monographs about the diseases of old age have been published by observers, who have drawn from this hospital the material for their works. We will only mention the remarkable memoir of Hourman and Dechambre[*] on the pneumonia of the aged, and the treatise on cerebral softening by Durand-Fardel.

These scattered fragments had to be united in a systematic manner in order to construct at last the pathology of old age. Such was the object which Prus tried to realise in his "Researches on the Diseases of Old Age," presented to the Académie de Médecine in 1840. But the French observer had been preceded in this direction by Canstatt in Germany. We owe to this author the first systematic treatise which has appeared on the diseases of old people.[†] Unfortunately this work, dated 1839, was composed under the influence of Schelling's teaching, which reigned so long on the other side of the Rhine, and which bears the ambitious name of the Philosophy of Nature. Imagination holds an immense place in it at the expense of impartial and positive observation. Still we find in Canstatt's work ingenious

[*] *Archives de médecine.* 1835—36.
[†] *Die Krankheiten des höheren Alters*, etc.   Erlangen, 1839.

and often true ideas, which will assure him an honourable place in science.

An entirely opposite method inspired the studies of Beau* and Gillette † on the diseases of the aged, as well as the clinical treatise published in 1854 by Durand-Fardel. We might mention, besides these systematic works, numerous monographs relating to special points in senile pathology ; but we could not hope to speak of them all, and besides, we shall have more than one occasion in the course of our lectures to speak of these works.

I shall end this short historical account by mentioning three interesting works recently published abroad, and from which we shall borrow largely. The first is the voluminous clinical treatise on senile diseases which we owe to the pen of Dr. Geist, physician to the Hospital of the Holy Spirit at Nuremberg. The second is a collection of clinical observations published by Dr. Mettenheimer, and made at the hospital for old people in Frankfort. The third is Day's work, published in London in 1849.‡

II. A common feature is visible in most of the writings which have just been mentioned : it is a manifest tendency to refer the peculiarities which distinguish the diseases of old age as much as possible to the anatomical or physiological modifications which the organism undergoes by the mere fact of old age. This is not surprising if one notices that nearly all these writings are of recent date, and belong on one side at least to the structural school. At any rate, the preliminary study of these modifications ought to throw the most vivid light on the history of senile maladies. We shall have to remark, among other things, that the changes of texture impressed on the organism by old age sometimes become so marked, that the physiological and pathological states seem to merge into one another by insensible transitions, and cannot be clearly distinguished.

We shall therefore attempt a rapid account of the anatomy and physiology of old age, but without forgetting that we have to

* *Etudes cliniques sur les maladies des vieillards.* Journal de Médecine de Beau. 1843.

† Article VIEILLESSE, of the Supplement to the *Dictionnaire des Dictionnaires de Médecine.* Paris, 1851.

‡ Geist, *Klinik der Greisenkrankheiten :* Erlangen, 1860.—Mettenheimer, *Beiträge zur Lehre der Greisenkrankheiten :* Leipzig, 1863.—Day, *A Practical Treatise on Diseases of Advanced Life,* 1849.

keep to a special point of view. We shall confine ourselves to indicating the most general features, and when we touch on details it will only be to deduce from them applications, which have a distinct bearing on practical medicine.

Certain general modifications immediately strike the attention. You all know the external appearance of the old man : the dry and wrinkled skin, the scanty grizzled hair, the mouth without teeth, the crooked sunken body : all these changes correspond to a general atrophy of the individual, for at the same time as the stature diminishes the weight of the body lessens, as Quételet has shown.* A more or less pronounced emaciation generally accompanies these varied phenomena. Still, one may meet with a different state of things. It is what they used to call the *habitus corporis laxus,* characterised by an accumulation of fat under the skin and in the abdominal cavity. But this state is generally transitory and soon gives place to the *habitus corporis strictus,* which is almost always present at the period of decrepitude.

The emaciation that we have to do with is the consequence of an atrophic process, which exerts its action not only on the voluntary muscles and on the various parts of the skeleton, but also on most of the visceral organs : the brain, the cord, the nerve trunks, the lungs, the liver, and lastly all the blood-forming organs, participate in this retrograde process ; the spleen and the lymphatic glands undergo a remarkable diminution of weight and volume, which increases with the advance of age.

But by a very curious kind of contradiction, the physiological reason of which does not appear to me sufficiently established, the heart and the kidneys † elude this law and preserve the dimensions of middle life. The heart may even undergo a real hypertrophy in some old people : ‡ that, it seems to me, is a pathological state following what is called the senile alteration of the arteries. The network of capillary blood vessels, on its side, becomes progressively spoilt, not only in the principal viscera,

---

* According to Quételet (book ii., chap. 2) a man attains his maximum weight about 40 ; he begins to diminish in weight at 60, and at 80 he has lost, on an average, 6 kilograms. In a woman the maximum weight occurs at 50. *Sur l'homme et le développement de ses facultés.* By A. Quételet, perpetual secretary of the Académie royale de Bruxelles. Paris, 1835.

† Rayer, *Maladies des reins,* vol. i., p. 5.

‡ It is hardly necessary to recall here the justly celebrated work of Bizot, inserted in the 1st volume of the Memoirs of the Société médicale d'observation de Paris.

but also in the substance of the skin and mucous membranes. These latter in the digestive canal lose at the same time part of their villous and glandular elements.*

In what does this atrophic action consist, which thus exerts its action on the organs and tissues ? It is firstly and principally a process of simple atrophy ; the parenchymatous cellular elements, the muscular, and perhaps also the nervous elements, diminish progressively in size, without presenting any essential modification in their structure : this is especially noticeable, according to Otto Weber,† in the muscles, the elements of which are of small and almost equal size, contrary to what obtains in adult life. The connective tissue, however, does not participate to the same degree in this work of slow destruction ; in the viscera we see this tissue predominating over the specific elements : this has been very clearly established by Dr. Bastien, so far as concerns the liver and the majority of the abdominal organs.

But at a more advanced stage the atrophy is accompanied by a degenerative process, that is, the elements undergo modifications in their chemical characters, and become the seat of pigmentary or fatty infiltrations, and of calcareous incrustations. This is what occurs, for example, in the cerebral cells, according to the statements of Prof. Vulpian,‡ the perfect exactitude of which I have often been able to demonstrate. According to Virchow, while the neuroglia tends to predominate in the encephalon over the nervous elements, it becomes usually permeated by a greater or less number of amylaceous bodies ;§ the tissue of the brain then undergoes a chemical change according to the researches of Bibra, confirmed by those of Schlossberger.‖ The fatty matters which enter into its constitution undergo a notable diminution, whilst on the contrary the proportion of water and phosphorus increases.

And yet, according to Vulpian,¶ fatty granules are formed in the primitive fibres of voluntary muscle by the mere fact of progressing age ; and this change may reach such a degree in the

---

* Berres, after Geist, loc. cit.—N. Guillot. *Researches on the Mucous Membrane of the Intestinal Canal. Journ. l'Exper.*, vol. i., p. 161. 1837—38.

† *Handbuch der allgemeinen und spec. Chirurgie*, t. i., p. 309. Erlangen, 1865.

‡ *Leçons de physiologie générale et comparée du système nerveux*, p. 645. Paris, 1866.

§ *Handbuch der sp. Pathologie*, vol. i., p. 316.

‖ See Geist, op. cit., p. 158.

¶ Loc. cit.

lower limbs, where it occurs especially, that it determines a more or less complete paraplegia. The involuntary muscular fibres do not escape from fatty degeneration, and you will have a frequent opportunity of satisfying yourselves that the muscular walls of the heart are almost always affected with it in women who die at an advanced age. With this alteration of the cardiac tissue are connected the phenomena of deficient cardiac contraction, which are so frequently observed in old people, even when they appear to enjoy good health.

Lastly, the coats of the cerebral arterioles are often filled with fatty granules, as Paget* and Prof. Robin† have noticed ; and Vulpian‡ has shown that this senile change is not peculiar to man, but is met with equally in old brutes, especially the dog.

It will not escape any of you, gentlemen, that these changes, when they have reached so pronounced a degree, pass the limits of the physiological state, since they are themselves capable of producing functional troubles which may be extremely grave. This is especially evident in regard to what is known as the atheromatous change in arteries, and the calcification which so often accompanies it.

From the point of view of its histological development, arterial atheroma§ tends to be widely separated from the usual forms of senile atrophy. The latter appear to be the result of a purely passive process ; the former, on the contrary, seems to consist, in the first phase of its evolution, in a more or less active proliferation of the elements which normally constitute the internal coat of the arteries. Fatty degeneration takes possession of these new-formed elements at a certain stage ; but this is a secondary phenomenon. The granules thus formed accumulate in the deepest parts of the internal coat, which are first and especially altered ; they stretch the most superficial layer, which still resists for a long time. Thus are formed those collections, rich in fat and cholesterin crystals, which have been called atheromatous abscesses. Sometimes they burst into the cavity of the arteries whose coats they occupy, and their contents, mingling with the blood, may be swept along by the torrent of the circulation, and may penetrate into vessels of small calibre,

---

* *On Fatty Degeneration*, etc. *Lond. Med. Gaz.*, 1850.
† *Mémoires de la Société de Biologie*, vol. i., p. 33. 1850.
‡ Loc. cit.   § Virchow, *Cellular Pathology*.

producing the often formidable symptoms of capillary embolism. At an earlier stage the atheromatous swelling merely causes a narrowing, and then complete obliteration, of the artery. Then in different parts of the system arise those changes due to faulty nutrition, which form one of the most characteristic chapters of senile pathology. We shall see, indeed, that most of the cases of cerebral softening and capillary apoplexy in the encephalon which are observed in old age are to be referred to atheromatous obliteration of the arteries ; * it is the same with visceral infarcts, senile gangrene of the extremities, and many other changes.

But here we encroach on the domain of pathology, which we wish to avoid for the present. I will now indicate in few words the physiological modifications, which correspond with the changes of texture of which I have just given a brief description. If it is true, speaking generally, that all the functions get simultaneously feebler, do not suppose that this proposition is in every case an exact one ; only the analytical study of the facts can teach us what is the real state of the case in this matter.

The generative organs and the muscular powers † undergo in old age a weakening so evident that we need not dwell on this point. As for the functions of the voluntary nervous system, it will suffice to recall to you the well known lines of Lucretius :

> " Præterea gigni pariter cum corpore, et una
> Crescere sentimus, pariterque senescere mentem."
> (*De Nat. Rerum*, ii., 446.)

The respiratory functions as a whole are similarly impaired, this being shown by the diminution in the quantity of carbonic acid exhaled, by the increase in the number of respirations, and by the reduction in the vital capacity of the lungs : this last result, according to the spirometric researches of Wintrich, Schnepf, and Geist, begins to appear about 35 and reaches its maximum from 65 to 75.‡

Most of the secretions are diminished, especially those of urine

---

* It is to be understood that we have not here to do with cerebral hemorrhages, which have also been attributed, without much evidence, to atheromatous change in the cerebral arteries. We shall afterwards have occasion for explanations on this point.

† See Empis, *Etudes sur l'affaiblissement musculaire progressif chez les vieillards. Arch. de Médecine*, 1862.

‡ Geist, op. cit., p. 102.

and sweat; and it is hardly doubtful that senile dyspepsia, on which our great naturalist Daubenton* has insisted in an interesting but little known work, depends in great measure upon the perceptible diminution of the gastro-intestinal secretions.

But what are we to think of the functional weakening of the circulatory system, when, according to Dr. Marey,† the heart in old people is more powerful than ever, and the arteries present energetic pulsations ? It seems demonstrated at any rate that in old age the pulse augments in frequency.‡

We know little of the degree of intensity which nutrition presents in the aged : still the employment of the thermometer has given us more precise notions with regard to the production of heat. Before the application of this instrument to researches of this kind, it was supposed that the temperature in old people was lower than in adults; but we now know that the heat of the central parts remains almost the same at all ages. It has even been maintained that the general temperature rises towards the end of life.§ My own researches tend to show that the only real difference which exists between the temperatures of the aged and the adult, is that in the former the temperature of the axilla is much lower than that of the rectum, whilst in the latter the difference is scarcely perceptible.

Here is an old woman of 103 who enjoys excellent health; temperature in the axilla is 37·4° (99·3° F.) ; in the rectum, 38° (100·4° F.), which is the maximum normal temperature in the adult.

Thus, gentlemen, if old age weakens most of our faculties, it is far from paralysing them all; and rigorous observation shows us that in certain ways the organs of the aged acquit themselves of their task with quite as much energy as do those of the adult.

III. Gentlemen, the preceding sketch has shown us that the progress of age establishes, by virtue of physiological modifications, a profound difference in pathological phenomena.

* *Mémoires sur les indigestions, qui commencent à être plus fréquentes chez la plupart des hommes à l'âge de 40 à 45 ans.* Paris, 1785.

† *Etudes sur la circulation*, p. 415.

‡ Leuret et Mitivié, *Sur la fréquence du pouls chez les aliénés.* Paris, 1832.—Geist, op. cit., p. 85.

§ Von Bärensprung, in *Canstatt's Jahresbericht*, 1851.—Geist, op. cit., p. 32.

We shall have, then, to study the subject from three different points of view :

1. There exist maladies special to old age, which depend in part at least on the general modifications which have taken place in the system. We will quote as examples ; senile marasmus, senile osteomalacia, senile atrophy of the brain ; certain alterations in the blood ;* senile heart-weakness ; lastly, arterial atheroma, the study of which constitutes one of the most interesting aspects of the pathology of old age.

2. Amongst the diseases which may exist at other periods of life, there are several which present a special character in old age ; such for example is lobar pneumonia, that great enemy of old people, and one of the principal causes of death in this hospital. We shall come back later to this part of the question.

3. Old age seems in some respects to create pathological immunities. Eruptive fevers, typhoid fever, and phthisis are little known at this age ; still we must not exaggerate the importance of these immunities, which are far from being absolute, as Rayer has demonstrated for typhoid, Murchison for typhus, and other authors for various maladies.† Who does not know, besides, that Louis XV. died of small-pox at the age of 65 ?

* The frequency of intravascular coagulations in old people seems to show that there exists in them a tendency to inopexia, and *purpura senilis* comes under the same rule ; for it is probable that this last affection depends, at least very often, on spontaneous rupture of the capillary vessels.

† See Rayer, *Gaz. méd.*, vol. x., p. 573 (1842) ; and Uhle, *Ueber der typhus abdominalis der alteren Leute,* in *Archiv für Physiol. Heilkunde,* vol. iii., 1859. These authors mention striking examples of typhoid in old people. Murchison tells us that no age is free from typhus : from 15 to 20 the proportion is 16 p.c. ; from 60 to 65 it is 2·5 p.c. ; from 70 to 75 it is 1·21 p.c. The case of most advanced age was an old man of 84. Relapsing fever is less frequent than typhus in old people, yet a few examples have been observed ; above 50 the proportion is 6·63 p.c. ; above 60 it is 1·6 p.c. Old women are more subject to these two diseases than old men are. For typhoid the proportion is 1·46 p.c. above 50 ; above 60 it is 0·5 p.c. These figures suffice to show that the relative immunity enjoyed by old people with reference to the continued fevers is far from being absolute. (A treatise on the Continued Fevers of Great Britain. London, 1862, pp. 61, 303, and 410.)

As to phthisis, Vulpian and I have noticed that tuberculisation, even the acute form, is more frequent at the Salpêtrière than is generally supposed. Moureton, one of Vulpian's pupils, has reported in his inaugural thesis nine cases of acute tuberculisation in the aged. Three of these persons were more than 80, and the acute phthisis was primary in all the cases except one. (Thèses de Paris, 1863.)

Every year at the Salpêtrière we observe several marked cases of cerebro-spinal meningitis. In 1852 I collected a certain number of cases of this kind ; they are to be found united in the thesis of Dr. Inglessis. (*Sur quelques cas de méningite cérébro-spinale observés à la Salpêtrière pendant le printemps de* 1852. Thèses de Paris, 1855.)

D

I think I have said enough, gentlemen, to convince you that there is a *senile* pathology; and in order to offer you a striking example of the modifications which age may give to morbid manifestations, we shall at the next lecture study the febrile state as it presents itself in old people, trying to bring into prominence the analogies and the differences which it offers as compared with fever in the adult.

LECTURE II.

THE FEBRILE STATE IN OLD AGE.

SUMMARY.—Deficient reaction in old age.—Organs seem to be affected in isolation.—Latent diseases.—The gravest lesions may pass unobserved.—Fevers in the aged.—What is fever?—Importance of clinical thermometry.—Rigors in the aged.—Temperature curves in lobar pneumonia.—Practical deductions to be drawn from them.—Defervescence, crises, critical perturbations.—Diseases in which the temperature sinks instead of rising.

GENTLEMEN,—At our last meeting I tried to make clear the peculiar stamp which old age impresses on all manifestations of disease. I depended chiefly on physiological facts; to-day we are going to pursue this study, resting exclusively on clinical grounds.

Not only are there in old people special immunities and pathological predispositions unknown in adults, but moreover we see that general reaction, which we are accustomed to meet with in presence of disease, undergo in them a complete transformation. At this period of life the organs remain in some degree independent of one another; they suffer separately from one another [isolément], and the different lesions of which they may be the seat scarcely influence the economy as a whole. Moreover, the gravest disorders manifest themselves by little-marked symptoms: they may even pass unobserved, and it is in old age that we notice the greatest number of latent maladies.*

Gentlemen, this point of view is important enough in practice to deserve being brought into relief; I will therefore give you a few appropriate examples.

Lay aside for a moment the study of physical signs, the importance of which is so great in every way; forget the difficulties presented by auscultation and percussion in old people; we shall soon have occasion to return to them. Let us occupy ourselves solely with the phenomena of sympathetic reaction, the often complete absence of which is well calculated to astonish us.

First, let us take as an example one of the most frequent

* " At an advanced age the organs seem to live and suffer in isolation, their sphere of activity appears more restricted. . . . . It must never be forgotten that at an advanced age the gravest lesions may coexist with a small number of slight, almost insignificant, symptoms."—Grisolle, *Traité de la pneumonie*, 1re. édition, p. 425.

D 2

affections in this hospital : I mean biliary gravel, which in the adult usually gives rise to phenomena of great intensity. You are acquainted with the formidable picture of hepatic colic, appearing with a series of alarming symptoms, which, once seen, it is impossible to forget. Well, you will learn with surprise that in the aged it is often difficult to recognise these symptoms, so much diminished are they in intensity. The most we find is a little heavy feeling in the region of the liver, some sickness, slight jaundice, delirium, and cerebral symptoms which are more apt to lead us into error than to enlighten us on the nature of the disease.*

Just as distension of the biliary ducts by the passage of calculi seems so little prone to give rise to general reaction, so is it with the excretory ducts of the kidneys, which may experience the contact of urinary gravel almost without pain ; thus the sharp pains of nephritic colic are almost unknown in our old people.

In another class of cases we may see diabetes make its appearance in subjects of an advanced age with very different symptoms from those which characterise it in the adult. The urine, often not abundant, may only contain glucose intermittently ;† and thirst, that significant symptom which most often puts us on the track of diagnosis at other periods of life, may be completely wanting in old people.

After having noticed such facts, you will learn without surprise that cancer‡ of the stomach and liver, as well as pulmonary tubercle,§ may remain in a latent state during the whole course

---

* "At the infirmary of the Salpêtrière few autopsies are made without coming across a greater or less number of calculi in the gall-bladder, yet hepatic colic is extremely rare at the Salpêtrière."—Beau, *Etudes sur l'appareil spléno-hépatique; Arch. de Méd.*, Avril, 1851, p. 401. " The fact is true for colic with all its development of pain ; but we must also recollect the diminution of sensibility ; and it is not rare to observe dull pains in the gastro-hepatic region, pains which the patients always refer to imaginary causes, but which may well depend on the presence of calculi as their real cause."—Gillette, op. cit., p. 898.

I quite share in this respect the opinions of Gillette, and I may add that according to my own observations, dull aching pains accompany the passage of urinary calculi more often in old people than in adults.

† Bence Jones, *On Intermitting Diabetes, and on Diabetes of Old Age. Medico-chir. Trans.*, 1853, vol. xxxvi.

‡ " It is in the aged that we encounter those degenerations of the stomach of deceptive course which are accompanied neither by sickness, violent pains, nor dyspepsia, at least these are not complained of."—Gillette, loc. cit., p. 898.

§ " Phthisis in old persons is remarkable for its slow and insidious form."—Gillette, loc. cit., p. 893.

of their development ; in these cases surprises are often in store for us at the autopsy.

But it is especially in lobar pneumonia, so frequent in this hospital, that we come across such a strikingly complete absence of general signs. I shall content myself with quoting a passage extracted from the important memoir of Hourman and Dechambre.*

" The old women do not even complain of malaise ; no one in the wards, neither guardians, servants, or neighbours, perceive any change in their condition. They get up, make their beds, walk about, eat as usual; then they feel a little fatigued, sink upon their beds, and expire. This is one of the *sudden deaths* in old age at the Salpêtrière. The body is opened, and we find a great part of the pulmonary parenchyma in a state of suppuration."

Do not these accounts seem very strange ? Must we say then that the laws, which regulate the connection of symptom with lesion in the adult, are completely inverted in the aged ? By no means. Let us remark first of all that facts of this kind, though they cannot be doubted, must yet be considered as exceptional. They are not, moreover, quite unknown in ordinary pathology. Pneumonia sometimes remains latent in the adult under certain peculiar conditions of the organism, and more especially in drunkards. We may associate with this type many other grave affections. We know, for example, that hemorrhagic small-pox may at the commencement assume a favourable aspect, which is abruptly belied by a fatal termination ; but it is especially in the group of pestilential fevers that facts of this kind are to be observed. Thus in epidemic yellow fever, pest, and typhus, there are cases where the profound way in which the organism is affected does not reveal itself by any symptom, which presages the gravity of the disease. The pulse may be natural or but little at fault, the tongue clean, the skin cool, or slightly hot in the region of the stomach and liver ; the mind may be unclouded, the strength preserved. All at once black vomiting comes on, and death takes place unexpectedly. An American physician, Caldwell, to whom we owe a good treatise on yellow fever, has designated by the picturesque name of *walking cases* those insidious cases, in which persons who are sick unto death fancy themselves scarcely ill, and continue to

* *Archives de Médecine*, 1836, vol. xii., p. 57.

attend to their affairs up to the last moments of their existence.*

These insidious forms are not, then, exclusively peculiar to senile pathology; but if we leave on one side these infrequent cases and consider only those of ordinary practice, we are led to recognise the general rule, that in the aged there is a want of correlation between the local lesion and the production of general symptoms. Such a tendency occurs in the infant, as Gillette† has ingeniously observed, only here it is in an inverse direction. At this age reaction is, as it were, exaggerated and tumultuous, the violent disturbance of functions by no means demonstrating a grave disease. In old people, on the contrary, the organism remains, so to speak, unmoved in presence of the gravest changes. It is, then, by deficiency that the reaction is abnormal, and the physician must redouble his attention and take into account the slightest indications, if he does not want to be surprised by completely unforeseen accidents.‡

But it is time to quit the very general point of view from which we have been looking, in order to approach the question which is specially to occupy us to-day. We want to study the febrile state in the aged, as compared with the febrile state in children and adults ; and in order to give more precision to the ideas I am going to express I shall take as an example lobar pneumonia, that affection febrile in the highest degree and common to all ages of life. Its development will enable us to determine the deviations which may be impressed by old age on one of the chief symptoms of most acute affections.

Fever, says Gillette,§ in a passage in which he has echoed the opinion of all the special authors who have preceded him, fever is characterised in old people by acceleration of pulse and dryness

---

* *Med. and phys. Mem. containing a particular inquiry into the origin and nature of the late pestilential epidemics of the United States.* Philadelphia, 1801.

† Loc. cit., p. 873.

‡ We must remember also that sympathetic phenomena in the old sometimes take a quite unusual turn. Thus pneumonia may assume an undevelopt form, and present itself sometimes with the appearance of cerebral apoplexy with complete resolution and coma, sometimes with the aspect of true hemiplegia with or without contraction of the paralysed limbs. I insist particularly on these pneumonic hemiplegias, of which Vulpian and I have met with several examples. They generally end in death, and we have been able to convince ourselves that they correspond with no encephalic lesion. In children pneumonia may appear under a cerebral form, characterised by eclampsia or coma.

§ Loc. cit., p. 874.

of skin, without rise of temperature being very marked. He then observes that the initial rigor is little marked or completely absent, as also are the sweats. The other accessory phenomena of the febrile state are all, according to the same author, more or less profoundly modified. In short, the description which he gives offers a striking contrast with what we know of the appearance of fever at other ages. Is this picture exact—does it faithfully represent the truth? I must say that it does not quite satisfy me; but in order to justify my difference of opinion it is necessary to touch on a preliminary question.

What is fever? What do we mean by the febrile state?

It is hardly necessary to warn you, gentlemen, that the definition we are looking for will be entirely descriptive; we have no intention of penetrating the intimate nature of the phenomenon which we want to characterise.

At the time of Hippocrates, when the examination of the pulse was not yet practised, elevation of temperature constituted the sole and unique element in fever. Of this the definition of Galen is sufficient evidence, *Calor præter naturam*;* such was this great physician's conception of the febrile state. Tradition for a long series of years respected the opinion of Galen; but ultimately it became modified, and we find Boerhaave, guided by the iatro-mechanic notions which prevailed in his time, declaring that " acceleration of pulse is the only symptom in fever which is ever present from beginning to end, and which alone is sufficient to make the physician recognise the presence of fever." † The question since that time has been often raised, and answered in very different senses; but it must be admitted that to-day the unanimous testimony of modern works has been in favour of the opinion accepted by antiquity. It has been recognised and proclaimed on all sides that the increase of animal heat is really the fundamental fact of the febrile state. Among the other phenomena which most generally accompany it there is not one, not even the acceleration of pulse, which appears in so constant and necessary a manner. Fever does not exist when the temperature remains at the normal standard, and frequency of pulse may reach extreme limits without there

* *De different. febrium*, cap. 1, *De generali febrium divisione*. There is another definition of Galen's, but it is found in a less authentic work, and the frequency of the pulse is here brought in.

† Aphorism 570.

being any febrile movement. We need but mention the excessive excitement of the circulatory system observed in certain cases of arterial palpitation, especially in exophthalmic disease and hysteria.* Can we say, on the other hand, that there is fever every time that the temperature rises? That is a point on which it is hardly possible yet to speak definitely. We see, in fact, the heat of the body rise in cases from which all febrile reaction seems absent; in tetanus, in the epileptic attack; and in cholera, especially at the moment of death, it may reach 42° or 43° (107·6° or 109·4° F.). There, no doubt, is an element which escapes us; but the increase of animal heat always predominates in fever over the other symptoms, and may even serve in many cases to determine its intensity.

It is the methodical employment of a means of investigation unknown to the ancients, which has in greatest degree contributed to make definite our ideas on this point. I mean clinical thermometry. Although critics have by no means spared it, this means of investigation has now made its way, and we can foresee that the time is not far distant when its use will be generally extended through ordinary practice.

It is said that the celebrated Dutchman, Swammerdam, in the seventeenth century, was the first to have the idea of determining the heat of patients with the thermometer.† Since then several physicians have devoted themselves to this kind of investigation. In 1754, de Haen called the attention of his pupils to the necessity of substituting the use of the thermometer for the application of the hand in estimating the heat of the body. We owe to him also the proof of an important fact, to which we shall often allude, because it is very often noticed in practice with the aged : it is, that at the very moment when the skin of fever patients is pale, purple, and chilly in consequence of the contraction of the superficial capillaries, the blood temperature rises many degrees above the normal. This happens in no transient manner, as in the initial rigor of fever, but, so to speak, permanently, and lasting all through the febrile state.

John Hunter was during the last century almost the only author who responded to this appeal. But in our days the works of Prof. Gavarret (1839), of Bouillaud, of Monneret, and

* Briquet, *Traité de l'hystérie*, p. 326.
† Requin, vol. i., p. 91.

many other French physicians, indicated the coming importance in practice of this means of investigation. But it is in Germany, and only in these last years, that real progress has been made in this respect. It may be said without exaggeration that in the hands of Bärensprung, Traube, Michael, of Wunderlich above all, clinical thermometry has undergone a radical transformation. In fact, it became no longer a question of showing that the temperature rises several degrees in fever, nor of determining its intensity in different diseases; it was necessary to follow the phenomenon day by day, almost hour by hour, from its origin to its termination, in the different phases of its evolution; to record even its minutest oscillations; and to show that the graphic tracings obtained by this methodic exploration furnish constant types for each kind of disease, with variations corresponding to the most important events of these diseases; for thus only could it be established that these tracings are of real importance in practice; that they enable us, better perhaps than anything else, to follow the progress of the morbid process, and to recognise its different incidents; that, consequently, they cannot fail to furnish valuable indications both for diagnosis and prognosis. Lastly, it had to be shown that the thermometric curves vary according to certain rules, certain laws, according as the disease has been left to itself or treated by the methodic employment of this or that therapeutic agent; for there was reason to hope that therapeutic experiment would find in this method a *criterium* of almost mathematical precision.

Such is the complicated task which the authors I have mentioned imposed on themselves, and if they have not in every case attained the end in view, it would be deeply unjust not to recognise that they have scattered numerous truths along their path.

This seems at last to be understood both in France and England, and numerous physicians in these two countries are occupied in this direction.*

I have attempted for nearly three years to repeat as often as possible on the people under my care in this hospital such

* Consult on this point the excellent theses of Maurice (Paris, 1855), Spielman (Strasburg, 1856), Hardy (Paris, 1859), and Duclos (Paris, 1864). In England important researches have been made by Sidney Ringer, whose labours are recorded in Aitken's work.

clinical observations as we are now considering. Hitherto thermometric investigation has been almost limited to children and
adults. The results which I have obtained will enable me to
present you with some brief considerations on the modifications
which, in old age, the temperature undergoes during the febrile
state at the different phases of its evolution, and to compare this
with the other periods of life. But I have it most at heart to
show you what advantage we can derive from thermometry in
our practice among old people. I need hardly remind you here
that my descriptions will refer especially to the pyrexia which
accompanies lobar pneumonia; I shall, however, often allude to
other forms of the febrile state.

I. Old people have but slight rigors, said Beau,* and we
have seen that Gillette reproduced almost exactly the same
opinion. This proposition is much too absolute; I have more
than once observed in old people violent and prolonged rigors at
the beginning of pneumonia, erysipelas, or synochal fever, a
very common affection at the Salpêtrière at certain periods of
the year. These rigors, characterised by convulsive tremblings,
by cyanosis and algidity of the limbs, appear with still greater
intensity in the attacks of symptomatic intermittent fever, which
so often accompany deep suppurations, phlebitis in the viscera,
and those inflammations of the biliary passages which the presence of hepatic calculi so readily determines in old age.†

And yet, in the ·midst of all these phenomena, at the very
moment when the external surface of the body offers every sign
of considerable coldness, the central temperature remains at a
very elevated point; by placing the thermometer in the axilla,
we cannot, it is true, perceive the full intensity of the reaction; ‡

* *Etudes cliniques sur les maladies des vieillards.* Journal de Beau, 1843, p. 292.

† If hepatic colic is not common at an advanced age, it is, on the contrary, very
common to find calculi, and especially intra-hepatic gravel, giving rise to suppuration
of the biliary passages in old people. This lesion is shown externally by a *symptomatic
intermittent fever*, in which the beginning of each attack is marked by a violent rigor;
in the interval the thermometer demonstrates that there is often complete apyrexia.
Death always takes place after these symptoms. Cornil has published in the Memoirs
of the Société de Biologie (1865) several cases of this kind collected from my practice.
It is known that Monneret had already mentioned the existence of fever of remittent
or intermittent type in affections of the liver. (*Archives de médecine*, 1861.)

‡ There is almost always in such cases a difference of some fractions of a degree,
sometimes of a degree, between the temperature of the axilla and that of the rectum.

but in the rectum there is a temperature of 40° to 41° (104° to 105·8° F.), as I have often had the opportunity of demonstrating for myself.

This sudden elevation of temperature at the beginning of diseases corresponds exactly enough with what we observe in the adult, and in this respect, at least, the old man yields in nothing to subjects of another age. But this rapidity of the invasion is only met with in certain maladies; there are others in which the febrile heat increases slowly and gradually; and in order to remain within the realm of senile pathology, we will take as examples broncho-pneumonia and catarrhal fever. It is rare, however, in affections of this last type, to see the temperature rise to the same degree as in lobar pneumonia; we shall soon have an opportunity of demonstrating this. Now, let us see what are the characters of the general reaction in this inflammation, which we have chosen as the type of the febrile affections of old age.

II. Shivering marks the onset of the disease, which follows from this moment a regular course of development. Then it becomes interesting to watch its daily progress with scrupulous attention, and to determine with the thermometer the least oscillations in the animal heat; for in the great majority of cases they correspond with great exactitude to the different phases of the disease.

A momentary amendment usually succeeds the initial rigors; the temperature sinks sometimes more than a degree, and the patient feels comparatively comfortable. But it is a deceptive calm, and the same evening or the next morning the disease resumes its course. The temperature goes up to 40° (104° F.); when it remains as high as that for several days, we are justified in thinking that we have to do with a severe case; when, on the contrary, it tends to sink progressively to 39° (102·2° F.), the prognosis is relatively favourable. The figures I have mentioned give the evening temperature, for the fever in pneumonia (even lobar) does not advance with rigorous continuity; there are diurnal remissions which are shown every morning by an average difference of half a degree. But in catarrhal pneumonia these oscillations are much more strongly marked; they amount to a degree, a degree and a half, and sometimes more. When you reflect that in this latter affection the temperature rises slowly by successive degrees, and hardly ever reaches the figures observed in lobar pneumonia, you will easily understand that the mere inspection of the thermometric tracings often enables us to distinguish between these two diseases, the differential diagnosis of which is often decidedly difficult.

I have placed before you several examples of this kind, most of which have been collected in our wards. A simple glance will make you grasp the differences which I am trying to bring out.*

The juxtaposition of these temperature curves will enable you at the same time to compare the tracings obtained in the adult and infant in both lobar and catarrhal pneumonia with those observed in the aged ; a rapid glance is enough to make you grasp their complete analogy.

Among the tracings I have collected, there are two intended to bring out the influence of therapeutic agents on the oscillations of temperature. The first of these figures shows how the administration of digitalis in large doses led at two different times to a notable lowering of the temperature. This phenomenon, which never occurs *spontaneously* at this period of the disease, may be similarly produced by tartar emetic or bloodletting. But this defervescence is usually only temporary, and each time that the administration of the drug is suspended, you see the temperature rise afresh.

The second figure shows the effects of rum administered in doses of 120 grams. During the early part of the disease the temperature sank slowly but progressively under the influence of this drug, to rise again as soon as the administration ceased ; the disease then resumed its natural course and ended in recovery. But that is a point to which we shall recur more at length in the course of these meetings.

The persistence of an elevated temperature for several days without well-marked diurnal oscillations, constitutes an important clinical character in lobar pneumonia, *especially in old age*. In the adult we might mention several affections (the eruptive fevers and exanthematic typhus, for example) which share this character. We scarcely meet with it in old people except in erysipelas, if we may judge by what we observe at the Salpêtrière. The clinical importance of this fact, therefore, cannot

---

* It has not been thought needful to reproduce these tracings. [TRANSL.]

be exaggerated, especially when one thinks of the difficulties which auscultation of the chest usually presents in old age. Indeed, in many cases we succeed in formulating the diagnosis of a pulmonary inflammation by thermometry long before the ear is able to perceive the stethoscopic signs which reveal its existence.

III. I have now to point out the peculiarities which exploration by the thermometer shows us in the period of decline of the febrile state, or, as they say in Germany, during the defervescence. Sometimes the fall of temperature which indicates the return of the normal state is accomplished in successive stages for a space of three or four days; this is the case in catarrhal fever and broncho-pneumonia; sometimes, on the contrary, it takes place abruptly, and in twelve, twenty-four, thirty-six, or forty-eight hours one sees the temperature sink from one to two degrees, or even more. Thus at least it generally happens in lobar pneumonia if the issue is to be favourable. Often this rapid decline of the febrile movement is preceded by a sudden rise of temperature, which is accompanied with an exacerbation of the symptoms more or less pronounced and often very alarming. This used to be called the "critical perturbation." Lastly, let us note that in defervescence the temperature sinks sometimes below the normal, and remains so for some hours, sometimes a whole day, returning ultimately to the level of perfect health. The goal is then overpassed, so to speak; but it is only rarely that I have seen this lowering of the temperature below the normal accompanied in old people by the more or less alarming symptoms of collapse, which not unfrequently are indicative of it at a less advanced age.

The defervescence in many cases is the signal for the critical phenomena which are to close the case; we see them appear either at the very moment when the temperature drops or a little later; the latter case is the most frequent.* In this respect there is no real difference between the old man and the adult; only the critical sweats, so frequent in middle age, are quite rarely observed in old people; critical diarrhœa, on the contrary, is a common enough phenomenon.

In the tracings I spoke of, you can follow the phenomena of

* See in this matter Traube's work, *Ueber Krisen und Kritische Tage.* Berlin, 1852.

defervescence in the infant, the adult, and the old man, and recognise the fact that at all periods of life they happen according to identical laws.

Hitherto we have only considered cases which end in recovery ; when the disease is going to end fatally, the temperature, which till then had remained within the ordinary limits, rises suddenly one or two degrees in a day, or even in a few hours. These are the circumstances in which death in the adult usually occurs in lobar pneumonia. It is the same for the aged in the great majority of cases ; but tolerably often in them we observe a mode of ending which seems to be exceptional at the middle period of life ; instead of rising, the temperature sinks progressively for a day or two down to about 38° or even 37·5° (100·4° or 99·5° F.) at the moment of the fatal termination. And this bad kind of defervescence occurs not only in cases where the patients have been subjected to the action of depressants, but even in those where the disease has been left to itself.

Gentlemen, I think I have shown you the importance of clinical thermometry in studying the diseases of old age, and the usefulness of the results to which it can lead us from the triple point of view of diagnosis, prognosis, and treatment. But what I had especially at heart to demonstrate to you is this, that the phenomena of fever observed at the most different periods of life are always at bottom the same, and follow identical laws. As in the adult, there is a general reaction in the aged ; but it is concealed, and we must seek for a manifestation of it in the central parts of the system.

It is, then, very important to distinguish here between the results of thermometric exploration in the axilla and in the rectum. In regard to temperature, the axilla corresponds to the surface of the body, the rectum to the internal viscera. It is true that in the majority of cases, the curves showing the heat at these two spots are almost parallel : in the adult one might almost say they coincide ; in the old person, that which corresponds to the temperature of the axilla remains a little below that of the rectum. But there are cases, and these often the gravest, where there is a great discrepancy between the two curves. The temperature of the external parts sinks, whilst that of the internal rises, and the difference may reach several degrees. You see, in such a case it would not do at all to depend exclusively on the results given by the thermometer in the axilla.

So far, gentlemen, I have hardly talked to you of any diseases but those in which the temperature rises above the normal. But there are a great number of affections (especially in old people) which give rise to the inverse phenomenon, and cause a real lowering of the temperature of the central parts. Without speaking of cholera,* the effects of which in this particular are universally known, I may mention, as examples, certain heart affections, pericarditis, senile gangrene, marasmus, and various forms of cancer. This algide state is a grave symptom, and demands prompt assistance. Now, it can only be revealed by the thermometer, which consequently is here called on to perform fresh services.

But I do not want to begin on this subject to-day ; I shall no doubt have occasion in the course of these meetings to show you the result of the researches which I have undertaken on the symptomatic value of algidity in old age.†

* During the last cholera epidemic which devastated Paris, I had the opportunity of observing that the temperature of the central parts remains at the normal throughout the disease, until it rises at the approach of death, as Doyère had already indicated. (*Mém. de la Soc. de Biologie*, 1866)

† See Lecture XX.

LECTURE III.

NODULAR RHEUMATISM AND GOUT——STATE OF THE BLOOD IN GOUT.

SUMMARY.—Frequency of chronic articular rheumatism at the Salpêtrière.—Its likeness to gout.—Doctrine of identity: silence of the physicians of antiquity on this point.—Necessity for undertaking the preliminary study of gout before that of chronic rheumatism. — Gouty diathesis : its general characters.—Regular and irregular gout : acute and chronic gout.—State of the blood in gout.—The chalkstones of gout are composed of sodium urate.—Uric acid exists normally in the blood.—It is found in excess in the blood of the gouty.—The thread experiment. —Uric acid does not exist in excess in the blood of rheumatics.—Gout is not the only disease which accompanies this alteration.—Accessory modifications in the blood-composition in the gouty.—State of the urine in acute gout, during the attack and in the interval between attacks : in chronic gout.

GENTLEMEN,—We have been studying in our two previous meetings the general characters which diseases present in old age ; to-day I intend calling your attention to one of the chronic affections most commonly met with in this hospital.

This is *chronic articular rheumatism*, which forms certainly one of the commonest infirmities of the female sex, at least among the poor ; indeed we find it in 8 p.c. of the infirm women at the Salpêtrière.

It seems to me then that this question from the practical point of view deserves to have your attention ; the more so that the morbid history of this disease offers us many difficulties to solve, many points to clear up. For long, indeed, this apparently unwelcome study has been neglected, and notwithstanding the great importance of some recent works, there remains much progress to be accomplished in this respect. Now, it is only observers placed in a hospital like that of the Salpêtrière who can undertake such a work ; indeed it is indispensable, in order to attain this object, to have before us a large number of patients, so as to be better able to compare among themselves the very different types which chronic rheumatism may assume.

But on the threshold of the question a difficulty stops us. Though rheumatism and gout, regarded in a general manner, come into contact on many sides, and seem in many ways to present a profound analogy, it must be admitted that in the chronic form of these two affections the resemblance becomes striking and apt to embarrass the observer.

We are led then, almost in spite of ourselves, to touch on a question of doctrine, and to ask ourselves if we ought to merge these two diseases into a common description, or establish a radical difference between them.

We know that the great physicians of antiquity pronounced in favour of the former of these two opinions; or to speak more exactly, they seem never to have queried whether there was a problem to solve in this matter. Under the name of *arthritis* or joint-disease (*articulorum passio*) they have left us the description of a disease in which we sometimes find the characters of gout, sometimes of rheumatism; and the ancient tradition maintained itself through the centuries till the time when Baillou diverted the term *rheumatism* from its primitive acceptation, and applied it to that group of symptoms which we know to-day as *acute articular rheumatism*. A little later chronic articular rheumatism in its turn acquired a long contested independence.

But the distinction established by Baillou, which has never obtained universal assent, is to-day vigorously combated by eminent observers; and although most physicians recognise a profound difference between gout and rheumatism, the doctrine of their identity has found some defenders among our contemporaries, whose names carry authority in science.

These disagreements, gentlemen, depend in great measure on the very nature of the case. More than once you will be brought to recognise at the bedside how difficult it is to distinguish gout from rheumatism, especially in their chronic forms; and the name " rheumatic gout " [*rheumatisme goutteux*], which is often applied to those obscure cases on the boundary line between the two affections, seems implicitly to involve an acknowledgment of powerlessness.

And yet I am thoroughly convinced that the words *gout* and *rheumatism* correspond to two essentially distinct morbid types which ought not to be confounded. This I hope to show you by studying these two diseases, one after the other, in order to bring them into a position in which we can compare them. Possibly we shall find them meeting in the matter of etiology; but that is a point to which we shall return later on; once developed, however, they follow a parallel course without ever coming in contact.

E

They are, to quote an eminent pathologist, two branches growing from a common trunk. Provisionally, we may accept this ingenious comparison, the exactitude of which is not quite proved; but let us notice that when once distinct from the common trunk, these two branches bear very different fruit.

We shall begin this study, gentlemen, with an account of gout. Thanks to the recent labours of which it has been the object, this affection is better known to us in many respects than rheumatism is; moreover, I consider it as in some ways a type of constitutional affections, a model disease. Indeed, through circumstances unhappily too exceptional in medicine, we have found here a *morbific material*, the presence of which gives rise to many different phenomena; we possess a clue to guide us through this labyrinth, and we can for a long period follow up to a certain point the logical sequence of the symptoms, which successively unfold themselves under this influence. I am far from pretending that gout is now known to us in its intimate essence; the primary causes here as elsewhere elude our investigations, and we can only flatter ourselves that we have got hold of one of the most important links in the chain; we have discovered a vice in the humours upon which depend the chief phenomena to be observed in the course of this disease. I hope, gentlemen, that the numerous details into which we are going to enter will not fatigue your kind attention. For when we are dealing with one of these affections which offer a material basis for our researches, with gout, syphilis, lead-poisoning, we must dig out the subject to the bottom; thus, at least, we may hope to dissipate in part the obscurity which still reigns over so many other points in medicine.

One word on the general characters of the diathesis that we are going to study.

Gout is a chronic and constitutional affection, most often hereditary, and always connected with a peculiar dyscrasic state; for the presence of an excess of uric acid in the blood constitutes one of the principal characters of the disease. It is incontestable that most of the morbid manifestations which give to gout its peculiar physiognomy arise from this special condition; this is the case, for example, with regard to the diseased joints.

You know, gentlemen, that from the anatomical standpoint, gouty disease of the joints is characterised by the deposit of sodium urate either inside the joints or in the neighbouring parts.

But independently of these joint affections, and of this special state of the blood, gout may give rise to numerous and varied visceral affections, sometimes structural, sometimes merely functional. There is even reason to think that in some cases, rare however, the diathesis merely produces internal troubles of this kind during the whole evolution of the disease, without ever producing those external manifestations on which we are accustomed to reckon.

This is what old writers used to call *irregular*, as opposed to *regular*, gout, which corresponds to the classical type of the disease. Yet even in it we come across visceral disturbances; sometimes they appear suddenly in the midst of an attack (*retrocedent gout*), or in the interval (*misplaced gout*); sometimes, on the contrary, it is by a slow, progressive, almost latent, development, that those profound organic lesions are formed, which are so often met with in gouty people. (Chronic Bright's, fatty heart.)

Thus, gentlemen, all this old nomenclature, bristling with odd terms, which former writers applied to gout, is really based on clinical observation; we find by rigorously studying the facts, regular, thorough-going gout, and irregular, undeveloped, retrocedent, misplaced gout, etc. It would no doubt be useful to reform this language, which has grown very antiquated; but I do not feel in a position to do this just yet, and shall continue to employ the terms made use of by my predecessors, reserving the right of making their sense more exact.

For example, gentlemen, you will hear me speak of *acute* gout and *chronic* gout. Now, gout is an essentially chronic affection which never can be acute; yet these two terms correspond with the two chief phases of the malady.

Again, the subject of gout may first experience articular attacks having the characters of an acute affection, and the recurrence of which is more or less regularly periodic; they may be limited to a small number of joints, and specially to the great toe; then it is *partial* acute gout. In *general* acute gout, which is so much like rheumatism, all the joints may be attacked, even the big ones; often, for example, we see it affecting at the same time, knees, elbows, and wrists.

In the interval of the attacks other disturbances may arise, which are dependent on the gouty diathesis; such, for example, is that dyspepsia which so often torments gouty people; such again is gravel, the appearance of which in certain patients alternates with that of the gouty attacks.

Pretty frequently in the course of an attack of acute gout functional troubles arise, which may be attributed to the retrocession of the malady; but visceral affections dependent on appreciable structural lesions are on the contrary rare enough.

Chronic gout may take this form from the outset, but in general only follows several attacks of acute gout. The patient, who formerly enjoyed long intervals of repose, finds the attacks growing more frequent in the course of the year, and getting nearer and nearer together; they increase in number without diminishing in length; at last they become continuous, superposed on each other; they become in some degree *subintrant*, to use a term borrowed from the history of paludal fevers; then the patient is a prey to almost continuous pains, with alternations of remission and exacerbation.

With these permanent symptoms permanent lesions correspond, at first in connection with the joints, then in the internal organs; it is especially in chronic gout that these profound visceral affections are found, and they are generally the determining cause of death. Besides which, when the disease is prolonged, we see that cachectic state supervening, which so commonly brings to a close all the great constitutional maladies; it is then that dropsies, anæmia, and marasmus develop; then that the patient falls into an almost complete atonic condition, and that nature seems no longer to respond to the therapeutic agencies with which we try to oppose the progress of the disease.

After having given you these preliminary notions, I will enter on the actual history of gout, beginning with the study of the anatomical changes which are its necessary accompaniments; and as in this general affection the state of the blood seems to be a matter of chief importance, I shall first of all direct your attention to this fundamental point.

Morbid hematology of gout. Since the time when Scheele discovered lithic acid—uric acid as we now call it—many authors have supposed that this substance might be developed in the liquids of the system in the course of gout. Wollaston was the first to demonstrate that the chalk-stones of gout were composed of alkaline urates; since then, Forbes Murray and Holland in England, Jahn in Germany, Rayer and Cruveilhier in France, have advanced the opinion that the blood of the gouty ought to contain uric acid. But it is to Garrod* that the honour is due of having furnished positive demonstration of this fact (1848).

Traces of uric acid exist normally in the blood, but during an attack of gout the blood may contain ·005 to ·017 p.c. of it. To demonstrate this proposition, however, it is necessary to go in for very delicate chemical operations which are not suited to clinical practice.

There is a simpler and more easily applied procedure which, without indicating the exact amount of uric acid in the blood, enables us to determine its presence there. This is, to put about 5 grams of serum into a clock-glass (not a watch-glass because its curvature is too abrupt); then to add a few drops of acetic acid, and drop in a bit of thread. After leaving the liquid at rest in a dry place for 36 or 48 hours, you will be able to notice on microscopic examination that rhomboidal crystals are deposited on the thread which you immersed in the liquid. These crystals are composed of uric acid.

To obtain this result certain precautions must be taken. In the first place the serum must be fresh, for the presence of albuminous substances develops a kind of fermentation in it; the uric acid then decomposes into oxalic acid, urea, and allantoin, as though some lead oxide were present.

It is also necessary to avoid drying the serum too much, for then crystals of ammonio-magnesian phosphate appear in the form of very elegant vegetations. But as this salt is pretty soluble, it is only necessary to add a little water to the preparation in order to dissolve it; then rhomboidal masses of pure uric acid make their appearance.

This experiment, which is not delicate enough to show the traces of uric acid which exist in normal blood, does very well for clinical purposes. It discloses the presence of 1 part of uric acid in 65,000 of blood. (Garrod.)

When no blood is at one's disposal, it may be replaced by the

* *Med. Chir. Trans.*, 1848.

serum from a blister, which will give the same reactions, provided one has taken care not to apply the irritant to a point
attacked by gouty inflammation, for all inflammatory action
causes the disappearance of uric acid.

The clinical importance of this experiment is easily understood, for in many cases it is an excellent means of diagnosis.
It enables us also to determine in what circumstances an excess
of uric acid is produced in the blood. This phenomenon is
permanent in cases of chronic gout, but its intensity increases
before the attacks, sinking again below the normal level. In
acute gout it is absent between the attacks, at least at the
beginning of the disease (Garrod)* ; it appears afresh some
time before the explosion. Lastly, in cases of other than
articular gout we see various incidents occur, which seem
connected with the same conditions; for analysis reveals the
presence of uric acid in the blood.

On the contrary, articular rheumatism, whether acute (Garrod)
or chronic (Charcot), is never associated with this particular
dyscrasia; in it, then, we have a valuable element of diagnosis
in doubtful cases, for it is only necessary to apply a blister to
the patient, or to draw a few grams of his blood, in order to
assure ourselves whether the phenomena observed depend on
gout or rheumatism.

Still, it would not do to regard this excess of uric acid as a
pathognomonic sign of the gouty diathesis; it may also be
shown to exist in Bright's disease and in lead-poisoning. It is,
however, probable that this latter condition predisposes to gout ;
at least this seems probable if we judge by the frequency of this
affection among the lead-workers of London. (Garrod.)

The presence of uric acid in the *humours* of gouty patients is
also shown by the composition of divers secretions, both normal
and morbid. I have found it in the cerebro-spinal fluid ; Garrod
has met with it in the serum secreted into the pleura and
pericardium. It is not known for certain whether it exists in
the intestinal secretions, but it has been found in the discharge
of pustular eczema (Golding Bird), and in the white dust which
often forms on the skin of the gouty ; and which is composed
mostly of sodium urate (Petit, O. Henry).† Anyhow it is certain

---

* See Reynolds, *A System of Medicine*, 1866, art. GOUT.
† *Journal de pharmacie*, Oct., 1841.

that sweat, whether spontaneous or artificially excited, contains no trace of it. (Garrod, De Martini, Ubaldini.)*

We have still to inquire whether the blood does not present other alterations in its chemical composition in gout. But this part of the question is still rather obscure.

It seems established, however :

1. That the proportion of corpuscles in acute gout remains at the normal standard, an evident contrast with the anæmia of rheumatism; whilst in chronic gout a diminution of globules takes place in the long run : this is gouty anæmia.

2. That in acute gout the fibrin increases in amount; at least the clots are buffy.

3. That the blood albumen diminishes in chronic gout, if there is any affection of the kidneys : in such a case one meets with an excess of urea.

4. That the alkalinity of the blood is always diminished, a condition which seems to favour the production of chalky deposits.

5. That the blood sometimes contains traces of oxalic acid.

To complete this study we must consider the state of the urine in gout; we want to know whether uric acid is to be found in greater proportion than usual, as has been maintained, or whether, on the contrary, there is a smaller quantity of it, as modern researches tend to demonstrate.

In order to solve this question satisfactorily, we have not merely to determine the proportional quantity of acid contained in a sample of urine, but to find out the total amount of uric acid eliminated by the kidneys in the twenty-four hours, and this not only for one day but for several; for the excretion of uric acid by the kidneys is intermittent.

It is then indispensable to have recourse to a methodic analysis, and it must be remembered that the presence of a free acid in the urine, or the small proportion of water in it, is enough to determine the formation of those sediments, to which an exaggerated importance is generally attributed.

After having taken into account all causes of error, Garrod has arrived at the following conclusions :—

In acute gout, during the attack, the urine is scanty and high-coloured, but the quantity of uric acid excreted in the twenty-

* *Union médicale*, April, 1860, No. 40, p. 24.

four hours is almost always less than normal (·25 gram instead of ·5 gram). There is thus a diminution in the excretion of this product which coincides with an increase of its proportion in the blood.

In the intervals the urine has not been examined; we may point out, however, that gravel is frequent, as well as crystalline deposits of uric acid, formed before micturition (Rayer); but the occurrence of this phenomenon is not sufficient to prove that there is a real excess of uric acid either in the blood or in the urinary excretion.

In chronic gout, the tendency to diminished excretion becomes more and more marked. During the attack the urine is pale and abundant; no deposits form in it on cooling, so long as there is no pyrexia : one can find only traces of uric acid. But from time to time there occur *discharges,* during which the urine contains a larger amount of this substance.

In the intervals these characters persist; often we find albuminuria, and the urine sometimes contains fibrinous cylinders.

To sum up, gentlemen, it is evident that in the gouty diathesis there is an excess of sodium urate in the blood and humours (to use the language of antique medicine); it is also sodium urate which forms those deposits in the joints, which in all times have been noticed in the gouty; but this excess of uric acid is not shown by its increased excretion by the kidneys; it seems on the contrary to coincide with deficient elimination.

LECTURE IV.

MORBID ANATOMY OF GOUT.

SUMMARY.—Local changes in gout.—State of the joints.—The joint-cartilage.—Deposits of sodium urate form by preference in non-vascular tissues.—State of the synovial membrane and ligaments. — Chalk-stones. — Their composition. — Inflammatory phenomena.—Dry arthritis.—Ankylosis.—Seat of election in gout ; joints that are attacked.—Chalky concretions around joints.—Concretions in the substance of the skin.—Tophus in the external ear.—Enumeration of chief points where chalk-stones may form.

GENTLEMEN,—At our last meeting we saw that at every period of its development gout is accompanied by an excess of uric acid in the blood.

I am going to show you to-day that the local changes in this disease depend for the most part on the direct consequences of this general change, and that the deposits which are met with in the midst of organs and tissues are nearly always formed of sodium urate.

The changes to which I am going to call your attention have been long known. Long ago it was known that in gouty people, tophi, chalky deposits, were formed round the joints ; but these facts were regarded as exceptional ; and as connected with the gravest and most inveterate cases. It was for Garrod to show that the *slightest attack of gout* leaves an indelible impress on the affected tissues, which are stamped for ever with the seal of the disease.

Let us begin by studying what happens in the diseased joints ; there we shall find that gout appears with constant and really characteristic anatomical characters.

I. Beginning with the first attack deposits of sodium urate form in the cartilages of the joints ; * they occupy its most superficial part, and are situated either between the cells or actually in their interior, as Cornil and I have determined. Usually they are found towards the centre of this free surface, as far as possible from the insertion of the synovial membrane, which, as you know, stops short at the circumference of the cartilage.

* Garrod, *On Gout*, p. 211. London, 1863.

You will easily understand the cause of this remarkable preference. The parts reached by the circulation are least exposed
to the formation of these deposits, which occupy rather the
tissues wanting in vessels; now the synovial membrane and the
bone have an eminently vascular structure ; so the gouty concretions form at the surface of the cartilage to get away from the
bone, and at the very centre of this surface to get away from the
synovial membrane.

At a more advanced period of the disease, when a chronic
condition has succeeded to the acute attacks, the synovial membrane itself is invaded : it is the outlying fringes of this membrane, less rich in vessels, which are first affected ; later,
incrustations are found on the synovial membrane itself.
According to Prof. Rouget it is in the epithelioid cells that the
deposits form; moreover, the whitish *débris* sometimes met with
in gouty joints is only sodium urate originating in epithelial
desquamation.

Lastly, we know that the ligaments themselves are sometimes
involved in this incrustation. But not even there does the morbid
process stop ; it may go further and invade parts outside the
joint ; the tendons and synovial bursæ may become the seat of
it ; and when the concretions form in the neighbouring areolar
tissue, they take the name of *tophi*. You know that they sometimes acquire considerable dimensions. But these extra-articular
lesions, which are associated with a more advanced degree of
saturation, are always consecutive to the alteration of the articular
cartilages, which may exist alone, but is never absent, when the
uric acid deposits have invaded the neighbourhood of the joints.
At least I am not acquainted with any exceptions to this rule.

Let us see now what is the composition of the material con-
stituting these *dépôts*. Seen with the naked eye it looks
amorphous and resembles plaster of Paris, but examined through
a microscope it seems entirely composed of acicular crystals : it
is true that disseminated heaps of amorphous matter are sometimes found in the affected cartilage ; but Garrod maintains that
by help of the polariscope it can be shown that these agglomera-
tions themselves have a crystalline structure.

Acted on by acetic acid, rhomboidal crystals of uric acid are
formed. It is by means of this reagent that one can demonstrate
the presence of the deposits in the cartilage cells. But we have

other means of determining the chemical composition of these incrustations. If the affected cartilage be first treated by cold water, then by alcohol, and then by hot water, it becomes perfectly transparent; and the reagents which have been used for the washings deposit crystals of pure sodium urate on evaporation; these crystals give sodium carbonate on incineration, and, treated by boiling nitric acid and then by ammonia, they give rise to the "purpurate of ammonia," or murexid, the colour of which is so characteristic.

We need dwell no longer on the chemical aspect of the question : it will be enough if I point out to you that the cartilage, when freed from its incrustations, shows a perfectly normal structure, and presents no change which is appreciable either to the naked eye or to the microscope. Such at least is the general rule.

As to the often muddy liquid which the joint-cavity sometimes encloses, it not unfrequently gives an acid reaction, and on microscopic examination it is seen to contain epithelial *débris* and acicular crystals.

II. We shall now mention other lesions which, though not constant, do not therefore deserve a less detailed description.

When one opens a gouty joint at a period near the attack, one almost always finds the synovial membrane red and injected; this condition never goes on to suppuration however; but an excess of liquid is often found in the joint.

In cases of inveterate gout one may meet with all the lesions of dry arthritis; erosion of cartilages, secondary ulcerations, osteophytic growths, have been mentioned by different observers, and I have myself seen several examples of them; but these are exceptional facts, the nature of which is not well known, but which deserve attentive study.

Must we recognise in these curious cases a kind of transition between gout and rheumatism ? Could they be the result of a sort of combination of the two diatheses ? or have we to do rather with a mere complication ?

That is a question, the answer to which, it seems to me, must be put off for awhile.

Ankylosis may result from the alterations we have been describing: sometimes there is a mere rigidity, which results from the incrustation of the ligaments; but real osseous ankylosis is met with too, as Garrod and Ranvier have noticed ; and this may happen after a first attack, as has been pointed out by Todd and Prof. Trousseau.*

III. Gout, as has been known since ancient times, does not affect all the joints indiscriminately. It is the metatarso-phalangeal joint of the great toe which enjoys the disagreeable privilege of attracting its most frequent visits ; then follow the fingers ; then at a great distance the knees and elbows : the hip and shoulder are usually avoided.

One sometimes, however, sees the great toe free from gout, whilst other joints are attacked; and this fact is of great practical importance, for it enables us to understand why acute gout affecting several joints is sometimes so much like acute articular rheumatism ; and we can thus account for the way in which certain observers have been led to regard these two affections : it is evident, for example, that an attack of gout simultaneously affecting knees and wrists, may be difficult to distinguish at the bedside from a purely rheumatic affection.

Among the rare and exceptional cases we may mention those in which gout attacks the vertebral column ; the temporo-maxillary joint (Ure) ; the arytenoid cartilages (Garrod) ; the auditory ossicles (Harvey) : from this last a new kind of deafness results.

IV. From this study of post-mortem anatomy we can deduce a certain number of considerations, the importance of which from the clinical point of view, cannot be contested.

1. Note first that the incrustation of the cartilages is in-separable from articular gout, and seems to exist from the very first attack.

2. In a gouty patient the joints which have been diseased are the only ones which present this lesion of the cartilage : some-times it is only to be found in a single articulation.

3. The incrustation of sodium urate lasts after the attack ; in the interval it may not be revealed by any appreciable deformity.

4. This lesion is peculiar to gout, and is never met with in articular rheumatism, acute or chronic.

We have still to inquire what relation there is between an attack of gout and the formation of a deposit. Is this last phenomenon the cause or the consequence of the incidents which

* Todd, *Practical Remarks on Gout*. London, 1843, p. 45. Trousseau, *Clinique médicale de l'Hôtel-Dieu*, vol. iii., p. 328.

accompany it ? A question difficult to answer, which we shall discuss farther on.

V. We have seen that deposits of sodium urate form outside the diseased joints. They are met with, (1) in the tendons, and specially the *tendo Achillis*; (2) on the periosteum, but never in the bony tissue ; (3) in the serous bursæ (those of the olecranon and patella) ; (4) in the subcutaneous areolar tissue ; (5) in the actual substance of the skin. These two last points deserve special attention.

The subcutaneous *dépôts* which form near joints are an important item in the symptomatology of chronic gout, for their presence is often evident during life. They are known as *tophi* or *chalk-stones*, an expression often abused ; it is exclusively applicable to the periarticular collections of sodium urate, and should never be employed to signify the bony nodes of chronic articular rheumatism.

These chalky masses at the first period of their development are of soft and doughy consistence ; later, they grow hard and acquire some solidity. Chemically they consist of sodium urate, mixed with urate and phosphate of calcium. Microscopically we find in them fine crystalline needles.

They form specially in the hands, and occupy the extensor surfaces ; we find them also round the great toe and at other points. They are ovoid nodulated lumps, sometimes sessile, sometimes stalked, and they may reach the size of a pigeon's egg. They occur round the joints without actually resting on them ; moveable laterally, they do not precisely reproduce the shape and outline of the bony ends near them. Their lateral pressure on the joints does not always alter the form of the latter. There is no symmetry in their distribution. The skin covering them is glossy, sometimes of a dull white ; one can see the subjacent deposits through it. These different characters enable us to distinguish chalk-stones from the characteristic deformities of nodular rheumatism, which we shall study later on. But we must not forget that there are some difficult cases in which the fingers get crooked, as they do in chronic rheumatism: the mere consideration of the joint-deformities is not in such cases sufficient to establish the diagnosis, if there are no external chalk-stones. In that case we must depend on the totality of general or local symptoms characteristic of the gouty diathesis: one may even come across cases in which a recourse to a chemical examination of the blood will be useful, if absolute precision in diagnosis is needed.

VI. The concretions which form in the actual substance of the skin are of special interest from a practical point of view. Foremost among them are those concretions in the external ear, pointed out by Ideler, Scudamore, and Prof. Cruveilhier: Garrod has been able to show their great clinical value.

These little deposits are generally situated on the edge of the helix; but they may occupy the anti-helix, or the internal surface of the pavilion; they pass through three phases of development; at first they are soft, then grow hard, forming little whitish masses; lastly they may drop, leaving behind them a small cicatrix, the existence of which may be demonstrated when the chalk-stone itself has disappeared.

In 37 cases Garrod met with external chalk-stones 17 times; 7 times in the ear only, 8 times in the ear and near the joints; once only near a joint without an accompanying deposit in the ear.

These tell-tale signs sometimes appear very early; I have been able in a dyspeptic case to predict an explosion of gout, thanks to the presence of a chalk-stone in the ear; yet the patient had had no joint troubles at the time when he consulted me. Garrod noticed these concretions forming in one of his patients five years before the appearance of any symptom in connection with the joints.* In this way we can understand their importance in diagnosis.

In the absence of concretions in the external ear you would examine, (1) the eyelids, (2) the wings of the nose, (3) the cheeks, (4) the palms, (5) the corpora cavernosa.

At all these points cutaneous deposits have been found, identical with those I have just described.

I have now to speak of the morbid anatomy of visceral gout. We shall devote our next meeting to this study.

---

* These exceptional facts cannot weaken the general rule. The joint troubles nearly always precede the formation of these external deposits.

LECTURE V.

MORBID ANATOMY OF VISCERAL GOUT.

SUMMARY.—Suppressed gout; *functional lesions* in gout.—In most of the cases in which an autopsy has been performed they depend on material changes.— Structural lesions most often met with in the viscera of gouty people.—Fatty degeneration of the heart.—Atheroma of the aorta.—Lesions of the bronchi.— Gouty nephritis.—There are two quite distinct kinds of it.—Gout of the kidney. —Gouty kidney of the English; lesions corresponding to this expression.— Deposits of sodium urate.—Bright's disease.—Interstitial nephritis.
    Morbid changes in animals like those of gout.—They do not exist in mammals. —Are met with in certain birds.—Lesions of the same kind in reptiles.—Experiments of Zalesky.—Consequences of ligature of the ureters in different animals.

GENTLEMEN,—If gout were a commoner affection in our hospitals, we should probably be better acquainted with the visceral lesions which may result from this disease. But, as you know, the opportunity for making post mortem examinations on gouty patients rarely occurs in France; the English authors have been better off in this respect, and have furnished us with some interesting details on this subject. But, speaking generally, it may be said that the question is little understood, at least so far as the anatomical lesions go. Gouty nephritis is the only exception to this rule; so we shall study it with special care, after having rapidly sketched the state of our knowledge touching the other visceral manifestations of gout.

I. We shall first have to consider those sudden modifications of the course of gout which have received the name of metastases or retrocessions.

It is evident that in such cases we must suppose that at first the lesions are quite superficial, especially when these events have not had a fatal issue. It does not seem likely that the diseased organ is the seat of a profound alteration, and one would be disposed rather to class troubles of this kind in the group of *functional lesions*. But here the control of morbid anatomy is almost completely wanting, by reason of the ease with which, in the majority of cases, the symptoms pass away.

Things do not always happen thus, however; death sometimes supervenes, and we may be called on to perform the autopsy : in such cases organic lesions have often been found, and we possess several creditable observations of this kind. Some of these facts relate to the gastric incidents of gout ; we owe them to Dietrich, Perry, and Budd. The patients have succumbed with the classical symptoms of gout which has retreated to the stomach, and there has been found an œdematous swelling of the submucous connective tissue of this organ as well as more or less profound alterations of the mucous membrane itself.

In other cases, when the patients have rapidly succumbed during an attack of gout, the ordinary lesions of cerebral hemorrhage, and sometimes even rupture of the heart, have been found.

If it were allowable to decide the point from these examples, we should be led to believe that even in the cases where functional troubles arise by reason of gout, they correspond with less superficial organic changes than is generally supposed.

But other lesions apparently dependent on this affection have been met with in subjects attacked by gout, whether acute or chronic, when an intervening affection or the progress of the disease has been the cause of death. We will rapidly pass them in review.

A. The muscular walls of the heart are often affected by fatty degeneration. S. Edwards, Lobstein, and some other observers, have found sodium urate in valvular concretions, but the accuracy of this fact is contested by Garrod.

B. The aorta is often the seat of atheromatous changes ; moreover, Bramson, Bence Jones, and Landerer have met with urate of sodium in its walls.

C. The presence of this substance has been noted by Bence Jones in the walls of the bronchial tubes.

D. Hitherto no special alteration has been found either in the brain, its meninges, or the cerebral arteries.

E. The kidney-changes of gout, usually described as gouty nephritis, must be divided into two kinds.

In the first place, we have the affection called gouty nephritis by Rayer ; it might be called *grit of the kidney*. It presents the characters of chronic interstitial nephritis, but is specially distinguished by sandy infarcts of uric acid, sometimes in a crystalline state. There may also be more considerable gravel. These deposits are found : (1) on the surface of the kidney and in the cortical substance; (2) in the pyramids and papillæ; (3) in the calices and pelvis; usually the concretions are larger at this last point.

These changes may be met with in cases other than those of articular gout; but it is indisputable that they are very common in this disease.

In the second place, we meet with *gouty* nephritis, properly so called; it is the *gouty kidney* of the English authors. Noticed by Castelnau in 1843, it has been well described by Todd and Garrod. Anatomically it is characterised by—

(1.) Infarcts of sodium urate in the form of whitish streaks; they are met with in the medullary substance (never in the cortex), and sometimes in the pyramids : microscopically, they are seen to be formed of crystalline needles, which, according to Garrod, occupy the intervals between the uriniferous tubes. But I think I have shown that they originate in and obstruct the actual cavities of the uriniferous tubes.*

(2.) By accompanying alterations of the kidney corresponding to the ordinary lesions of Bright's disease.

There is at first a tubular nephritis† which reaches two different degrees. In the first, the kidney keeps its ordinary volume, but the cortical substance thickens and gets a yellow tint. The tufts of Malpighi are injected; the uriniferous tubes are filled with epithelium cells, distended, opaque, and full of fatty or albuminoid granules. In the second stage we find atrophy of the cortical substance, and that granular state of the kidney which belongs especially to Bright's disease.

But besides the tubular nephritis, we also find the interstitial nephritis which corresponds to the gouty kidney of the English authors. It is characterised especially by a thickening of the connective tissue between the tubules, with proliferation of nuclei; the kidney is diminished in volume; it is wrinkled, granular, and nodulated on the surface : the cortical substance is notably atrophied. In this affection the kidneys are never found lardaceous.

According to Garrod, these changes are found in every case of inveterate gout examined after death. They may be present early on and have been met with after seven or eight attacks.

* Charcot and Cornil, Memoirs of the *Société de Biologie*, 1864.
† Loc. cit.

F

In a case observed by Traube the symptoms of this renal affection showed themselves one year only after the first manifestations of gout. This would be a visceral form of the disease.

Although the alterations of the renal tissue, barring the deposit of sodium urate, differ in nothing from those of ordinary Bright's disease, the symptoms of this gouty albuminuria are remarkable for their benignity and their slight intensity. We need not insist on this point, which belongs to symptomatology.

Several incidents which figure often enough in the series of gouty symptoms may be referred to this group of causes. Thus *dyspepsia* is often aggravated, if not altogether caused, by this morbid state of the kidneys, and œdema is often a consequence of it. One may observe the convulsive or comatose form of uræmia in gouty people, which evidently depends on the state of the kidneys. Cerebral apoplexy and hypertrophy of the heart may also reckon as distant consequences of the renal lesion.

II. Here ends our account of the anatomical lesions characteristic of the gouty diathesis. But before leaving this subject, I think it well to bring before you certain facts of *comparative and experimental pathology*, which seem to me calculated to throw much light on the questions we have already raised, and which we shall next consider.

May gout occur in animals? And supposing that it may, does it produce effects like those which afflict the human species?

In a recent work on comparative pathology, Gleisberg replies in the negative. He rightly observes that most of the affections spoken of as gout ought to be referred to chronic rheumatism. Anyhow, it is incontestable that in certain animals an affection much like human gout is developed, and is characterised like it by deposition of urates in the different tissues.

It is not in mammals that we find our points of comparison, as analogy would have led us to suppose, but in birds and certain reptiles kept in captivity and placed under special conditions. You will be less surprised at finding in these two great classes of animals an affection so resembling gout, if you reflect that in them the work of disintegration, as Davy and other chemists have shown, does not produce urea, but ammonium urate. It is only this latter product which is found in the urine.

The authors of various works on ornithology will tell you, gentlemen, that lesions very like those of gout may exist in different birds. Aldrovandi tells us that falcons are liable to have swellings composed of lumps of gypseous matter round their toes. This disease is incurable.

There are analogous facts in regard to parrots. Bertin of Utrecht found in *Psittacus grandis* uratic swellings in the neighbourhood of the joints, and analogous infarcts in the joints and kidneys.

Lesions of the same kind have been noticed in reptiles ; Pagenstecher has seen the kidneys and joints affected in this way in *Alligator sclerops*. In serpents these changes may take place in the kidneys ; in the tortoise Bertin has also found articular and renal lesions.

It is curious to meet with lesions in all respects so like those of gout in animals so little allied to man. But a more remarkable fact still is that these lesions may be artificially produced by physiological experiment. This is shown in an interesting work published at Tübingen by Zalesky.

This observer tied the ureters in fowls, geese, and in certain snakes (*Coluber natrix*). The first morbid phenomena are evident in from twelve to fifteen hours after the operation. Life lasts two or three days. After death, sodium urate is found in the following viscera :—

(1.) The kidneys contain it in the medullary, but not the cortical, part. The ureters also contain it.

(2.) The lymphatics, the serous membranes, the areolar tissue, the capsules of all the organs, are impregnated with it.

(3.) The gastric follicles contain a notable quantity.

(4.) It is found in the valves of the heart.

(5.) The joints present considerable accumulations of it both inside and out.

The muscles contain no deposit of urate of sodium, but the muscle-juice contains much uric acid. The brain and its membranes appear to be completely free from it.

As to the liquids of the system, the blood contains notable quantities of uric acid, and after death we find clots of alkaline urates.

Lastly, the gall-bladder contains an enormous quantity of sodium urate—a fresh coincidence with human pathology; for in man, according to Frerichs, calculi are sometimes found in the gall-bladder, which are composed of sodium urate.

That we might accept these statements without reserve, it would be necessary to renew and vary the experiments. We should have to study, for example, the effects produced by ligature of a single ureter, and find out whether, after a certain space of time, we should not arrive at the same results. It is not for this reason any less true that the experiments of Zalesky are of great interest, and deserve to be taken into serious consideration.

Gentlemen, although this excursion into the domain of comparative pathology may seem to you a little foreign to practice, the importance which I attach to these facts need not astonish you : we shall meet with them again when we come to discuss the physiological theory of gout.

LECTURE VI.

THE SYMPTOMS OF GOUT—THE URIC DIATHESIS—ACUTE AND CHRONIC GOUT.

SUMMARY.—Two chief forms of gout : acute gout, chronic gout.—Gout is always at bottom a chronic disease, but the acute attack has a quite different aspect from the permanent state.—Uric acid diathesis.—Group of symptoms which characterises it.—Urinary secretion less abundant and richer in solid material.—Microscopic grit.—Acute gout.—Prodromata.—Invasion of the articular pains.—General symptoms.—Chief characters of acute gout.—Secondary phenomena.—Deviations from the regular type.—General acute gout.—Indolent or asthenic gout.—Recurrence of the attacks.—Insensible transition of acute, into chronic, gout.—Gouty cachexia.—Gravity of the intercurrent affections.—Chronic gout succeeding acute gout.—Gout chronic from the beginning.—Development of chalk-stones.

GENTLEMEN,—The anatomical changes in gout have hitherto exclusively occupied our attention. We have studied the modifications which both the solids and liquids of the system undergo under the influence of this affection. I have now to bring before your notice the symptoms which depend on the existence of these changes.

We showed at the beginning that gout, being now acute, now chronic, appears under two principal forms, each of which deserves a special description. It must not be forgotten, however, that in all cases gout is an essentially chronic disease. In short, the first attack is the earliest manifestation of a constitutional state, which subsequently may remain latent for some years, but which sooner or later is revealed by fresh symptoms. If cases of transient gout exist which are marked by a single attack, facts of this kind are very exceptional and do not invalidate the general rule.

Still, the aspect of an acute attack is so different from that of the disease when regarded as a permanent condition, that we are forced to respect these terms which are consecrated by custom, and which, in spite of their inexactitude, undoubtedly correspond with real facts.

We shall therefore study first acute gout and then chronic gout, conforming thus to the universally accepted tradition. But before dealing with this subject it will be best to call your attention to a morbid state which sometimes shows itself before the appearance of the articular phenomena, and which in patients already attacked by gout, often enough fills up the intervals between the attacks. You are already thinking of the uric acid diathesis. Let us for a few moments consider this general state, our knowledge of which has been chiefly contributed by the English.*

Uric Acid Diathesis. The fundamental point is a peculiar dyspepsia, the commonest symptoms of which are flatulence and distension of the stomach, gastric acidity and consequent pyrosis. At the same time there is a bitter taste in the mouth, and the tongue is dry and furred : almost always constipation is to be noticed.

The liver seems also to participate in the disturbance of the digestive apparatus ; it is often swollen, and reaches beyond the margin of the false ribs ; sometimes one notices a half icteric tint, and the scanty stools are grey and discoloured.

Fairly pronounced nervous phenomena accompany this dyspeptic state, and may even exist independently of it. We find uncalled for lassitude, prostration, headache ; sleep is interrupted ; often the patients get hypochondriacal. In women this state may be complicated by manifestations of hysteria.

In certain people cardiac palpitations and bronchial catarrh may also appear. These phenomena, of no great importance in themselves, acquire a more serious meaning by reason of the other circumstances which go along with them. But what specially characterises this peculiar state is, that it gets worse periodically and is very susceptible to errors in diet ; this is a feature of its connection with gout, the importance of which cannot fail to strike us.

What happens to the urine in such a case ? Generally speaking, it is less abundant and richer in solid material ; the urine is scanty, but very acid and highly coloured ; it is loaded with sediment, which generally forms after emission, but which may be already formed in the bladder ; it is common in such cases to find crystals of uric acid in the urine ; this is the "*gravelle microscopique*" of Rayer.

---

* Todd, *Practical Remarks on Gout,* etc. London, 1843.—Budd, *On the Organic Diseases of the Stomach,* etc. London, 1855.

When the uric acid diathesis shows itself before the articular phenomena of gout, one may sometimes observe from the beginning an excess of uric acid in the blood. But the group of symptoms which I have just described is met with especially during the intervals between attacks ; one then finds rheumatoid pains developing in the muscular masses, and in the joints which are the seat of election of the inflammatory symptoms. These pains appear as abrupt twinges, and in the absence of articular inflammations they are one of the most characteristic symptoms of gout, the explosion of which they may sometimes precede.

No doubt there are cases where things may remain in this state, and in which the predisposition which gives rise to the uric acid diathesis never reaches the last phase of this morbid development, just as in some cases gout is developed from the beginning; but usually it is from this morbid basis that actual gout grows up. We shall now study its development.

Acute Gout. Suppose that an attack of acute gout is on the point of declaring itself in a person who hitherto has never experienced the assaults of this disease. In the majority of cases special prodromata will announce the approaching fit ; sometimes this is an extreme exaggeration of the symptoms of the uric acid diathesis which have just been described ; sometimes, on the contrary, it is an abnormal feeling of well-being, a peculiar excitement ; sometimes phenomena that are new in the experience of the patient are produced—an angina, a sciatic or muscular pain, for example. But it must be remembered that in a certain number of cases prodromata may be completely wanting ; the attack then breaks out abruptly without any warning.

The invasion of the articular pains is sudden and violent, and almost always takes place at night. The patient feels all at once a characteristic pain, compared by some to a sting, by others to a blow with a stick ; many individuals imagine that they have had a sprain, and the diagnosis is sometimes difficult just at first. This sensation is most often felt in the metatarso-phalangeal joint of the great toe. Soon the affected spot gets red and swollen ; the veins of the affected limb are distended, and the limb assumes a purplish colour, and is sometimes covered with ecchymoses, according to Gairdner; at the same time there develops a real or apparent fluctuation, due in the former case to the presence of an excess of fluid in the cavity of the joint.

The general symptoms which accompany these local manifestations are fever, erratic shiverings, and a nervous irritable state; the urine is notably diminished in quantity, and deposits abundant sediment on cooling.

Towards morning the pain and most of the other symptoms are better, only to grow worse again in the evening or during the night; this state lasts five or six days when medicine intervenes, a week to a fortnight when it does not. Thus there is a kind of chaplet of little attacks, strung together, but separated by intervals of remission.

From the first days a well-marked œdema of the inflamed parts appears and soon extends over the whole limb, the swollen parts retaining the impression of the finger: the decline of the attack is marked by superficial desquamation. At last all is right again, and the patient enjoys a repose which will only be disturbed at the next crisis.

In brief, the most salient characters of acute gout are the following:—

1. The sudden invasion and the special character of the pain. A Frenchman quoted by Watson,* comparing this sensation, which he had often experienced, to the effects of strong pressure, said that at the first turn of the screw it was rheumatism, but that at the second it was gout.

2. The œdema of the limb at the onset of the attack, desquamation at its decline.

3. The absence of suppuration.

4. The special seat of the symptoms which are localised by preference in the great toe.

5. The febrile reaction, the intensity of which is proportional to the number of joints affected, contrary to what we observe in acute articular rheumatism.

Lastly, we must bear in mind the subsequent phenomena. The most striking fact is the relief experienced by the patient at the end of the attack ; this feeling of relative comfort probably corresponds with the destruction of a certain quantity of uric acid.

* *Principles of Physic*, etc., vol. ii., p. 752.

Along with this modification of the general state we must note the modifications which supervene in the local state. Most frequently, after a first attack, there remains no interference with the movements of the joints, but sometimes we find a prolonged rigidity or an indefinite persistence of the œdematous state. These, according to Garrod, are the results of injudicious treatment, such as, for example, the application of leeches to the diseased spot.

In some cases, happily very exceptional, there is ankylosis from the beginning (Todd, Trousseau, Garrod) ; at other times there is a premature formation of chalk-stones.

Such, gentlemen, is the most ordinary type of an attack of regular acute gout. I might no doubt have traced you a more animated sketch of it, if I had not compelled myself to follow an analytical method, but you can readily console yourselves for this by reading the immortal description which Sydenham has given of it, or the eloquent pages devoted to this subject by Trousseau.

Let us see now what deviations may occur from the regular type which I have just described.

Let us first consider the irregularities with reference to the seat of the articular symptoms. Generally, or more correctly speaking, in the immense majority of cases, it is the great toe which is affected, sometimes on one side only, sometimes on the two sides successively. Scudamore showed that in 512 cases of gout, the great toe was affected 373 times at the first attack, either alone or along with other joints ; and out of these 373 cases there were 341 in which the symptoms were limited to one joint.

It is evident that, from the diagnostic point of view, this singular preference is of the greatest importance. In this respect there is a well-marked difference between gout and articular rheumatism.

But there are cases in which the great toe is only attacked secondarily ; the disease appears at another point, the knee for example. Traumatic influences here seem to play an important *rôle ;* as in the case of rheumatism, a wound or blow predisposes the injured joint to become the seat of gout: we shall see this later on in reference to etiology.

There are exceptional cases in which the great toe remains

quite free, both at the first and at subsequent attacks.   Garrod points out cases of this kind, and I have myself observed a few. Gout may then, from the onset, affect the knee or any other joint.

Lastly, there is a form of the disease which deserves our special attention, for it presents the greatest analogy to acute articular rheumatism, at least in its outward appearance ; I mean *primary general acute gout,* which from the beginning affects several joints at once ; a large number, both great and small, may be affected simultaneously.   The attacks then have a longer duration, and last for two or three weeks, sometimes even being prolonged for several months.   This is what Trousseau calls gout in successive paroxysms.   How often have not these symptoms been referred to acute articular rheumatism.

But gout is not variable merely in regard to the seat of its manifestations.

The intensity of the chief symptoms, the pain and the general reaction may be remarkably diminished.   This is often the case in women and feeble patients.   This is the mild or asthenic form of acute gout, the prognosis of which is less favourable, and which readily passes into a chronic state.

But gout, as I have already pointed out, is an essentially chronic affection, even in its acute form.   It is therefore indispensable to study the attacks in their relation to one another, following them step by step at each recurrence, and noting the characters which the new attacks present.

Recurrence of the attacks.   At its origin, gout seems to grant pretty long intervals of rest to its victims ; there is but one attack every two or three years.   Later, they recur annually : then they appear twice in the year, spring and autumn, a fact which already indicates a modification in the character of the disease, for the first attacks generally happen at the end of winter (Trousseau).

At last, the intermediate period getting less and less, the attacks recur every three or four months : here we have already a transition to the chronic state.

Remember also that accidental conditions may intervene to disturb this regular progress ; traumatic lesions, severe inflammations, erysipelas, may sometimes accelerate its course, and suddenly provoke unexpected recurrences.

Characters of the fresh attacks. For a long time there occurs no striking change in the group of symptoms which characterises the attacks. Limited to one or two joints, the arthritis continues to occupy the same seat; the general symptoms remain equally intense, and the intervals between the attacks are free from any morbid manifestation.

But as the disease progresses it imperceptibly changes in character, and shows a more and more marked tendency to assume the chronic form. One then sees the large joints attacked one after another, and this almost always in the following order: first the toes, the insteps, the knees, then the hands, the wrists, the elbows, and in some rare cases the shoulder and hip. It is then that the patient, struck by the indubitable analogy, fancies readily that his disease has changed its nature and been transformed into rheumatism.

At the same time the attacks, though longer, are diminished in intensity: they take a subacute form, and are accompanied by a less intense febrile reaction ; the intervals are less free and the non-articular phenomena of gout are more and more marked; the patient suffers more than formerly from dyspepsia, palpitations, and various nervous troubles ; in a word, the disease, at first concentrated, has ended by spreading out ; it gains in extension what it loses in depth. But it has already become chronic gout. We shall proceed to study the characters of this latter affection.

Chronic Gout. This form of gout is essentially characterised by the general depression of the powers of the system with which it is accompanied, seeming to justify the expressions *atonic*, *asthenic*, gout, applied to it by some authors. A marked enfeeblement, a tendency to the cachectic state, always appear in different degrees, when the disease has arrived at this point. Moreover, intercurrent affections are of quite exceptional gravity in such cases; bronchitis, pneumonia, typhus, take an unusual course, and this last affection is almost always fatal (Schmidtmann, Murchison); in this respect a connection may be established between gout and diabetes, which will be justified later by other analogies.

We know already that in chronic gout there is a permanent

alteration of the blood and urine, which explains to us, up to a certain point, why the intervals between the fits are filled up with more or less serious non-articular symptoms,—palpitation, dyspepsia, nervous troubles. It is also by reason of this change that the tendency to certain structural visceral affections of kidneys, liver, heart, and vascular system in general, seems to develop.

But chronic gout, though generally following acute gout, may appear as such from the beginning, and then presents rather different characters.

1. When chronic gout follows acute gout, it affects the joints almost constantly; but the local symptoms become less acute, the pains less intense; at last, as I have already indicated, the upper limbs begin to experience the influence of the disease. It is at this time that we observe articular deformities, at this time especially that chalky concretions form; these latter we shall soon consider specially.

At the same time the change which has taken place in the constitutional state is evidenced by a less intense reaction at the time of the attacks, and in the intervals by more marked visceral symptoms.

2. When, on the contrary, gout is chronic from the beginning, chalk-stones often form early on, especially in the hands; this is the *primary chronic form* of gout, in which the local symptoms depend almost exclusively on the presence of larger or smaller deposits.

Grave visceral affections early appear in a certain number of cases of this kind.

Todd has seen albuminuria appear two years after the onset of the disease, and two years later the patient experienced epileptiform symptoms and died comatose. In another patient, whose case is reported by Traube, there was albuminuria one year after the first symptoms, and the body was already covered with chalk-stones.

We shall now consider the clinical characters of these concretions which are already known to us from the anatomical point of view. Indeed, chalk-stones, once formed, have a kind of independent existence, and consequently deserve a study to themselves.

Their diagnostic importance cannot be exaggerated, for they give rise to special deformities which belong exclusively to gout; moreover, their occurrence is much more frequent than was formerly supposed. Scudamore said they were to be met with in 10 p.c. of the cases; that was a good deal, but now, reckoning concretions of the external ear, it may be affirmed, as is done by Garrod, that they exist in half the cases.

Their formation, which was very well described by Moore, in 1811, comprises three periods. Subsequently to an attack,* during an interval of remission, and sometimes with no pain, a fluctuating liquid raises the skin, as was observed by Cœlius Aurelianus. Secondly, these deposits solidify, and assume the form of hard, indolent, more or less rounded masses, which grow bigger at each attack, and even in the intervals. Lastly, in the third period, the skin ulcerates and gives passage often to considerable quantities of chalky matter.

When this elimination occurs without inflammatory action, the cretaceous masses become bare; and in England gouty old men may often be seen to mark their points in playing with the chalk-stones which ornament their hands, and which leave on the green-table a white mark like a chalk line. At other times more or less active inflammation develops, there is swelling, with red or purplish colouration and threatening of gangrene : then it opens; pus escapes along with chalky matter composed almost entirely of sodium urate. In consequence of this, ulcers, which are difficult to heal, sometimes form. The urate of sodium being infiltrated through the meshes of the connective tissue, the wound cleans with difficulty, and the cicatrices have a tendency to open afresh.

Sometimes the joints themselves may be involved, but, a fact well worthy of remark, without any serious danger for the patient.

The discharge of this material soon leads to a local or general amendment. Garrod has even shown that if one attempts to repress this action by astringent applications, the articular pains sometimes reappear in the neighbourhood of the ulceration or at a more distant point.

In its last phase gout induces a cachexia, the principal

---

* I knew a gouty patient who never had a pain anywhere, however transient, without a tophus immediately forming th-re. (B. Ball.)

elements of which are profound anæmia, extreme muscular weakness, especially of the lower limbs, and an intense depression of the nervous system; the patients become incapable of undergoing the slightest fatigue, and cannot bear the least noise.

Here, gentlemen, ends the clinical history of regular gout. This form of the disease, as you have been able to convince yourselves, is specially characterised by a marked and often exclusive preference for the joints. This type is the one you will most often meet with in practice, and which you will find the easiest to recognise. One cannot say this of the anomalous, irregular, or larval forms of gout; they often borrow the aspect of the most various affections, and those most foreign to the gouty diathesis, and the physician who has neglected to practise specially the diagnosis of cases of this kind, is liable to commit errors involving the most regrettable consequences. This subject then is well-deserving of our attention for some time, especially since this study will enable you to grasp one of the most essential differences between the spirit of ancient medicine and of contemporary science. We shall commence this study at our next meeting.

LECTURE VII.

SYMPTOMS OF VISCERAL GOUT.

SUMMARY.—Partiality of the ancients for the study of the metamorphoses of disease. —Importance of larval gout from this point of view.— Scepticism of the moderns. —Definition of visceral gout.—*Functional* troubles; *organic* lesions.—Gout, larval, misplaced, retrocedent.—May visceral gout exist independently of any articular affection ?

Affections of the digestive canal. — Spasm of the œsophagus. — Dyspepsia, cardialgia, gouty gastritis.—Hepatic manifestations of gout.—Circulatory system : lesions of the heart and vessels.—Sudden death.—Cerebral manifestations of gout.— Its influence on diseases of the spinal cord has not yet been clearly demonstrated.— Respiratory system ; gouty asthma.—Urinary passages : often affected in gout.— Functional troubles of the kidneys.—Gouty nephritis.—Indication of some other non-articular affections dependent on gout.

GENTLEMEN,—As I told you at the close of our last meeting, the study of visceral gout will now occupy our attention. As I have already mentioned to you, the subject came vividly before the minds of our predecessors, and you will readily perceive the reasons for this. Accustomed to general views, and little anxious to analyse clinical facts minutely, the physicians of past ages have always had a marked partiality for the study of the metamorphoses which affections of long duration undergo. From Galen to Roderic a Castro, who in the 17th century published a curious work with the odd title " Quæ ex quibus," and from him down to Lorry, a great many authors have endeavoured to describe the transformations of diseases (*mutationes morborum*). Gout occupies an important place in these writings, and has been invoked more than once, when it was desired to prove that a disease may assume the most varied forms without losing its identity.

It is generally admitted now-a-days that our predecessors exaggerated the number and frequency of the transfigurations which pathological states may undergo ; and at the present time this study, which was once so flourishing, has somewhat fallen into oblivion ; or more correctly, it is regarded from quite another point of view.

As for what specially concerns larval gout, it must be agreed that the ancients saw it everywhere, even where it did not exist.

But I am not able to range myself with those physicians, who, under the present influence of too radical a reaction, have gone so far as to deny the existence of this form of gout. Such scepticism is too sweeping. Visceral gout is relatively not a frequent affection, but it does exist; I hope at least that I shall prove this to you. What we have to do is to determine by attentive analysis in what it consists, and what are the limits which it is convenient to assign to it.

It does not seem needful at this stage in our progress to justify in your eyes the importance of this subject, which demands your attention from a double point of view; for with reference to general pathology, this very obscure and much debated question of metastases and retrocession is most intimately related to the subject in hand ; and as to special pathology, the history of these visceral manifestations enables us to grasp both the profound resemblance which connects rheumatism with gout, as well as the differences which separate them.

But before reaching clinical ground to deal with the description of particular facts, it seems to me indispensable to define as far as possible what is meant by the expression—*visceral gout.*

The term must not be indiscriminately applied to all the diseases with which a gouty person may be attacked. These affections, of which some are purely accidental, whilst others have but a distant relationship with gout, are modified no doubt by the nature of the ground in which they grow ; but they are not to be placed among the direct consequences of this disease.

We shall then reserve the term *visceral gout* for the morbid phenomena which develop in our internal organs under the immediate influence of the gouty diathesis ; and in this pathological series we shall distinguish two natural groups : the first comprises the *functional* troubles which arise from this general state; the second includes the *organic* lesions which may develop under its influence.

It is especially to the first of these two groups that the expressions are applicable of larval, misplaced, and retrocedent, gout, expressions one meets with in authors at every step ; and in order to preserve a homogeneous character for this group of pathological facts, we should only include in it those visceral affections, which in all essential respects are analogous to the articular lesions of gout, and play the same *rôle* in the pathological drama as they do, except for the locality which they occupy.

Let me quote here a few examples, in order that you may better grasp my thought. An individual, long dyspeptic, suddenly experiences an attack of gout ; and lo ! he is cured of his dyspepsia, at least apparently ; but the joint symptoms once more quiet, the stomach becomes affected again as before. That, gentlemen, is an incontestable case of visceral gout, in which the stomach seems to replace the joints in the series of morbid manifestations, and, as it were, is called to suffer in their place. It is known, likewise, that a patient affected with epileptiform convulsions may become gouty, and that recovery from the nervous symptoms may sometimes ensue ; Garrod has collected several instances of this.

In cases of this kind the visceral affection seems to consist in a purely dynamical disturbance ; at most there is a superficial modification of the tissues. You will see, moreover, that the gravity of these manifestations is dependent on the seat which they occupy.

But here we nearly always find wanting those crystalline deposits of sodium urate, which in the cartilages and fibrous tissues record to some extent the history of the preceding attacks. However, the anatomical elements may be impregnated with urate of sodium, as I pointed out above, without showing any crystalline deposits. These affections are very mobile in character ; they appear and disappear suddenly ; they may coexist with the articular symptoms, or may precede, or follow them ; but in the majority of cases the two alternate. When the visceral affection precedes the articular gout, and constitutes for a longer or shorter time the only manifestation of the diathesis, it is called *larval gout;* when, on the contrary, it follows the articular symptoms, it is called *retrocedent*, provided, at least, that the metastasis has been excited by the manifest intervention of an external cause,—cold, for example. Lastly, it is said that gout has *retroceded of its own accord*, when the disappearance of the symptoms has taken place spontaneously.

The study which we have undertaken here presents one of the most difficult problems to solve. May visceral gout occur in subjects whose joints have never been, and are never going to be, diseased ? In other words, may larval gout exist independently

G

of articular gout ? The thing is at least probable, but with how many difficulties is not the demonstration of it surrounded !

Still, it is to be noticed that these phenomena may occur in a subject whose parents were gouty, and on that account manifestly predisposed to gout. That is a preliminary presumption in favour of the hypothesis which we are endeavouring to defend. In the second place, the visceral affection often presents itself in one of the forms which it habitually assumes when coexisting with articular gout. Thirdly, there are cases in which the affection of the joints exists in a rudimentary state, and is shown by painful twinges. Lastly, the uric acid diathesis, characterised by the group of phenomena which I have previously described, may be present and give to these visceral manifestations of gout a stamp of authenticity which will hardly be called in question when the *presence of uric acid in the blood* has been determined.

We have now to consider the second group—that of organic lesions—which in the end almost always succeed the affections of the first kind, and occupy the same locality. But I am far from recognising an absolute distinction between these two groups of phenomena, and I willingly believe that the functional disorders are but the first stage of those modifications of structure which give rise to permanent troubles.

I have tried, gentlemen, to reduce to quite simple notions the very complicated nomenclature of gouty affections ; and that these notions may be impressed on your minds with still greater clearness I will sum them up in the following table :—

$$\text{Visceral Gout}............\left\{\begin{array}{l}\text{Functional }\left\{\begin{array}{l}\text{Larval (previous)}\\\text{Retrocedent (subsequent)}\end{array}\right.\\\text{Structural, with permanent lesions.}\end{array}\right.$$

I. We shall successively study the two forms of visceral gout which we have recognised, in each of the organs and systems which may become its seat. We shall begin with the alimentary canal, for it is here that affections of this kind particularly develop. It has been correctly said that " gout is to the stomach what rheumatism is to the heart." *

A. We will say but a word on quite a rare affection of the œsophagus, noted by Stoll and Garrod : I mean spasmodic constriction of this tube, which opposes the passage of the

---

* Ball, *Thèse pour le concours de l'aggrégation*, p. 158.

alimentary bolus. An attack of gout leads to a removal of this state.

B. Let us now consider gastric gout, a subject I have dipped into already, when telling you of the dyspepsia common to gouty subjects and of the nervous symptoms accompanying it.

Larval gout of the stomach precedes the fits, and may appear before any articular affection : in a great many cases, as soon as the joints are attacked, the gastric troubles undergo a notable amendment.

In a patient whom I have myself observed, there were digestive troubles before the first attack of gout ; the diagnosis was based on the presence of a chalky concretion in the external ear, and the subsequent course of the symptoms quite confirmed our view of the case.

In another case there had been previously a single attack of articular gout. Intense dyspepsia had subsequently shown itself, and after vainly invoking the aid of regular science, the patient thought he must call in homœopathy. Unlooked for success crowned this mode of treatment, and he was already congratulating himself on having had recourse to the new Medicine, when all at once came an attack of gout in the foot, and explained this miraculous cure ; here there was a visceral manifestation of the diathesis.

Gout that has retroceded to the stomach differs from larval gout by its sometimes greater gravity. It is in such cases that we often have the opportunity of observing those grave symptoms which sometimes end in death.

Gout, it is maintained, may retrocede of its own accord; this is the spontaneous metastasis of Guilbert. But most often this displacement has been excited by the intervention of a direct cause; the regular course of the disease has been interrupted by a vivid emotion, an attack of indigestion, or by inappropriate treatment; weary of suffering the patient has been imprudent enough to plunge the limb into iced water (Lynch, Parry), or to take a special remedy, colchicum for example (Trousseau, Potton of Lyon). Then the pain and swelling of the joints yield as by enchantment ; the patient is congratulating himself on the treatment he has adopted, when all at once the formidable phenomena of gout retrocedent to the stomach burst out.

We must distinguish here, as Budd and Scudamore have done,

two symptomatic types. In the first the disease appears in a *cardialgic* or *spasmodic* form, and there is then a sharp pain with feeling of cramp in the epigastric region, this distressing sensation being allayed by pressure; there is at the same time a marked distension of the stomach, with sickness, which is often uncontrollable, and a general state of more or less gravity : then we observe algidity with cold sweats come on; the pulse is small, frequent, irregular; there is a tendency to syncope. In such a case, especially since Cullen's time, stimulants are employed and alcohol in large doses can be borne.

In the second type, the disease takes an inflammatory form. There is sharp epigastric pain, especially on pressure; repeated vomiting, sometimes blackish or bloody ; a more or less intense febrile reaction, and as a consequence of all this, a state of general prostration. But here stimulants are not tolerated and blood-letting is spoken well of.

In cases where health is to be recovered, the whole set of symptoms suddenly disappears, either under the influence of treatment or spontaneously, and the gouty inflammation re-appears in the great toe. Most people believe in the efficacy of stimulant applications to the joint first affected, in order to recall the gout to the spot from which it seems to have been displaced ; but there are scarcely any well-authenticated facts recorded in corroboration of the utility of this treatment.

But science possesses eight or ten cases in which these symptoms have terminated in death. At the autopsy which has occasionally been performed, a thickening of the submucous connective tissue has been met with ; the gastric *mucosa* was œdematous and covered with hemorrhagic erosions, while the cavity of the organ has occasionally contained a black liquid. The lesions taken together seem to indicate a change of considerable duration, in spite of the sudden onset of the malady.

However, these cases which are so terrible are fortunately very rare ; Scudamore only quotes two or three of them, Garrod and Brinton have never met with any. Quite recently Budd and Dittrich have published two examples.

But when of less intensity, gout retrocedent to the stomach is not a rare affection ; it is met with especially where there is asthenia, gouty cachexia, and in people who have abused specifics, applications of leeches and of cold.

It may, however, be asked whether the existence of this disease has not been too readily admitted in a certain number of cases. It is easy, in fact, to commit errors of diagnosis in this matter ; and hepatic or nephritic colic, the digestive disturbance of albuminuria, perhaps even poisoning by certain remedies (especially colchicum) may have simulated gout of the stomach more than once. Simple indigestion coming on suddenly in a gouty patient might easily be confounded with an attack of retrocedent gout, by reason of the occasional gravity of the symptoms caused by the special predisposition, which the uric acid diathesis has established. Thus Watson observed that we should often speak of " pork in the stomach " instead of " gout in the stomach." Scepticism has been pushed to an almost complete denial of stomachic gout, and Brinton, after a long discussion of this point, ends by concluding that no doubt a little gastric irritability may exist in gouty people, but all that goes beyond this must be attributed to simple coincidence.

In this matter I am of a contrary opinion, and after having made ample allowance for errors in diagnosis, I think that the various affections invoked for this purpose are far from accounting for all the facts. We have seen above that physiological experiment succeeds in producing in animals phenomena analogous to those of the uric acid diathesis ; and we know that in such cases the gastric juice and the follicles of the stomach are loaded with sodium urate. Without assuming an identical condition to account for the symptoms of stomachic gout, I think that superficial lesions might be very well caused in the digestive system under the influence of retrocession, and this view is quite confirmed by the results of autopsies performed on gouty patients whose organs have long been affected. In cases of this kind Todd has often met with enormous dilatation of the stomach, and Brinton himself confirms these results by his own observations ; this would be a case of that paralysis and enfeeblement of the stomach which Scudamore had long pointed out in the chronic cases of this disease.

It is, however, probable that in the long run permanent lesions are produced in the cases in which these manifestations occur, which seem so purely functional ; and the fatal cases of which we have just spoken seem to furnish a proof of this.

C. Two forms of intestinal dyspepsia correspond with the two

forms of stomachic gout which I have just described : the first
is characterised by spasmodic colic ; the second is a real enteritis.
These phenomena may occur independently or be associated with
the various troubles of which the stomach may become the seat.

II. " *The liver is rarely healthy in gout*," said Scudamore, and
daily observation is demonstrating the justness of this opinion.

There no doubt are affections of the liver which are connected with the gouty dyspepsia, as well as transient swelling
of this organ preceding the attacks, as has been noticed by
Scudamore, Galtier, Boissière, and Martin-Magron.

But we do not yet know positively whether there are any permanent affections of the liver resulting from the gouty diathesis.
Scudamore thought that in the long run the spleno-hepatic system
felt the influence of gout and became the seat of permanent
lesions.   It is known besides from modern physiological work
that the liver and the spleen are probably the organs in which
uric acid is produced.

But the anatomical characters of this visceral affection, if it
exists, are not yet known to us ; and the hepatic lesions met
with in the gouty almost always depend on alcoholism.

Still, biliary gravel sometimes co-exists with the uric acid
diathesis and gout (Prout, Budd, Wunderlich, Willemin), and
in the gall-bladder we sometimes come across calculi of uric
acid, as Stöckhardt, Faber, and Frerichs have noticed.   Perhaps
the patients who supplied these concretions have been gouty.

III. The influence of gout on heart affections cannot be contested, but we have no longer here, as in rheumatism, to do
with endocarditis, pericarditis, or valvular affections.   These
lesions, when they occur in the gouty, appear especially to
depend on alcoholism or Bright's disease.

But the great point here is fatty degeneration of the muscular
tissue of the heart ; Stokes, Quain, Gairdner, Garrod unite in
asserting this.

At the commencement, this affection exists to but a slight extent, and is only indicated by functional troubles : palpitation,
dyspnœa, feebleness and irregularity of the pulse (Hervez de
Chegoin).   Retrocession of gout to the heart is not frequent
(Scudamore, Garrod) ; still, there are some examples of it, and

some of these patients have died from cardiac causes. But in that case the lesions we are going to study were already developed.

In the second stage fatty degeneration of the heart is present. The symptoms of this lesion are always the same, whatever their origin (Stokes, Garrod). They simulate functional troubles ; in fact, there are no well-marked physical signs, and we arrive at a diagnosis mainly by a process of elimination.

The impulse of the heart is weak, almost imperceptible ; the first sound is dull, and sometimes there is a murmur caused by fatty degeneration of the muscles of the valves. The precordial dulness is often augmented. The pulse is soft, compressible, intermittent, sometimes very slow, especially during an attack (20 or 30 beats). Lastly, the presence of arcus senilis has been pointed out (Canton) in patients suffering from this change in the muscular tissue of the heart.

The rational symptoms are also well calculated to mislead the observer. The attacks are paroxysmal in their mode of development ; there are violent palpitations, dyspnœa, a tendency to syncope ; we may notice cerebral symptoms taking the form of apoplexy, although there has been no intra-cranial hemorrhage (Law, Stokes) ; sharp pains are felt in the precordial region and radiate along the arm, thus simulating angina pectoris, which itself is often considered as an affection of gouty origin.

Then, sudden death is here very frequent : thus in 83 cases of fatty degeneration collected by Quain, death took place unexpectedly 54 times, to wit, 28 times by rupture, and 26 times by syncope. Many of these cases were those of gouty people.

It is clear then that in many cases in which death is attributed to gout retrocedent to the heart, there has only been fatty degeneration of this organ. Quain and Gairdner have seen death occur in these circumstances without rupture ; death with rupture has been observed by Cheyne and Latham. The fatal termination has often supervened during the attack of gout, which seems to act by disturbing the action of the heart.

Let us add, lastly, that the atheromatous state of the arteries which often coexists with these lesions of the heart may give rise to cerebral hemorrhage ; then we see real, and not false, apoplexy.

IV. A change has taken place in our ideas with regard to the connection which multiple joint affections have with affections of the nervous system : formerly most symptoms of this kind were attributed to gout ; now rheumatism, on account of modern researches, has acquired the first place. Yet gout still plays a part ; but it is interesting to notice that the two diseases proceed in parallel lines in this respect, and that all the forms of cerebral rheumatism are met with again in gout.

Thus rheumatic headache, pointed out by Van Swieten, and more recently studied by Gubler, has its analogue in gouty cephalagia, which has long been known, and which in recent times has been carefully described by Lynch,* Garrod, and Trousseau.

The acutely delirious, or meningitic, form of cerebral rheumatism, is also found, according to Scudamore, in the gouty. Rheumatic apoplexy, or the apoplectic form of cerebral rheumatism, mentioned by Stoll and well studied by Vigla, occurs in gout, according to Lynch and Prof. Trousseau, in the form of stupor.

The convulsions which occur in cerebral rheumatism may also be met with in gout ; only in rheumatism they assume especially the choreic form ; in gout they are rather epileptiform, as Van Swieten, Todd, and Garrod have observed.

Lastly, it is known that there is a form of rheumatic insanity, which has been studied by Burrows, Griesinger, and Mesnet ; the same thing happens in gout, according to Garrod ; but it is rare, at least in France ; Baillarger, whose experience carries weight in such a matter, has told us that he never met with a single example of it.

Note a point of difference, however, for *aphasia*, which does not exist in rheumatism (except on account of heart disease and consequent embolism), is met with on the contrary in gout. It must be added that cerebral symptoms have less gravity in gout than in rheumatism ; but their alternation with the joint symptoms is more marked ; that retrocession is more evident ; and, lastly, that though a larval form of cerebral gout is pretty often found, it is very rare in rheumatism.

You must not confound these cerebral symptoms of gout with

---

* We commend Lynch's memoir to the attention of our readers ("Some Remarks on the Metastasis of Diseased Action to the Brain in Gout," etc., *Dublin Quarterly Journal*, 1856, p. 276.)

delirium tremens, coming on at the time of an attack (Marcet), nor with the delirium of acute intercurrent affections ; nor, lastly, with the nervous symptoms which may be roused by dyspepsia, affections of the heart, and uræmia, which last is much more common in gout than in rheumatism. In this matter prolonged observation, attentive study of the patient for a long period of time, are the only means of avoiding every error.

V. The influence of gout on diseases of the spinal cord is a matter still under discussion. Todd and Garrod point out the occurrence of slight symptoms, a sort of *paresis*, alternating with the attacks ; but it would not do to confound with a lesion of the spinal cord that muscular weakness which succeeds violent attacks of articular gout, and which may almost simulate real paraplegia.

It is true that Graves has reported a case in which at the autopsy hardening of the cord was found ; but this example does not appear to me very satisfactory. We must not forget, besides, that if there are spinal cord affections dependent on gout or rheumatism (a point which has not yet been proved),* there is no doubt that very marked articular affections may develop in consequence of lesions of the spinal cord, even of traumatic ones.†

VI. The respiratory apparatus may also become the seat of certain manifestations of gout, which we will rapidly pass in review.

1. *Gouty asthma.* Among the thoracic affections which may be thus spoken of, there is a form of what is called *nervous* asthma ; the lungs are then perfectly free during the intervals between the paroxysms, and there is a manifest alternation of the chest symptoms with those affecting the joints. Dr. Vigla has reported an interesting example of this to the *Société de médecine des hôpitaux.*

But there is a second form of gouty asthma which depends on permanent lesions and especially accompanies emphysema :

---

* It has now been clearly demonstrated that there is a rheumatic myelo-meningitis. Two cases with autopsy reported quite recently from the practice of Prof. Béhier furnish irrefragable proof of this occurrence.

† Ball, *Thèse de concours pour l'aggrégation,* 1866, p. 87.

here also we meet with alternations of exacerbation and re-mission, corresponding to the disappearance and return of the articular symptoms. These cases are pretty rare : Patissier has seen 2, out of 80 patients ; Garrod 1, out of 40 ; and Hyde Salter, to whom we owe a treatise on asthma, also reports one case.

2. Some old authors describe a gouty pleurisy. Probably they were cases of simple pleurodynia, as we shall see later.

3. Does gouty pneumonia exist ? Some observers have spoken of it, but well-authenticated facts are wanting. Scudamore has twice seen gout appear after recovery from pneumonia. It may be asked whether this was not a fortuitous coincidence. At any rate, according to the same author, these two affections may coexist without exerting any influence on each other. We shall return later to this point.

VII. Affections of the urinary passages are common in gout, and become almost the rule at a certain period of the disease. They are rare, on the contrary, in the different forms of chronic articular rheumatism. This is a distinctive character which it is important to make clear.

But all that relates to uric acid calculi and gravel, must, according to the rules which we have hitherto followed, be excluded from our consideration of visceral gout ; it is true that such events occur frequently in gouty cases, but they do not belong exclusively to them.

But there are affections directly due to gout, and these we shall now describe.

A. The kidneys may be attacked with a functional disturbance which offers evident analogies to articular gout. It comes on at an early stage of the disease ; its symptoms are, a sharp but transient pain, which evidently alternates with the articular gout, and which may be localised in either kidney ; and albuminuria of short duration. It may happen that during the whole period of this complication no gravel is passed.

This manifestation of gout is not exceptional; Garrod has observed several cases of it, and I have myself seen one with Dr. Clin. The patient in question was a physician, and was consequently able to give a trustworthy account of what he was experiencing.

B. Permanent affections of the kidneys become almost the

rule in chronic gout; there is an albuminous nephritis with anatomical characters which leave no doubt as to its origin, namely, infarcts of sodium urate in the renal tissue. We have already described these alterations when treating of the morbid anatomy.

Once developed, the albuminous nephritis of gout differs but little in its symptoms from ordinary Bright's disease. We generally find the urine clear and pale ; it contains a variable but nearly always quite small quantity of albumen ; there is but little urea, and the salts are diminished in quantity ; microscopically, we meet with fibrinous cylinders dotted over with epithelial cells or loaded with. granules. There may be œdema of the face and lower limbs ; but this symptom is often absent. We find also, as in ordinary Bright's disease, dyspepsia and diarrhœa. But, as I have already indicated, the progress of the disease is slower, and its prognosis less grave, than that of ordinary albuminous nephritis.

Still, uræmia has sometimes been observed during this affection : Basham, Todd, Deschamps (of Bordeaux), and other observers, have reported several examples of its occurrence ; I myself called attention to this point several years ago, and Fournier has made its importance clear in his remarkable graduation thesis on uræmia.

C. Gout of the *bladder* has been noted by various authors : Scudamore has spoken of it, and Todd has tried to define its characters ; * a large number of those cases which the English call *irritable bladder* should be referred to it.

At first, as we have already seen in the case of the kidneys, there is a transient affection, a functional trouble, characterised by sudden and violent pain in the bladder, by tenesmus, and by discharge of blood and muco-pus from the urethra, even when there is no complication with calculi (Todd) ; these phenomena may alternate with the articular affections.

But at a more advanced stage we find a permanent lesion, with catarrh of the bladder, and other phenomena of the same kind. Prof. Langier has kindly communicated to me a case which shows the reality of vesical gout, independently of all complication with stone.

* Todd, *Clinical Lectures on certain Diseases of the Urinary Organs.* London, 1857, p. 359.

D. Lastly, gouty *urethritis* has been spoken of, with discharge of pus from the urethra. But have not the authors (Scudamore especially) allowed themselves to be misled ? Perhaps it was really gonorrhœal arthritis. Such at least is the interpretation which may be put upon some of Scudamore's cases.

VIII. *Non-visceral, non-articular gout.* Independently of the internal diseases which may develop in the course of gout, there are other manifestations of the same malady, which, without attacking internal organs, are yet localised elsewhere than in the joints : muscles, tendons, nerves, skin, and some other parts of the system may be affected.

A. In a first group we will place together the affections of this kind which affect ligaments, tendons, and fibrous tissues in general.

We have already seen that when the joint-cartilages have been saturated with sodium urate, the ligaments and tendons are found impregnated with this substance. The symptoms of this state of things are generally mixed up with those of articular gout; sometimes, however, they may have an independent existence. We know, for example, that the fibrous tissue in front of the knee may become the seat of pains very like those of acute gout; this is the *goutte prérotulienne* of Rayer. It may be asked whether gout can exist in a larval form in the tendons and ligaments ; may it precede articular gout or replace it entirely ? That is still an obscure point, which requires fresh investigation.

B. *Muscles.* Gouty patients often experience during the attacks painful cramps in the muscular masses of the limbs ; they are very subject to lumbago, and may experience very sharp pains in the side of the chest, in fact a stitch : the intercostal muscles or the fibrous tissue of the thoracic walls are probably the parts affected (gouty pleurodynia). By the patients these sensations are often called *rheumatic pains,* but in reality they belong to gout.

C. *Nerves.* Pains have also been observed in the course of the nervous trunks, especially of the sciatic and the trifacial, during the progress of gout. Their characteristic is to appear abruptly and vanish likewise, alternating with the articular symptoms.

D. *Cutaneous affections.* Brodie and Civiale long ago noticed that there is an evident relation between psoriasis, gravel, and uric acid calculi. It is certain that psoriasis is often met with in patients belonging to gouty families, and that it may occur along with gout in one and the same individual. This is a fact which the observations of Holland, Garrod, and Rayer have placed quite beyond doubt. Eczema has also been seen along with, or alternating with, the most characteristic attacks of gout.

Such at present are the only cutaneous affections the connection of which with gout is really established. But under the name of *arthritides* Bazin and his school have collected a great many different eruptions supposed to have some relation to rheumatism and gout, two affections which he confounds together as *arthritis.* It must be admitted that the observations brought to support these opinions leave much to be desired, and that gout is here completely left in the shade. The facts collected by Bazin relate exclusively to rheumatism.

E. *Ocular affections.* Morgagni had already pointed out the conjunctivitis which sometimes occurs during a first attack of gout ; several authors have noticed it since then ; but of all the ocular maladies which have been brought into relationship with gout, that which best merits a reference to this diathesis is no doubt *iritis.* Lawrence and Wardrop have reported cases in which the alternation of iritis with well characterised gouty attacks could not be questioned ; and Prof. Langier has told us of a case in which this phenomenon was perfectly evident. It is extremely remarkable to find the iris thus affected in gout, since we know that articular rheumatism, especially when subacute, nodular, or gonorrhœal, gives rise to the same complications. Lastly, Garrod in a recent article * has described a gouty affection of the eye which had not previously received attention : I mean inflammation of the sclerotic, with whitish deposits of sodium urate on the surface of this tunic.

F. *Affections of the auditory apparatus.* We have already sufficiently insisted on the chalky concretions of the external ear, so that we need not return to them here ; we have also pointed out the change in the auditory ossicles. Now, I think it certain that patients affected with chronic gout are liable to

* Reynolds's *System of Medicine,* article " Gout," by A. B. Garrod.

become deaf; it would be very interesting if we could refer this new kind of deafness to the lesions which we have just mentioned, but I know of nothing definite on this point, and new researches would be necessary to make our notions exact in this matter.

We will conclude here our account of non-articular and visceral gout, and at our next meeting consider some affections which offer a certain degree of relationship to gout.

LECTURE VIII.

AFFECTIONS WHICH MAY BE ASSOCIATED WITH GOUT.

SUMMARY.—Phenomena which seem allied to the gouty diathesis.—Uric acid anthrax.
—Malignant inflammations and erysipelas.—Dry gangrene.

Intercurrent affections in gout.—Injuries, phlegmasias, typhus, syphilis, &c.—
Course of inflammations in the gouty who are not cachectic.—Critical gout.—
Action of drugs, lead, mercury, opium, &c.

Concomitant affections of gout.—Its affinity to diabetes.—Greater or less frequency of this affection.—Diabetes, obesity, and gout are often met with, if not in
the same individual, at least in persons of the same family.—Confirmatory observations.—Practical consequences.—Gravel.—Urinary concretions.—Uric acid,
oxalic acid.—The formation of a uric acid sediment does not always prove that
its excretion is increased.—Gravel sometimes depends on the presence of an excess
of uric acid in the blood.—Real or supposed relationship between gout, scrofula,
and phthisis; between gout and cancer; between gout and rheumatism.

GENTLEMEN,—The limits with which I have thought it wise to
circumscribe our account of non-articular gouty affections have
prevented my speaking to you of certain occurrences which
appear to arise more or less directly from the gouty diathesis.
The moment is come to say a few words about them.

I. In many of the diseases which impress a profound modification on the " crasis " of the blood, a special predisposition to
malignant inflammations and to gangrene has long been noticed.

Albuminous nephritis is an example of this kind of thing: in
albuminuric patients one often notices gangrenous erysipelas
and diffuse inflammations come on in the dropsical regions,
either spontaneously or as a result of incisions or punctures.
Thus the punctures and scarifications which in other dropsies
are a means of relieving the patient, are distinctly contra-indicated in cases of this kind (Rayer).

Diabetes offers us a second example of this unfortunate predisposition. The English physicians had long noticed that
carbuncles, dry gangrene, and diffuse inflammations readily
appear in diabetes; when Marchal of Calvi, without a knowledge
of the work of his predecessors, had the merit of calling attention
to this subject, which before his time had been scarcely studied
in France.

Now, we meet with an analogous series of phenomena in the uric acid diathesis and in confirmed gout.

This pathological coincidence, already perceived or indicated by Morgagni, Thompson, Schönlein, Ure, Carmichael, and Prout, has been illumined lately by the labours of Marchal, who has clearly distinguished the diabetic symptoms from those dependent on gout, which had not been done by his predecessors.*

The phenomena of this kind relating to the uric acid diathesis may be divided into three chief categories :—

1. *Gouty carbuncle,* occurring *before* the attack of gout, is considered as accidental by Garrod and Trousseau ; but symptoms of this kind, occurring in the actual course of the disease, appear to depend on the gouty diathesis. Ledwich and Marchal have reported several such cases.†

2. The *phlegmonous inflammations and erysipelas* which may occur in the gouty have been mentioned by Prout.‡ It is known besides that the operation for cataract succeeds badly in these patients, because the eye almost always becomes inflamed.§ Connected with these facts is the suppuration of the eyeball, which occurred in a case of chronic gout,‖ and the non-union of fractures. In a case in which the external malleolus was fractured an attack of gout came on ; the fragments came apart, the skin ulcerated, and the bone was bared ; but everything got right again after the cessation of the attack.¶

3. *Dry gangrene,* pointed out by Carmichael, Rayer, and Marchal, comes on especially in debilitated subjects attacked with the chronic form of gout and presenting tophi.**

II. We shall now speak of the intercurrent affections of gout.

It is no longer a question here of affections which are subordinate to the gouty diathesis, but rather of complications

* Morgagni, *De sedibus et causis morborum,* lib. iv., epist. iv., § 24, et seq.—A. R. Thompson, *History of a Case of Dry Gangrene,* in *Med. Chir. Trans.,* vol. xiii., 1827, p. 178.—Schönlein, *Pathologie und Therapie,* vol. iii., p. 248. The author ascribes to arterial ossification the gangrene of the extremities which, according to him, is often observed in gout.—Ure, *Researches on Gout, Med. Times,* 1848, vol. ii., p. 145.— Carmichael, *Dublin Quart. Journ.,* 1846, vol. ii., p. 283.—Prout, *Stomach and Renal Diseases,* p. 211, 1848.—Marchal (de Calvi), *Recherches sur les accidents diabétiques ;* Paris, 1864.

† Trousseau, *Clin. Méd.,* vol. iii.—Garrod on *Gout,* 2nd ed., p. 285.—Ledwich, *Dub. Med. Journ.,* vol. xxv., p. 43.—Marchal, loc. cit., p. 38, 283.

‡ Loc. cit., p. 211.   § W. Budd, *Library of Medicine,* vol. v., p. 213.

‖ Critchett, *Med. Times,* 1858, vol. i., p. 62.   ¶ O'Reilly, *American Med. Times,* p. 39.

** Carmichael, loc. cit.—Rayer, *Oral Communication.*—Marchal, loc. cit., p. 39.

which may supervene in the course of the disease. How are intercurrent affections modified by gout? In this respect we may establish a parallel between Bright's disease, diabetes, and the disease now occupying our attention. Injuries in gout are followed by the consequences which we have just indicated; and here we have a point of contact between these three affections. Inflammatory diseases, according to Prout, often assume an adynamic character in gouty people, especially when they are strumous and fat; it is in this manner, says he, that the greater number of them die.* This is another analogy with albuminuria and diabetes. Typhus in gouty people presents an exceptional gravity; it is always fatal according to Schmidtmann and Murchison.† Syphilis, according to Wells, is very severe in patients attacked with gout; it readily assumes a scorbutic character.‡

These symptoms in cachectic gouty subjects are explicable, according to Garrod,§ by the impermeability of the kidneys. A rapid tissue metamorphosis often calls for an enormous elimination, which cannot take place when the renal secretion is deficient. But it is probable that the problem is more complex than the English author seems to suppose ; the constitution [crase] of the blood must play a great part here. It may at least be affirmed that under the influence of such a diathesis, the mechanical, physical, and chemical phenomena of life must proceed with greater difficulty than in the normal state.

But when no cachexia exists, the termination of these diseases is far from being so fatal, and things proceed almost as if under ordinary conditions. It must be noticed, however, that inflammatory action almost always excites the gouty predisposition and brings on the attacks. We have already pointed out the

---

* This passage has often been alluded to in the course of our lectures : we will give it in full :—" Such a combination is by no means unusual in corpulent middle-aged individuals of a gouty strumous habit ; and is always to be viewed with some anxiety. I have generally noticed that such individuals die of some sudden and overwhelming attack of internal inflammation rapidly assuming the adynamic form ; or of apoplexy. They seem also to be subject to the severer forms of erysipelas ; and to diffuse inflammation in general of the cellular tissue. Indeed the greater number of instances of fatal diffuse inflammation arising either spontaneously or from simple innocuous punctured wounds, which have fallen under my notice, have happened in individuals whose urine occasionally contained sugar, as well as deposited lithic acid gravel."— p. 211. *Stomach and Renal Diseases*, by Dr. Prout, 1848.

† *Obsér*, t. iii., p. 379.—*Continued Fevers of Great Britain*, 1862.

‡ Spencer Wells, *Practical Observations on Gout*, etc., London, 1854, p. 87.

§ Garrod, *Reynolds's System*, vol. i., p. 855.

H

effects of injuries in this respect.   With regard to inflammations three forms may be distinguished :—

1. The intercurrent affection (pneumonia, pleurisy, angina, erysipelas) lasts a longer or shorter time, and then gout appears. Scudamore and Day* have reported examples of this.   This appearance of gout is generally regarded as a favourable phenomenon ; it is called *critical gout.*   We know that the same sort of thing may happen in rheumatism.

It may be asked whether under such circumstances the explosion of gout has not been determined by the intercurrent affection : if this is the case, the appearance of gout would not be a critical phenomenon.

2. The inflammatory affection takes its course in company with gout, without experiencing any notable modification.   This sometimes happens in the case of angina and pneumonia.†

3. There is a sudden suppression of the external symptoms of gout at the moment that the intercurrent affection appears. This is a grave case ; we must try and recall the gout to the extremities, but failure usually attends our efforts.

III. The action of certain drugs, as one might suppose *a priori,* has special characters in gouty people.   Thus *lead,* administered in medicinal doses in order to arrest hemorrhage, has produced a rapid saturation with the metal, accompanied by the blue gum line and saturnine colic.   *Mercury,* according to Garrod and Price Jones, brings on salivation more quickly in gouty people than in others.‡   I may add that *opium* should only be administered with the greatest care in patients attacked by chronic gout, when any indications of renal disease are present, for this drug may in such cases determine cerebral symptoms, the intensity of which is out of proportion to the dose employed.§

An interesting fact to notice, which belongs to the same order of events, is that turpentine ceases to be eliminated by the urinary passages.   Hahn, quoted by Guilbert, administered this

---

* Scudamore, *On Gout,* p. 21.—Day, *Diseases of Advanced Life,* p. 317.—Patissier, *Rapport sur les eaux de Vichy,* 1840 (obs. 50, 52).—Parry, *Collection,* vol. i., p. 246.

† Scudamore, loc. cit.

‡ Garrod, loc. cit., p. 354 and p. 578.—Price Jones, *Med. Times,* 1855, vol. i., p. 66.

§ Todd, *Clin. Lect. on Urinary Diseases,* p. 343, London, 1857.—Charcot, *Gaz. Méd.,* Nos. 36, 38, 39.

drug for seventeen months to a gouty patient, without producing that characteristic odour of the urine which is usually manifested in such a case.   Was this patient albuminuric ?*

IV. We shall now consider those concomitant affections of gout which have a more intimate relationship with this disease than those on which we have just been dwelling, and which are still more intimately connected with the totality of the modifications which the system undergoes.

Hunter laid down the principle that when the organism is attacked by a certain diathesis, no other general affection can coexist with it; in other words, a constitutional affection once established in an individual, allows no rival disease.

To this principle is related the doctrine of *antagonisms*, a doctrine exaggerated no doubt by the Vienna school (Rokitansky, Engel), but which yet contains a basis of truth.

But besides antagonisms there certainly exist affinities; and it is especially relations of this kind that I wish to bring before you clearly.

A. *Gout and diabetes.*   The notion of a more or less direct connection between diabetes and gout seems scarcely to go back beyond forty years.   Scudamore, far from divining this affinity, maintains that these two diseases depend on quite opposite causes.   But a German author, Stosch of Berlin, who in 1828 published a treatise on Diabetes, points out in this work a *metastatic diabetes*, coming on after the cessation of gout; in this connection he quotes two English authors, Whytt and Fraser.   Two years later Neumann mentions a *diabetes symptomatic* of gout. †

More recently, Prout, who seems to have taken a glance at all questions of this kind, mentions attacks of gout and rheumatism among the most frequent causes of diabetes.   Nothing is commoner, says he in another place, than to find a little sugar in the urine of the gouty ; they are not aware of it till the usual symptoms of diabetes, polyuria, thirst, emaciation, are plainly declared.‡   Another English observer, Bence Jones, has also shown that uric acid gravel predisposes to diabetes.§

* Guilbert, *De la Goutte.* Paris, 1820, p. 100.
† *Pathologie*, vol. i., p. 607.   ‡ Prout, loc. cit., p. 34, p. 33.
§ Marchal (de Calvi), loc. cit., p. 233.

In France, Rayer has many times pointed out to his pupils the connection which exists between uric acid gravel, gout, and diabetes. On this matter, the thesis of A. Contour,[*] and the lectures of Cl. Bernard may be consulted. The eminent physiologist has shown, in short, that diabetes may alternate with the symptoms of another disease, and particularly with *attacks of gout* and rheumatism.[†]

We have ourselves had the opportunity of observing a case which entirely confirms Cl. Bernard's observations. In a man of 56, long a sufferer from gout, the use or rather the abuse of a specific remedy (*liqueur de Laville*) had lessened the intensity of the attacks, which at last disappeared almost completely ; but, following a slight attack which was promptly put an end to, there appeared thirst, polyuria, exaggerated appetite, emaciation, loss of strength, and the other phenomena which characterise diabetes. When this individual came to consult me for the first time, his urine contained a considerable quantity of sugar. An appropriate diet, which he took for more than a year, brought about a notable amelioration in his condition ; but the diabetes having considerably diminished we observed some slight attacks of gout again come on.

Marchal has also considered the connection between these different diseases in reference to diabetic gangrene, beginning in 1856. Later, he published a book in which this subject is studied with remarkable ability.[‡]

According to this distinguished observer, there is a *uric acid* or *gouty diabetes ;* this conclusion agrees with previous observations and with actual facts. But perhaps it is to be regretted that Marchal has extended the influence of this form of diabetes and that of the uric acid diathesis in general a little too far. The considerations which he offers us on this point are scarcely applicable to the favoured classes of society, at least in France.

There is no doubt that a relationship exists between diabetes on the one hand and gout and uric acid gravel on the other; but the frequency of this relationship varies according to the circumstances in which the observer is placed. Thus Griesinger, who

---

[*] Contour, *Thèses de Paris,* 1844, p. 49.

[†] *Leçons de physiologie expérimentale,* etc., p. 436, 1855.—*Diabètes alternants.*

[‡] *L'Union Médicale,* 1856, No. 29. *Recherches sur les accidents diabétiques,* etc., loc. cit., p. 469, 409 (1864).

studied diabetes among patients of all classes, only found three gouty among 225 diabetic ; * on the contrary Dr. Seegen, who practises at Carlsbad, and whose patients belong consequently to the wealthy classes, has met with three cases of gout in 31 of diabetes. The proportion you will see varies from 1/10 to 1/75.†

One must not, however, confine oneself to collecting cases in which gout becomes transformed into diabetes in the same individual ; it is also necessary to do what has been done with so much success in affections of the nervous system, namely, study the hereditary transmission of the symptoms, and their distribution among different members of the same family.

In the same person one rarely sees gout and confirmed diabetes coexisting, but these two affections alternate with one another. Uric acid gravel or gout opens the scene ; and in general the gout vanishes the moment that the diabetes appears. Rayer had already noticed that gout changes into diabetes ; and Garrod rightly remarks that *when diabetes appears gout ceases.*‡

It must be added that *corpulence* often precedes the development of diabetes.

The prognosis may sometimes be as grave in such a case as when we have to do with ordinary diabetes ; gangrene and pulmonary phthisis may supervene. Still, it must be remembered that gouty diabetes is most often relatively mild, especially if the patient adopts an appropriate diet. Then we have the latent form of diabetes (Prout). I might quote cases in which the recovery has seemed to coincide with the return of gravel or of gout ; this is what made Prout say that in diabetes the appearance of uric acid gravel is a favourable sign ;§ yet these two affections may coexist without improving each other.

We shall now consider the relations between gout and diabetes, as occurring in a family composed of several individuals. Thus we may see a father who is gouty, diabetic, and phthisical, procreate a gouty son (Billard de Corbigny,)‖ or perhaps a diabetic father a gouty son (Charcot).

* Griesinger, *Studien über Diabetes, Archiv für physiol. Heilkunde*, 1859, p. 16.

† P. Seegen, *Beitrage zur Casuistik der Meliturie.*—Virchow's *Archiv*, Bd. 21, 30, 1864.

‡ Garrod, *Reynolds's System*, vol. i., p. 825. See also Gulstonian Lectures on Diabetes, *Brit. Med. Journ.*, 1857, p. 319.

§ Prout, loc. cit., p. 25.

‖ *Gazette des Hôpitaux*, 1852, p. 212.

I have myself had the opportunity of seeing a very remarkable case of this kind, which was mentioned to me by Dr. Réal, and in which gout, scrofula, diabetes, and corpulence were found to appear in most of the members of the same family. Below are the facts in a tabular form :—

TABLE I.

Father, Brewer, distiller	....	....	Large man	Diabetes	Died phthisical at 43
Mother	Lymphatic	Sciatica	....	....	....
1st son, Brewer	{ Scrofula { Keratitis	Articular Rheumatism(?)	Corpulent	Diabetes at 50	Still living (60)
2nd son, Brewer..........	....	Gout at 25	Corpulent at 35	Diabetes	Died delirious
3rd son	Lymphatic	Gout at 30	Corpulent	Diabetes	Died of an accident
4th son (alcoholic habits)	....	....	Corpulent	....	Died of cirrhosis
5th son	Keratitis	Gout	Corpulent at 35	Diabetes	Died phthisical at 48
A daughter	....	Gout	Corpulent	....	Still living
Daughter of last........	....	Gout	Corpulent	....	Still living

Here is evidently a more or less intimate relationship between these different diseases, reproduced in this way to different degrees in all the members of a family.

I have observed the following combination :—

TABLE II.

Father gouty............ { 1st son—Gravel
2nd son—Diabetes
3rd son—Gout, Phthisis
Daughter—Gravel

One might easily multiply examples of this kind ; but I think I have told you enough to show you that there is a relationship, regulated by still unknown laws, between the uric acid diathesis, diabetes, and gout.

The practical consequences of these facts are easy to appreciate. We must carefully examine the urine of the gouty; and when we recognise this particular form of diabetes, we must institute a treatment which is suitable to its origin.

B. *Gout and gravel.* The uric acid diathesis comes in contact with gout on all sides. It is not therefore surprising that gravel, which is often a manifestation of this diathesis, is pretty often met with in gouty subjects. The relationship between these two diseases has always been recognised. " Thou hast gravel and I have gout," wrote Erasmus to Thomas More, " we have married two sisters." Sydenham, Murray, Morgagni, have pointed out the same affinity, and to me it appears incontestable.

But at the same time there is a certain antagonism between

the two diseases ; it is rare in fact to meet with them simultaneously ; they have rather a tendency to alternate with one
another. Most often gravel precedes gout, and disappears when
the latter is developed ; * but one may observe the inverse order,
and find the gout completely disappear when the calculi form ;
I have witnessed a case of this kind. Moreover, when we find
gout and gravel coexisting, we must not suppose, as is too often
done, that they have appeared simultaneously ; for frequently the
stones have been long accumulated in the kidneys before expul-
sion and the consequent symptoms of nephritic colic.

It is important to notice that the chemical composition of
urinary concretions in gouty people is not always the same.
Usually one finds them consisting of uric acid ; but they may
also contain ammonium urate, and are sometimes composed of
calcic oxalate. However, the oxalic gravel is closely related to
the uric ; it is known, indeed, that uric acid may be regarded as
a compound of urea, allantoin, and oxalic acid.

Moreover, these urinary deposits may alternate. In gouty
patients who have stone, Gallois has sometimes found that the
calculi were composed of concentric layers, in which uric acid
and oxalates appeared alternately ; a manifest proof of the
changes which successively took place in the composition of the
products of renal excretion.†

Let us note also that these two acids may be met with in the
blood of the gouty,‡ in their sweat, and in their urine, outside
the periods in which gravel is found ; a new proof of the correlation which exists between these different morbid manifestations.

But I must again remind you that the formation of a urinary
sediment composed of amorphous urates or of crystalline uric
acid, shortly after micturition, does not prove that the excretion
of this acid is absolutely increased. A notable diminution of the
urinary water, or a marked acidity of the urine, are sufficient to
cause the precipitation of these sediments without there being
any actual increase in the amount of uric acid. On the other
hand we now know, thanks to the labours of Bartels,§ that urine,

---

* Scudamore, loc. cit., p. 531.

† De l'oxalate de chaux dans les sédiments de l'urine, etc., Mém. de la Soc. de Biologie
Paris, 1859, p. 74.

‡ Garrod, loc. cit., p. 127.

§ Harnsaure Ausscheidung in Krank.—Deut. Archiv für klin. Med., Bd. i., Heft. i.,
p. 13. Leipzig, 1865.

which has preserved perfect clearness long after emission, may contain a considerable proportion of uric acid. To be aware of the real state of the case, it would be indispensable to analyse the whole quantity of urine passed during the 24 hours, and even to repeat this examination for five or six consecutive days, according to the directions of Parkes and Ranke;[*] for it has been shown that the excretion of uric acid undergoes most marked variations, not only at various periods of the day, but also from one day to another.

It seems, however, a not unlikely thing that uric acid should exist in excess in the blood when the urinary sediments form not only after but before emission, and still more so when calculi form. But this event may be brought about by causes entirely independent of the uric acid diathesis; a purely local inflammation of the urinary tract is sufficient to determine it (Brodie, Rayer).[†] I have more than once been able to demonstrate the complete absence of uric acid in the blood-serum of non-gouty patients, who were habitually passing more or less bulky concretions of uric acid.

I have, however, no wish to deny absolutely the correlation between these two orders of events; far from this, it has been shown that in certain subjects gravel is associated with the existence of an excess of uric acid in the blood. Dr. Ball has told me of the case of a man aged 64, who frequently passed small calculi of uric acid after violent nephritic colic. A blister having been applied to the epigastric region, the presence of a notable quantity of uric acid was made out in the serum derived therefrom. The patient, however, had never had any symptoms of articular gout, and was not albuminuric. No doubt this case is to be classed near those in which we find gravel precede the appearance of gout, and then alternate with this disease.

In fact three groups of cases of this kind may be made out. Sometimes gravel precedes gout; this is the most frequent case: sometimes the gout precedes the gravel, a rarer case : sometimes, lastly, these two states coexist, which is more exceptional still. Out of 500 gouty patients, Scudamore only met with 5 who had stone ; and Brodie maintained he had never seen gravel in a gouty patient who had chalky concretions.

[*] Parkes, *On Urine*, p. 218.—Ranke, *Ausscheidung der Harnsaure*, München, 1858.
[†] Lectures on Diseases of the Urinary Organs.—*Maladies des reins*, Paris, 1839, vol. i., p. 94, 197, 198.

The symptoms occasioned by gravel mix themselves up with those of gout. There may be emission of sand with the urine and transient albuminuria; there may be renal gravel, which Rayer mentions by the name of gouty nephritis; but we know that there is another form of gouty nephritis, characterised by the deposit of urate of sodium in the tissue of the kidney (*gouty kidney* of English authors). And gouty patients may suffer from ischuria; there may be a gouty pyelitis, nephritic colic, and irritability of the bladder. All these symptoms, which may coexist with gravel, are not necessarily the result of it, and they may simulate it, as we have seen above.

C. *Gout, scrofula, and phthisis.* Is there a real relationship between gout, scrofula, and phthisis? We are little disposed to affirm this absolutely; and it is true that scrofula is common in patients suffering from nodular rheumatism; it is therefore allowable to query whether we ought not to refer to this last affection what has been attributed to gout. But Prout, who had carefully examined this point, admits that scrofula and gout are often associated, and that children born of gouty parents are liable to phthisis.*

This last affection, uncommon in acute articular rheumatism (Wunderlich, Hamernjk),† is common in persons with chronic rheumatic arthritis. In the gouty, on the contrary, it is rare, although diabetes, the close relationship of which with gout we have indicated, is, so to speak, a door ever open to the attacks of phthisis. However, in a young man who had chalky concretions round several joints, Garrod noticed phthisis of rapid course develop; but this case should be considered exceptional. ‡

D. *Gout and cancer.* Does gout exclude cancerous affections; or, on the contrary, does it favour their development?

My former master and predecessor at the Salpêtrière, Dr. Cazalis, believes in the existence of a close relationship between these two diatheses.

For myself, I can confidently affirm that in nodular rheumatism the occurrence of cancer and cancroid is not exceptional. I have not had occasion to meet with examples of them in cases of well-authenticated gout; but Rayer has noted the existence

* Prout, loc. cit., p. 492.
† Wunderlich, *Pathologie und Therapie*, vol. iv., p. 578.
‡ Garrod, *On Gout*, p. 578.

of both diseases, if not in the same individual, at least in the same family; and a case published some years ago in an English journal,* proves that these two affections may be present in the same individual. It was a case of cancer of the penis, with cancerous nodules in the lungs and liver, in a gouty patient 68 years of age, who had large chalk-stones and a gouty nephritis with characteristic infarcts of sodium urate in the kidneys. This case would suffice of itself to demonstrate that there is at least no absolute antagonism between gout and cancer.

E. *Gout and rheumatism.* The connection there is between articular rheumatism and gout has, as you already know, led many observers to declare the identity of these two diseases. We shall be better prepared to pronounce upon this point when we have studied rheumatism; so we will reserve this discussion for another lecture.

* Budd, *Lancet,* 1851, p. 482.

LECTURE IX.

ETIOLOGY OF GOUT.

SUMMARY.—Study of the conditions which determine the development of gout.—
Method which it is convenient to follow in researches of this kind.—Inconvenience of the premature intervention of chemical and physiological theories.—
Need of distinguishing between acquired facts and the hypotheses we seek to
apply to them.

Historical account of gout.—Antiquity of this disease.—Authors who have
mentioned its existence.—Decrease of gout in the present day.—Permanence of
its characters.—Modifications which have taken place in our hygienic customs and
their probable consequences.

Medical geography of gout.—It occurs especially in England and London.—Is
met with, however, to a less degree in several other countries.—Disappears almost
completely in hot countries.

Analytical study of the causes of gout.—Individual causes: Spontaneity;
Heredity; Sex; Age; Temperament and Constitution.—Hygienic causes:
Climates; Excessive feeding; Want of exercise; Intellectual work; Venereal
excesses; Fermented drinks, ale, porter, wine, cider.—Exciting causes.

Appendix.—English beers.

GENTLEMEN,—We have hitherto studied gout from the point
of view of the lesions which accompany it, of the symptoms
which characterise it, and of the affinities which connect it
with other diseases. We have now to look for the conditions
which determine its development. I shall show you in a few
words the method I propose to follow in the course of these
investigations.

We shall begin by an empirical study of the facts with which
direct observation furnishes us, apart from any theoretical
preconceptions; we shall then try to interpret these facts from
the point of view of modern physiology; in other terms, we shall
strive to follow in their successive evolutions the modifications
which the organism undergoes, when influenced by the causes
to which experience leads us to refer gout. We shall then
inquire how the changes thus brought about in the system can
determine the different phenomena, which constitute the clinical
history of this affection. In a word, we shall try to give ourselves a notion of the *morbid physiology* of gout. Such is
indeed the crowning act in every study of disease.

But remember clearly that the rigorous and systematic

separation of the two points of view which we have pointed out is more needful than ever in the question now occupying our attention; for here, especially, the premature and rash intervention of chemical and physiological theories into the interpretation of morbid phenomena might contribute to throw unjust discredit on this kind of study.

He who could succeed in harmonising the pathology of the ancients with the physiology of the moderns, said Boerhaave, would surely be of all physicians the most worthy of praise.* But the *modern* physiology of his time scarcely corresponded with the science which we now know by that name; and a few centuries hence our own physiology may well be no longer in harmony with the knowledge of the day. We ought then to use the greatest reserve, and only advance in this path with infinite precautions; for what was wanting to our predecessors was by no means a feeling of the importance of physiology in medical studies, but more exact and extended views about the difficult problems which they sometimes tried to solve without having fully measured their depth.

It must also be admitted that our knowledge of the products of disintegration is still obscure in spite of the progress realised in the study of nutritive functions, and uric acid itself is no exception to this rule. We know little of the conditions which determine its regular formation, and of the pathological circumstances which may modify this. So it is easy to see that the pathogeny of the uric acid diathesis is still in a rudimentary state, and that consequently it is at the present time impossible to formulate a complete theory of gout: the more needful is it to set up here and there a landmark, which shall serve perchance to direct the researches of the observers who shall come after us.

We shall begin this analysis by a rapid glance at the history and geography of gout; for since we are dealing with an eminently constitutional affection, which is intimately connected with the general state of the individual, it is indispensable, if we would grasp its characteristics firmly, to study the whole of the climatic and social conditions which seem to predispose the

* "Nec in medicum plus laudis redundare posset, quam ex eo labore, quo veterum pathologiam redigeret ad neotericorum physiologiam."—Boerhaave, *Med. stud. medic. Pars* ix., *Pathologia,* p. 573.

human race to it. To contemplate a disease from this point of view is to construct the outline of its etiology.

I. HISTORICAL PATHOLOGY OF GOUT. To trace the vicissitudes which diseases have undergone in the course of centuries, and to search in history for the causes of these changes, is the chief aim of historical pathology : thus investigations of this kind enable us to appreciate not only the pathogenic influence of external causes, but also the working of those conditions which are inherent in mankind.

But, that it may be possible to apply this method to the study of a disease, it is necessary that the attention of our predecessors should have been long directed to it. It is only under those circumstances that one can expect to gather together a rich harvest of historical documents. Now, such conditions are scarcely realisable except in the case of epidemic affections which once committed great ravages, and of certain chronic diseases, which in all times have attracted the attention of observers. A few examples will enable you to readily grasp my meaning.—The Plague, which used to be so formidable, appeared for the last time in France at the beginning of last century (1721); moreover it is tending to become extinct in the countries which have always been its chief foci. One may very properly inquire, then, what were the conditions which formerly favoured its development, and which apparently have now ceased to exist.—Leprosy existed at Martigues at the end of last century ; since that period it has disappeared from French soil; it is becoming rarer and rarer in Europe and seems inclined to take refuge in Norway, as gout does in England.—It is easy to understand the attraction there is for the philosophical physician in the history of an affection, which is about to vanish, after having played so great a part, and occupied such a place in the business of legislators in every age.*

Among the affections, an historical study of which offers a

---

* The rigorous measures which completely isolated the leper in the midst of society, were maintained in all their severity during the middle ages. They have perhaps contributed to the extinction of leprosy. Certain pathologists will prefer to invoke the spontaneous course of the disease; we willingly accept this term (*spontanéité morbide*), provided it be understood that it in no way prejudges the fundamental question, and only serves to express a deficiency in our knowledge.

really scientific interest, gout is evidently in the foremost rank. It is certain that in former times this disease prevailed in an almost endemic manner among the most favoured classes of society ; at the present day we see it becoming gradually extinct, and yet from the remotest times it has undergone no change in the development of its symptoms ; for we find this fully described in the writings of the ancients.

I shall tell you concisely the principal data for the solution of this question with which history furnishes us.

Antiquity of Gout. Gout has without question been known in Europe from the most ancient times : the writings of Hippocrates show this. But it was during the reigns of the early Cæsars that it seems to have reached its acme. In this respect we possess a wealth of information which leaves nothing to be desired. The productions of physicians, the works of historians, the satires of poets, are full of allusions to this disease.

As to the first century of the Christian era, Aretæus and Celsus on the one hand, Ovid and Seneca on the other, have given us ample information about the pathological conditions of the Roman world in this respect. For the second century Galen (130 A.D.) and the interesting dialogues of Lucian of Samosata,* furnish us with precious details from a hygienic and medical point of view. In the third century an edict of Diocletian exempts gouty persons from the public burdens, when they are suffering from articular deformities so considerable as to interfere with the ordinary functions of life,—a circumstance which seems to demonstrate both the extreme frequency of gout at that period and the immutability of its chief symptomatic characters.

From the third to the sixth century things seem to have continued in the same state, if we may judge by the writings of Oribasus, Alexander Trallianus, Aëtius, Paulus Ægineta, and several other physicians. In the middle ages, the Arabs, continuing the medical traditions of antiquity, teach us that gout had scarcely lost ground since the former period ;† and the

---

* *Tragodopodagra; Ocypius, the man with light feet.* According to some critics this last poem is not Lucian's.

† It must not be forgotten, however, that the statements of the authors of this period are not always worth much. Too often they copied from each other, without

authors of the Lower Empire, Actuarius, Demetrius Pepagomenus, etc., bring us to the 13th century. Lastly, in
modern times we find abundant evidences which leave no doubt
as to the general diffusion of gout in Europe.

So you see, gentlemen, an unbroken chain of historical
proofs shows us that for more than twenty centuries this
disease has maintained its sway in the countries where we now
live. But it is only necessary to glance around to convince
oneself that gout is tending to become rarer and rarer. We
must here enter on a few details.

Diminution of gout in the present day. It is especially since
the commencement of the present century that this retrograde
movement of gout has been manifest. The facts collected by
Corradi * teach us that even in England, according to Owen and
Fuller, the frequency of this disease has diminished, and that
the same thing has happened in Holland and Belgium according
to Coley, and in Switzerland according to Prof. Lebert. It has
almost disappeared in places where it used to be prevalent ; for
in our days it is scarcely met with in Rome and Constantinople.
It is evident then that in this respect things are greatly
changed. That is no doubt the reason why the writings which
have appeared on this subject for the last 60 years have been so
few ; for, except in England, material for new researches into
gout are rarely furnished for our observation.

And yet in spite of its decadence, this affection, as you will
see, has undergone no change in the development of its
symptoms.

Permanence of the characteristics of gout. It is only
necessary to compare the descriptions left us by antiquity,
with those which we find in modern authors, to convince ourselves that from the clinical point of view gout has always
conformed to the primitive type. Ocypius, the man with light
feet, resembles exactly in this respect the patients observed by
Van Swieten sixteen centuries later.

As to etiology, we always find the same conditions ; Suetonius

troubling to make personal observations. The Arabs especially have largely borrowed
from the medical literature of the Greeks ; and as gout is often discussed in the
works of the ancients, they have certainly appropriated a considerable part of the
labours of the latter.

* *Della odierna diminuzione della podigra*, etc., de'. Dre. Alfonso Corradi.
Bologna, 1860.

called gout *morbus dominorum;* Sydenham expressed the same idea in rather different language. As to the influence exerted on the development of this disease by excesses at table, it has always been among the most universally accepted traditions.

Let us add also that the Greek and Roman physicians, who so accurately described the characters of gout, hardly mentioned the existence of articular rheumatism, and several authors consider it a new disease, or at least almost unknown to the ancients. Such was the opinion of Sydenham, reproduced later by Hecker and Leupoldt.*

I shall have occasion later on to show you by unexceptionable proofs that there is much exaggeration in this view, and that rheumatism really existed among the great nations of antiquity; but there is certainly a very remarkable contrast between them, sufficient at all events to show that the general physiognomy of gout has never varied.

What conclusion shall we deduce from the facts I have just described? Shall we admit with Corradi that the decrease of gout results from the softening of our manners and a better hygiene with respect to food? It is certain that our manners have much changed. The suppers of Lucullus disappeared many centuries ago; we have no longer the heroic appetite of knights of the middle ages; it is no longer the fashion, as at the banquets of the Burgraves, to collect

" Round an entire ox, served on a golden dish."

We are accustomed to a less abundant and less exclusively animal diet, and to less prolonged meals; moreover, the abuse of fermented drinks has much diminished even in England, where the habits of last century left much to be desired in this respect.

II. MEDICAL GEOGRAPHY OF GOUT. Medical geography is, just like historical pathology, one of the most productive means of investigation in etiological researches. It teaches us the different regions of the globe in which certain diseases are prevalent, and thus enables us to study, on a vast scale, the cosmic, telluric, and even anthropologic conditions which may favour or retard their development.

* Hecker, *Rede über die aufeinander Folge der Dyscrasien,* etc., *Med. Vereinzeit,* 1837.—Leupoldt, *Geschichte der Medicin,* Berlin, 1863, p. 66.

As for gout, geography shows us that in the present day it only exists at a single spot on the globe as a generally distributed disease; you know I mean England. But this only applies to England, strictly so-called; for neither Ireland nor Scotland is in this respect in the same condition as the southern portion of the United Kingdom. Moreover, it is especially in London that this prevalence of gout is manifested; it is in this city that we see it flourishing, not merely among the wealthy classes of society, but also among the general populace, even among workmen who are least favoured so far as the material conditions of life are concerned. I shall try to explain to you directly the reason for this remarkable choice of a habitat. For the moment, we need only notice that gout exists in other parts of the globe, although to a much less degree. One meets with it in some parts of France, especially in Lorraine and Normandy, provinces always renowned for their good cheer. It exists also in Germany, and countries where beer is the ordinary beverage of the people.

It is certain, moreover, that this affection is only prevalent in temperate regions. Near the equator and in the tropics gout is almost unknown. In India it sometimes attacks the English, less often, however, than in their own country; but it spares the indigenous population. In Egypt it only attacks Europeans, and the wealthy Turks who take no heed to the precepts of the Koran; but the Fellahin seem to enjoy complete immunity.

And in Brazil gout is almost unknown, though the diet of the inhabitants is highly animalised (Dundas). I borrow most of these details from Dr. Hirsch of Berlin, who has published a good work on this subject.*

The influence of climate is here shown in the most evident manner; it is no question of race, for the negroes of the English army, when they are placed in the same conditions as the whites, are liable, like them, to contract gout. Some observations reported by Quarrier† seem to prove this.

Articular rheumatism behaves very differently in this respect: it seems to occur in all climates, and is often met with in India in the acute, as well as in the chronic, form; thus, to make use of Mühry's ‡ expression, rheumatism is an ubiquitous disease.

* *Handbuch der historisch-geogr. Pathologie.* Erlangen, 1859.
† *Edinburgh Medical and Surgical Journal*, 1808, vol. ii., p. 459.
‡ *Klimatologische Untersuchungen*, Leipzig, 1858, p. 212.

That is a striking difference between these two parallel diseases, and it is important to make it clear.

We have just sketched the main outlines of the historical pathology and the medical geography of gout. But we must now leave this bird's-eye study and descend from our very general point of view, to occupy ourselves with the minute analysis of the particular circumstances which may give rise to this disease. I shall have occasion in the course of this study to point out facts hitherto little known in France, but which deserve in every way to have your attention.

ANALYTICAL STUDY OF THE CAUSES OF GOUT.

I. INDIVIDUAL CAUSES. 1. *Spontaneity.* It is indisputable that gout may develop spontaneously; facts reported by all authors demonstrate this, and I have myself met with cases of this kind. So that there are in the actual constitution of certain persons conditions which favour the development of gout; external circumstances have only to bring them to light. There is nothing in this to astonish you; for the excessive formation or diminished elimination of uric acid seems to be the fundamental condition of this diathesis; now uric acid exists normally in the blood; and however little it be increased in quantity, the complete series of pathological events may unfold itself.

2. *Heredity.* The definition of gout, as all modern authors have formulated it, always includes the notion of heredity. Physicians with hospital practice have shown the frequency of hereditary transmission in this case; still more is it to be recognised in private practice. Here are some figures which will give you an approximate idea of the importance of this condition :—

Scudamore met with hereditary predisposition in 309 out of 523 cases of gout.

Patissier (report) in 34 out of 80 cases.

Garrod in 50 out of 100 cases.

Hereditary gout often develops early on, before the usual period. It is from 30 to 35 that one generally sees spontaneous gout appear, but hereditary gout does not always wait so long to show itself. Often it declares itself at the same age in all the members of a family. Garrod tells that in one of the great houses of England, the eldest son of the family, at the moment when he receives the heritage of his ancestors, is attacked by gout ; this inheritance has been bequeathed for four centuries.

3. *Sex.* The influence of sex on the production of gout is not less evident than that of heredity. Women in this respect enjoy a relative immunity which it is impossible to contest. Out of 80 cases, collected by Patissier, there are only 2 belonging to the female sex. It is at the time of the menopause that the symptoms usually develop, as Hippocrates pointed out.

In this respect, as we shall soon see, chronic rheumatism differs fundamentally from gout. There are, however, exceptions to this rule, and we sometimes see women become gouty at an early period ; but in such cases you may almost always recognise hereditary influence.

Let us add, lastly, that it is especially the asthenic forms of gout which prevail in the female sex.

4. *Age.* It is from 30 to 35 that, according to Scudamore, the classic age of gout extends. We rarely observe it before the twentieth or after the sixtieth year. Garrod has, however, met with one case in a patient of 9, and once in a young man under 17. He also reports some cases in which this affection appeared in old men of 60 or 70.

Rheumatism, on the contrary, appears earlier, and is generally observed before 35.

5. *Temperament, constitution.* An attempt has often been made to bring together the characters of a special constitution, predisponent to gout. But the study of facts shows us that it respects no temperament, and may appear as readily in enfeebled patients as in vigorous men ; only, the type of the disease is modified by the general condition of the organism. The sthenic form is met with especially in sanguine and plethoric individuals ; the asthenic form in women and nervous subjects.

II. Let us now leave the study of causes dependent on the individual, and consider those which depend on his environment. Let us occupy ourselves with hygienic conditions, and especially with diet ; among them we shall find precious facts for the solution of the problem we are trying to clear up.

1. *Climate.* Medical geography has already shown us that

I 2

gout scarcely occurs but in the temperate zones of the globe. Unknown in Brazil, Africa, and equatorial regions, it nevertheless sometimes attacks Europeans, who carry into hot countries the customs of cold ones; that is why in the East Indies the English are sometimes liable to it.

2. *Excessive feeding and want of exercise.* It has always been recognised that a too nutritious diet and too luxurious life—two causes which often act in concert—directly predispose to manifestations of gout; that is, no doubt, the reason why it predominates in the wealthy classes, and is less often met with among the general public. This is what is expressed in familiar terms, when people say that gout comes from an excess of income over expenditure. We shall soon see that facts do not always allow so simple an explanation; but it is at any rate certain that a too animalised diet favours the development of this affection, and that great eaters are often among the number of its victims.

3. *Influence of the nervous system.* The influence exerted by cerebral causes can no longer be denied. Intellectual labour, moral emotions, great intensity of thought, have always occupied an important place in the etiology of gout. This is what justifies the ingenious dictum whereby Sydenham consoled himself for being gouty: " Divites interemit plures quam pauperes, plures sapientes quam fatuos," said he, in speaking of this disease. There is no doubt that, in England at least, the most distinguished politicians become its martyrs. One may quote, among others, the example of the two Pitts. We know that the first of these two great ministers, Earl Chatham, was not a devotee of Bacchus. It is true that we cannot say as much of his son, William Pitt, who never made a speech in the Commons without having warmed up his eloquence by abundant potations.

4. *Venereal excesses.* The abuse of sexual intercourse may evidently act in such a way as to favour gout, owing to the consequent disturbance of the nervous system; but we may resort to a simpler explanation, for we know that excesses of this kind are closely associated with revelling, and it is to the influence of this latter circumstance that we ought, perhaps, to attribute the chief part.

5. There are two other causes which now demand our attention; I mean the influence of fermented drinks and of lead-poisoning.

The action of fermented liquors is so manifest, that Garrod is able to say, that man without these beverages might never have known gout.

The influence of lead-poisoning in this respect is much more limited; but from the pathogenic point of view this aspect of the question is of very great interest.

We shall successively study these two groups of facts.

A. *Fermented drinks.* From our present point of view, a radical distinction must be made between spirits (rum, brandy, whiskey, gin, &c.), which contain from 40 to 70 per cent. of alcohol, and simple fermented drinks (wine, beer, cider, &c.), the alcoholic strength of which varies from 4 to 20 per cent. It seems at first sight as though the more alcohol a beverage contains, the more should it predispose to gout; but this is not the case, and you will perhaps be surprised to learn that the use and even abuse of distilled liquors seems to exert no influence in this respect. In fact, gout is scarcely met with among populations who drink brandy. In Sweden, where alcoholism is so common, according to Magnus Huss, we do not find this disease. It is the same in Denmark, Russia, and Poland. In Scotland and Ireland gout is rare among the lower classes; in Edinburgh, in a long hospital practice, Bennett[*] and Christison only met with one or two cases. Now in these countries the only alcoholic drink which the people use is whiskey.

In London, on the contrary, gout is very common among the working classes, and is frequently met with in the hospitals. Now the only essential difference which one can find in this respect between the north and the south of the United Kingdom, is the enormous consumption of strong beers (ale, stout, porter) which goes on among the workmen of the capital.[†]

The truly remarkable influence of these drinks is recognised by all the English authors, commencing with Scudamore; he tells us that gout is much more common in London among the general populace since the use of porter has become habitual. The testimony of Watson, Budd, and Todd corroborates this assertion: Todd said that most of those who are addicted to the drinking of beer, and especially of porter, suffer sooner or later from gout.

[*] Clinical Lectures, 2nd ed., Edinburgh, 1858, p. 916.
[†] See Appendix, at end of Lecture.

An example borrowed from Budd* makes evident the influence exerted by drinks of this kind. There is in London a body of labourers whose work is to remove sand from the Thames. This operation is performed during low tide, and the hours of work consequently occur sometimes by day, sometimes at night. The labourers, who are exposed to every vicissitude of weather, are obliged, besides, to employ great muscular force. So, to obtain a better yield (observe the practical character of the English), these men are allowed a large ration of porter. Each of them drinks two or three gallons a day! Except for this enormous consumption of liquid, their diet is that of the lowest classes in London. Now gout is exceptionally frequent among these poor people, who share this melancholy privilege with the peers of the realm ; and although their number is not very considerable, several of them are each year admitted as gouty patients into the Sailors' Hospital. And yet they are generally unfortunate Irish peasants, in whom no hereditary predisposition could have been in operation.

Garrod has also arrived at the same results. He has shown that the employés of the great breweries are often attacked with gout; and yet nothing in their antecedents could explain this morbid predisposition, unless it were their abuse of ale, especially of porter.

Yet these two liquors are not remarkable for their alcoholic strength. According to Mulder,† Scotch ale contains 8 p.c., porter 5 p.c. This quantity is less than that of our French wines, and does not exceed that of German beers, which scarcely produce any such effects, in spite of the enormous consumption of them in the ale-houses.

Hence we see that *a priori* reasoning cannot be applied to the question before us, and that the influence of fermented drinks on gout is far from corresponding to their alcoholic strength. Circumstances of a different kind, which have been overlooked till the present day, probably come into operation, and for each kind of drink we must trust to the results of direct experiment.

We shall now inquire into the action of wines. We must give the first place to the spirituous wines (port, sherry, madeira, marsala), of which so much use is made in England among all

* Tweedie, *Library of Medicine,* vol. v., art. "Gout."
† Mulder, On Beer.

classes of society. They contain a considerable quantity of alcohol, varying from 17 to 20 p.c.

The lighter wines (Rhine, Moselle, Bordeaux, Champagne) are far from exerting the same influence.

But the same cannot be said of Burgundy, which, however, contains scarcely more alcohol than the last mentioned.

Red hermitage and Burgundy, the latter especially, said Scudamore, contain gout in every glass.

Cider itself, an apparently little-dangerous drink, seems also to favour the development of this affection. According to Garrod it is sweet cider, which has undergone only partial fermentation, which possesses this disagreeable property.

I think we have sufficiently demonstrated the influence which certain drinks may exert in this respect. Let us go on to another subject.

B. *Lead-poisoning.* Garrod showed that out of fifty-one patients in his hospital practice there were not less than sixteen who followed the profession of painters or plumbers ; and later researches have but confirmed this remarkable result. Lead-poisoning has therefore been placed among the predisposing causes of gout.

This coincidence once noted, evidence flowed in from all directions in support of it. Among authors prior to Garrod, we may quote Musgrave, who has seen gout follow colica Pictorum ; Falconer, who has made the same observation ; Parry, who in his record of observations established the fact that gout is common in patients with lead palsy ; lastly, Todd, who reports several cases of gout observed in analogous circumstances.*

Since the publication of Garrod's book, several English authors have pointed out facts of this kind ; we may mention specially Burrows and Begbie.† But in England, the action of the dietetic causes, which we have just enumerated, must be recollected. In France, where lead colic is so common, how comes it that gout is so rare among the people ?

Well, there are among the *saturnine* several gouty persons, in whom poisoning by lead is the only cause one can invoke. I

* G. Musgrave, *De arthritide symptomaticâ*; Genovæ, 1752 ; c. x. art. 5, p. 65.—C. H. Parry ; London, 1825, vol. i., p. 243.—Todd, *Practical Remarks on Gout,* p. 44, London, 1843.

† W. Falconer, *Brit. Med. Jour.,* 1861, p. 464.—Begbie, *Edinb. Med. Jour.,* Aug., 1862, p. 128.—Charcot, *Gazette hebd.,* 1863, p. 433.

have myself had occasion to observe a very remarkable case of this kind; and Dr. Bucquoy has just made a similar observation at the hospital of la Charité.

We have still to determine the cause of this strange coincidence. Garrod has shown that impregnation with lead causes an accumulation of uric acid in the blood, especially in advanced cases where paralysis exists; this fact has been ascertained in non-gouty cases of plumbism, where albuminuria does not seem to have occurred; for the urine has been examined with the result of showing that the proportion of uric acid had sensibly diminished; but in these analyses the presence of albumen is not mentioned. Garrod inquired whether in this case there was increased production of uric acid or defective excretion of this product. He leans towards the latter hypothesis, and here is the experiment on which he depends: after having examined for several days the urine of a certain number of patients suffering from various diseases, in order to determine the normal amount of uric acid, he subjected them to the medicinal action of acetate of lead, and observed that the excretion of uric acid diminished.

It would seem, then, that it is by paralysing the action of the kidneys, at least so far as the excretion of uric acid goes, that lead acts in favouring the manifestation of gout; but can this disease declare itself under the influence of this cause alone? Perhaps, in some very exceptional cases; but if there are co-operating causes the effects of lead will be far more obvious.

III. EXCITING CAUSES. Incapable by themselves of producing gout, the conditions we are going to enumerate have great influence in provoking the development of the attacks.

1. *Alcoholic drinks.* In gouty people, the ingestion, even in very small quantities, of certain wines, champagne or port for example, is enough sometimes to induce a violent attack of gout, or in other cases a simple swelling of the great toe. Thus Garrod has said: Whenever a few glasses of wine are sufficient rapidly and invariably to give rise to inflammation of a joint, that inflammation is certainly gouty in its nature.

2. *Indigestion;* gastric troubles act in the same way;

3. *Damp cold;* suppression of sweat, also;

4. The same may be said of immoderate *intellectual labours,*

to which I have already directed your attention as predisposing causes of gout ;

5. *Traumatic causes ;* operations, fractures, etc., may act in the same way; I have seen a wound produce simultaneously an attack of trismus and a fit of gout ;

6. *Debilitating causes ;* hemorrhages, blood-letting, grave diseases, also exert an influence on the production of the attacks. This is the more interesting to notice, that people like to fancy gout a disease of plethoric people. But Todd has proved that it readily attacks debilitated subjects.*

We shall devote our next meeting to the study of the theory of gout.

APPENDIX TO LECTURE IX.

ENGLISH BEERS.

We have so frequently in these lectures had to consider the influence exerted by ale and porter in the development of gout that it seems to me needful to give here some information on the processes employed in the manufacture of these liquors, as well as on their principal characters. I have therefore asked Dr. Ball to send me a brief account of these points to lay before the reader. The information contained in it will be the more useful, as it is not to be found at present in any other medical work.

There is no doubt that from very early times, the nations who were not acquainted with the use of wine, had discovered the means of employing germinating barley in order to procure alcoholic beverages.† Long before leaving their forests, the

---

* I have lately attended a former officer of the Confederate army, who during the war of secession in the United States was made prisoner by the Northern troops. Shut up in a damp, unhealthy prison, and with very insufficient food, he became gouty; he is so still, and yet he had no hereditary antecedents likely to predispose to gout, and till then had never shown any symptom of this disease.

† Herodotus and Diodorus Siculus tell us that the Egyptians were acquainted with the manufacture of beer; Pliny and Tacitus give the same evidence with regard to the Germans : " Potui humor ex hordeo aut frumento in quamdam similitudinem vini corruptus."—Tacitus, *De situ, moribus, ac populis Germ.*, cap. xxiii.

Germanic tribes possessed this art; so we are not surprised to find beer naturalised in England ever since the Anglo-Saxon conquest. The laws of Ina, King of Wessex, which were promulgated in 728, refer to *ale* and *alehouses*; and since that time beer has never ceased to be the national drink of the English.

But in this long series of centuries the public taste has varied more than once, and the brewers have been obliged to follow the fashion, when they did not anticipate it. In the middle ages hops were not used in beer, which seems to have had an insipid sweetish flavour; the attempt was often made to remedy this defect, by adding infusions of bitter and aromatic herbs. In 1524 the Flemings introduced the use of hops into England, but the practice was not legally authorised till 1552. The name of *ale* was then given to the sweet beverages prepared from malt, and that of *beer* was reserved for the liquors impregnated with the bitter principle of the hop. But in the 17th century all vestige of this distinction had disappeared, and hops were universally employed in the English breweries.

The origin of *porter* is much more recent. It was in 1730, according to Malone, that people first began to make use of it. About this period the workmen of London used to drink in the alehouses a mixture of beer, ale, and small-beer which they called *three threads*, because the retailer for every pint that he drew for the consumer was obliged to go to three different casks. To avoid this inconvenience the brewer Harwood formed the idea of producing a drink which should unite the tastes of these three liquids; he succeeded wonderfully, and the success of the new beverage among the lower classes of the capital got it the name of *porter*, which it has kept to this day.

To gratify the popular taste, the makers used formerly to communicate a very deep colour to this drink by the prolonged roasting of the grain; but it was soon perceived that by doing this, most of the saccharine matter contained in the malt was destroyed, and the richness of the liquid in fermentible bodies diminished. They then had recourse, in order to colour the porter, to a number of artificial processes, which were prohibited in 1816 by an Act of Parliament; and at the present day the only ingredients which can be used in the making of beer are water, malt, and hops.

But it was then discovered that the complete roasting of the malt, while destroying the sugar which it contains, gave rise to a very soluble colouring matter ; ever since then, this substance, which came within the meaning of the Act of 1816, has been largely employed in the manufacture of porter.

At present this liquor is a mixture of several kinds of beer, which is kept a long time after the mixing in order to push the fermentation to its extreme limits and convert all the sugar into alcohol ; but as, to begin with, the barley was strongly roasted, it contains little glucose even at the time when the action commences, and consequently can never be so rich in alcohol as the other varieties of beer. But its essential characteristic is a tendency to acetic acid fermentation ; for all the sugar having been destroyed, one more step suffices to convert the alcohol into vinegar. Theoretically this transformation ought never to occur, but practically porter delivered for consumption is often acid, as I have many times been able to assure myself.

The name of *entire* is generally given to the mixed beers ; that of *stout* is applied to a liquor prepared with more care and intended for more delicate consumers, but which shares the general characters which we have just described.

Under the name of *ale* are included all the other varieties of beer, which are not deeply coloured, and are not prepared from strongly heated barley; they are therefore richer in saccharine matter and in alcohol; and as the fermentation has not been pushed far enough to destroy all the sugar they contain, they have a very different flavour from that of porter, and have no tendency to acidify.

We may, then, divide the beers made use of in the United Kingdom into two great classes. Some are rich in colour but poor in alcohol, deprived of sugar, and ready to undergo acetic acid fermentation ; they are besides impregnated with a principle obtained by roasting the grain,—a fact not unconnected perhaps with their pathogenic properties. To this class belong the drinks known under the generic name of porter, and the use of which is so predisponent to gout.

The others, on the contrary, poor in colour, are rich in alcohol, and contain no trace of acetic acid.

It is evident that in this short notice we cannot include all the varieties to which fancy, accident, or local custom may have given rise. In England the beer of one county is not like that of neighbouring districts, and every famous brewer has secrets, which stamp a special character upon his products. It is enough to have offered the reader a general view of the subject, without stopping for the minute study of details.

LECTURE X.

PATHOLOGY OF GOUT.

SUMMARY.—Rational theory of gout.—It can scarcely be formulated in the actual state of science.—Cullen.—Discovery of *lithic acid* (uric acid).—Influence of this occurrence on modern work.—Researches of Garrod.—He showed that uric acid exists in excess in the blood of the gouty.—Origin of this excremental product. —It is hardly yet understood.—Are urea and uric acid immediate products of disintegration ?—Experiments of Zalesky.

Experimental researches.—Effects of fasting.—Animal diet.—Exercise.—Contradictory results on this point.—Influence of beverages ; experiments of Bocker.

Theory of the attack of gout.—Articulations affected by preference.—Fibrous tissues, cartilages.—Preference of gout for the great toe.—Invasion of one joint after another.—Tophi.—Deposits of sodium urate in the cartilages.—Pain.— General reaction.—Visceral symptoms.—Insufficiency of our actual knowledge on this head.

GENTLEMEN,—After having passed in review the various causes which are connected, more or less closely, with the production of gout, we have still to seek for the rational theory of this affection, and to bring together the facts of physiology and those which clinical observation furnishes us. We must not, however, flatter ourselves with obtaining complete success in this direction ; for if we are acquainted with the morbid principle in which the series of pathological events here centres, we are far from grasping all the links of the chain ; the conditions which influence the formation and elimination of uric acid are still unknown to us, and no doubt will long escape us.

But to understand properly the present state of the question, it is necessary to follow the different phases through which it has passed up to our own days. Let us see, then, what the opinion of our predecessors was in this matter.

The theories formulated about gout during the whole of the 17th century, and part of the 18th, are essentially connected with Humoralism ; with a few variations, it is the doctrine of Sydenham. There exists a morbific matter in the economy : it is the result of imperfect coction, conducted either in the *primæ* or *secundæ viæ;* and the efforts of nature to eliminate this *peccant matter* (phlegm, bile, tartar) constitute the symptoms of gout.

But a reaction against the former ideas became manifested from the time of Cullen. This celebrated author maintains that the existence of a morbific matter in the blood is by no means demonstrated. He regards the tophi, invoked by the humoralists in support of their ideas, as quite accidental occurrences. Gout, for him, results from a kind of plethora with loss of tone in the extremities.

The progress of chemistry began to modify this view up to a certain point. In 1775 Scheele discovered *lithic acid* (uric acid) in urinary calculi and urine; in 1793 Forbes Murray, on account of the relationship between gout and gravel, put forth the opinion that uric acid exists in the blood of the gouty; in 1797 Tennant and Wollaston established the fact that tophi are composed of urate of sodium.

Cullen's theory, however, continued to maintain itself in England. Scudamore went on regarding gout as a kind of plethora with no relation to the excess of uric acid in the blood; for him, chalk-stones are an exceptional phemonenon in gouty people: he had only found them 45 times out of 500 patients. Barlow and Gairdner shared this opinion, and more recently Barclay* has returned to this view, relying, I must say, much more on fancy than on observation; however, Parkinson, Home, and Holland have gone in for the uric acid theory.

In France gout has only been studied by a small number of authors; but those who have considered this question have admitted the presence of uric acid in the blood, at least theoretically, and have quite understood the importance of this capital fact. In this connection we may especially mention Andral, Rayer, and Cruveilhier.† The last considers the deposit of tophaceous matter in and around the joints as the characteristic lesion of gout. Now this chalky matter is urate of sodium. Cruveilhier found himself brought back, almost in spite of himself (he says), to the opinion of Sydenham and the older observers; he regarded sodium urate as the material cause of gout, and he did not doubt that the first attack coincides with a secretion of this substance, which is repeated at each subsequent attack.

In spite of the great interest possessed by the works I have

---

* *On Gout and Rheumatism*, p. 3, et seq. London, 1866.

† Andral, *Précis d'anatomie pathologique*, 1829, vol. i., p. 553, and vol. ii., p. 387.— Rayer, *Traité des maladies des reins*. Paris, 1839, vol. i., p. 243.—Cruveilhier, *Atlas d'anatomie pathologique*, 4ᵉ livraison, planche iii.

just pointed out, the period of positive knowledge dates, in my opinion, from Garrod's researches in 1848. This observer, so often quoted in the course of our lectures, has shown : 1st, that in acute and chronic gout an excess of uric acid exists in the blood ; 2nd, that from the first attack sodium urate is deposited in the joints ; 3rd, that during the attack there is a sensible diminution in the excretion of uric acid by the kidneys.

Those are the fundamental facts which may serve as the elements of a pathogenic doctrine ;. but they do not as yet make a physiological theory of gout possible. Yet some attempts have been made in this direction. I will point out to you their chief results :—

I. The presence of an excess of uric acid in the blood does not constitute gout,* but only creates a marked predisposition to this disease. We must, then, study the different circumstances which may increase the proportion of this excremental product. But at this first step the difficulties begin.

What is the origin, what are the sources, of the uric acid excreted ? Authors do not agree on this point.

A. The theory of direct combustion, formulated by Liebig, seems to offer an easy solution of the problem. It is in the blood itself, and at the expense of the albuminoid matters (fibrin, albumin, globulin), not sufficiently oxydised to be transformed into urea, that uric acid originates : there is an excess of income over expenditure ; too much has been eaten, too little exercise taken ; thence comes the development of gout.

But it has now been shown that under such conditions it is especially the urea, and not the uric acid, which increases. Moreover, these two products, according to the researches of Bischoff and Voit, result from the disintegration of the elements composing the tissues, and are never formed directly in the blood.

B. Which, then, are the organs, which the tissues, at whose expense uric acid forms ? Here again we find ourselves in the presence of contradictory results.

Urea comes from the muscles, it is said ; uric acid from the parenchymatous viscera ; it has, in fact, been met with in the brain and liver ; in the spleen (Scherer) ; in the lungs (Cloetta).

---

* Albuminuric nephritis and saturnine cachexia are also among the number of diseases in which there is an excess of uric acid in the blood.

Some pathological facts tend to confirm this notion: thus in splenic leucæmia, Uhle and Ranke have found an actual excess of uric acid in the urine; in affections of the liver Harley has arrived at the same result.

Other physiologists make the urates originate in the cartilages and fibrous tissues. Organic activity is in them less active by reason of their slightly vascular structure, as Bartels has pointed out,* and consequently oxydation goes on less completely in such situations. The researches of Prof. Robin† have led him to a similar opinion. He admits that in the fibrous tissues the albuminoid matters are transformed into gelatin; this substance in its turn decomposes by disintegrative action into *uric acid* and *urates*. Hence we see that if the activity of disintegration in these parts becomes exaggerated, there will result a saturation of the blood by these products—in other words, a uric acid diathesis.

Robin has found uric acid in normal fibrous tissue;‡ and the pathological state is in his view a simple exaggeration of what exists in a state of health. He thus explains why the joints are the chief seat of the lesions of gout: their richness in fibrous tissue exposes them to the first attacks of this disease.

Without underrating whatever may be plausible in these explanations, I will point out that the theory, according to which uric acid and urea are regarded as the immediate products of disintegration, is no doubt well worthy of consideration, but that it is after all a mere hypothesis. It is especially founded on the presence of these two substances in the normal blood, but in mammals they are only found there in the minutest proportions, whilst they seem completely absent from the blood of birds and reptiles.§ The presence of urea and uric acid in the tissues is also mentioned in support of this idea. But as to urea, the fact is only true in reference to a state of disease; in normal conditions one only finds creatin and creatinin in the muscles; in the case of uric acid the fact is better demonstrated.

In any case, the researches of some modern observers seem to

* *Deutsche Archiv für klinische Medizin.* Leipzig, 1865, Bd. i., Heft i., p. 13.

† *Dictionnaire de médecine,* de Nysten, 1865, p. 678.—Programme du cours d'histologie, 1864, p. 90.

‡ We have received a verbal communication from M. Robin to this effect.

§ Zalesky, *Untersuch. über den mämisch. Process.* Tübingen, 1865. The recent researches of Gréhaut seem to invalidate the results obtained by Zalesky.

upset this hypothesis.   Urea and uric acid, according to Zalesky, are formed in the kidneys themselves, and probably at the expense of creatin.   Tie the ureters of a dog and you will get an accumulation of urea in the blood ; there will be none if you extirpate. the kidneys.   In reptiles, ligature of the ureters causes an accumulation, not of urea, but of uric acid ; but removal of the kidneys produces nothing of the kind.   Zalesky concludes from this that urea (in animals who secrete it) and uric acid are formed in the kidney itself, and do not exist beforehand in the blood.

We do not find, therefore, in this direction any really important datum, any solid foundation whereon we could establish a rational doctrine.   We must then resort to other means of investigation.

II. The purely experimental investigation of the conditions which cause the proportion of uric acid in the renal excretion to vary, furnishes us at least with some interesting results.

The proportion of uric acid increases after a meal (Bence Jones).   Fasting diminishes this proportion by one-half; a vegetable diet acts in the same manner.

As to the effects of a purely animal diet, all the authors since Lehmann agree on this point.   There occurs an increase of uric acid and urea, especially of this latter substance.

Hitherto theoretical deductions seem tolerably harmonious with the results furnished us by observations as to the etiology of gout.   But we shall soon meet with contradictions when we pursue this study further.

It is generally admitted, for example, that exercise is one of the best means of preventing the uric acid diathesis.   The experiments of Lehmann confirm this view.   He has accurately shown that muscular activity has the effect of augmenting the quantity of urea, and diminishing the proportion of uric acid. The results have been confirmed so far as relates to the urea, but contradicted in the case of uric acid.   Beneke, Genth, and Heller[*] have found that exercise prolonged for three hours resulted in an increase of the quantity of this product.   Ranke[†]

[*] Beneke, *Nord See Bad.*, 1855, p. 85.—Genth, *Untersuch. über den Einfluss des Wassertrinkens auf dem Stoffwechsel;* Weisbaden, 1856.—Heller, *Heller's Archiv ; Neue Folge.*

[†] Ranke, *Aussch. der Harnsäure;* München, 1858, p. 240.

and Speck admit that unaccustomed activity would have this result. In short, whenever the activity is violent, or of long duration, there is rather an increase than a diminution of the uric acid.

In reference to the activity of the respiratory functions, it is generally admitted that the more active they are, the more the quantity of uric acid diminishes, while the proportion of urea increases. But we must say this view does not rest on any very positive fact.*

Concerning the influence of drinks we cannot yet draw any conclusions, in spite of the interesting experiments of Böcker.† According to this observer, alcohol and spirituous liquors lessen the formation of urea and uric acid; wines, on the contrary, as the already venerable experiments of Liebig have proved, tend to increase it; beer, when it does not act as a diuretic, diminishes the quantity of urea and increases that of uric acid, though very slightly; lastly, tea and coffee lessen the proportion of uric acid. If we admit that in these experiments the quantity of uric acid passed in the urine corresponds with its total formation in the system (which is probable, since the subjects made use of to establish these results were in good health), it would be proved that alcohol and spirituous drinks act quite otherwise than beer and wine in this respect, a fact in harmony with the results of clinical observation.

In brief, the data supplied by modern chemistry and physiology do not throw much light on the leading phenomenon of gout, namely, the presence of uric acid in the blood.

But since this fact has been experimentally demonstrated, can we, accepting it as a starting point, deduce therefrom the other symptoms of the disease? Such was the aim of Garrod's efforts. You shall learn the results of his labours, but observe that, in them, it is no longer a question of the general theory of gout, but only of the theory of the attacks.

III. We have seen that different circumstances predispose to an attack, and bring about its occurrence. The result of the former is an accumulation of uric acid in the blood, either by

---

* Consult Parkes, *On the Urine*, pp. 50 and 320.
† Böcker, *Beitrage zur Heilkunde*, vol. i., p. 240.

directly favouring its formation (abundant meals, abuse of certain drinks), or by diminishing its excretion (lead-poisoning, painful emotions). The latter affect the solubility of the uric acid in the blood, by diminishing the alkalinity of the liquid; such causes are, the influence of cold, which suppresses the acid secretion of sweat, and the use of acid substances—vinegar, &c.

We may, then, suppose that an excess of uric acid suddenly thrown into the circulating current accounts for the nervous troubles, the dyspeptic and other premonitory symptoms, which immediately precede the fit of gout.

The local symptoms of the disease are, up to a certain point, susceptible of the same explanation. We will pass in review the most important of these events, and consider them from this point of view.

The joints are specially affected in gout. This is a point of contact with other dyscrasias, which readily exert their action on the joints. We see this in purulent infection, in glanders, in the therapeutic employment of arsenic; lactic acid introduced into the veins seems also to act upon the joints (Richardson).

The fibrous tissues, and especially the cartilages, are specially susceptible to gout. We may attribute this disagreeable privilege to their slightly vascular structure, and the comparatively slight alkalinity of their substance—two circumstances which evidently favour the formation of those crystalline deposits which characterise the malady.

Gout specially affects the metatarso-phalangeal joint of the great toe. That possibly is connected with the fact that this joint is one of the most remote from the circulatory centre; it is also no doubt connected with the fact that this joint, which is so often called on to support the entire weight of the body, has often had some injury prior to any gouty manifestation; and we know that traumatic causes often have the effect of determining the invasion of gout.

One can explain, to a certain extent, the successive invasion of the joints, for when abundant deposits have formed in the cartilages of a joint, one may assume that there is saturation at that point; then the other joints begin, and follow a more or less regular order.

The formation of tophi also depends upon the saturation of the cartilages; thus it is always a secondary phenomenon.

The question may be put whether the deposits of sodium urate are the cause or the effect of the local inflammation. Garrod leans towards the former opinion. He points out that the inflammation caused by the deposits seems to have the effect of destroying the urate of sodium, and that after an attack the blood contains a less considerable proportion of this salt. Moreover, the deposits which form externally are not preceded by any inflammatory action, and if they do occasionally give rise to symptoms of this kind, it is entirely by acting as foreign bodies (external ear).

Thus the formation of these deposits in the cartilage would precede the first attack; and the formation of new deposits, either in the same joint or in fresh ones, would occasion the local phenomena characterising the subsequent attacks.

But why that acute pain which introduces the series of articular symptoms? It cannot be attributed to the inflammation: the local inflammation is quite as intense, but certainly less painful, in articular rheumatism. According to Garrod, we must attribute it to the actual presence of the deposits in the substance of the cartilage, and to the stretching thus determined; for it is only when the gout is *intra-articular* that the suffering is so acute; when the deposit occurs outside this is not the case.

Lastly, the symptoms of arthritis appear, and the general reaction is a consequence of the local events; its intensity is known to be generally proportionate to the number of joints invaded, and to the degree of the local inflammation.

Such, gentlemen, is the state of our knowledge on this subject. I have thought it my duty to devote myself to a discussion which has frequently been barren, in order to show you how much progress remains to be realised in this matter.

In reference to visceral gout we have already pointed out the results of Zalesky's interesting experiments; they have demonstrated to us that ligature of the ureters in certain animals induces the formation of deposits of sodium urate in the gastric follicles. It is very possible that in man, when the blood is saturated, the gastro-intestinal liquids get loaded with urates. Analogous phenomena may no doubt be produced at other spots. In the animals on which he experimented, Zalesky found a large proportion of sodium urate in an extract of muscle substance. It is easy to understand the great importance of these facts in reference to the visceral complications of gout; but a point less easy to explain is the occurrence of those sudden metastases which transfer the morbid action from one point to another: from the big toe to the stomach, and from the stomach to the joints. On this point, certainly, science has not said its last word.

I might now speak to you of the therapeutic measures with which gout may be combated. But I prefer to put off this subject to the time when we shall take up the treatment of chronic rheumatism; by bringing together the two accounts we shall find the materials for a comparison no less instructive than remarkable.

LECTURE XI.

CHRONIC ARTICULAR RHEUMATISM, AND ITS ANATOMICAL LESIONS.

SUMMARY.—Chronic articular rheumatism is an essentially hospital affection.—Its nature.—Its relationship to acute rheumatism.—Chief varieties of this disease.—Progressive chronic articular rheumatism (rheumatic gout).—Partial chronic articular rheumatism.—Heberden's nodosities ; must not be confounded with gout.

      Anatomical characters of chronic articular rheumatism.—Necessity of carefully studying the local lesions.—Unity of this disease.—Mention of the first works relating to the subject.

      Fundamental characters of chronic rheumatic arthritis.—Change in the synovial membrane ; in the cartilages ; in the fluid from the joints ; in the bony tissue.—Histological study of these various lesions.—Modifications corresponding to the chief clinical forms of the disease.

GENTLEMEN,—After having thoroughly examined the natural history of gout, we shall proceed to study an affection so like it, that the two diseases have frequently been confounded together. I hope, however, to show you that this union is not well founded, and that a special place must be reserved for chronic articular rheumatism, which is now to become the subject of our lectures.

For this purpose we shall be in a very favourable position. Whilst gout, which in France is not one of the diseases commonly met with in hospitals, and which, moreover, is uncommon in the female sex ;—whilst gout is almost unknown at the Salêptrière, chronic rheumatism on the contrary is one of the commonest diseases in this establishment. Indeed this affection prevails among women and the least favoured classes of society. And thus the proportion of persons admitted into this hospital for this kind of malady, is about $\frac{1}{15}$ of the total number of inmates.

Most of the authors who have made a special study of this disease, have made their observations in establishments like the Salpêtrière. In England the workhouses have supplied the materials for the interesting publications of Colles, Smith, and Adams. You know it was at the Salpêtrière where Landré-Beauvais produced the monograph which we have already had occasion to quote. So that we are entering upon a really clinical study in this case, and I shall often have occasion to place before you not only anatomical specimens, as I have often done hitherto, but also the patients who are attacked by the lesions I am going to describe.

I. The name which I have selected for the disease in question involves a pathological interpretation to which I fully adhere, but which all the authors do not admit.

Among the opponents of the opinion which I hold some declare that we have to do with a special affection, completely independent both of gout and of acute articular rheumatism; it is the *rheumatoid arthritis* of Garrod, the *rheumatic gout* of Fuller. Others consider the various forms of nodular rheumatism as coming under the head of gout.

I shall endeavour, gentlemen, to justify the opinions which I hold, and to show you that at the bedside one sometimes sees chronic articular rheumatism develop directly out of acute articular rheumatism, exactly as chronic lobar pneumonia may follow acute pneumonia. Still, it is true that one finds the chronic form of articular rheumatism almost always develop spontaneously, and without passing through the acute form ; but this negative fact cannot invalidate the connection which we are seeking to establish.

In reference to the relationship between gout and chronic rheumatism, we shall later on establish a radical distinction between the two diseases.

II. Chronic articular rheumatism presents itself under various aspects, which are apparently so opposed to one another that some authors have fancied that there were several different affections to deal with. I, on the contrary, only recognise different forms of one and the same disease.

To quote but one example of this, I may tell you that several authors readily admit that nodular rheumatism is nothing else than poly-articular rheumatism in a chronic state, but they refuse to recognise the rheumatic origin of the affection when it is localised in a single joint, slowly and insidiously producing there the grave and profound changes of *morbus coxæ senilis*.

I hope to show you that it is quite impossible to establish a real distinction between these different forms of rheumatism, and that it is often possible, on the contrary, to prove that they all take origin from one and the same source.

It is, however, indispensable from the clinical point of view to study separately the chief varieties of chronic rheumatism, as if there were really several distinct diseases; this is the only means of avoiding all confusion. After this preliminary procedure I shall endeavour to make clear the common bond which unites them.

The types of chronic articular rheumatism are very numerous, but we shall give our chief attention to the following forms :—

1. *Progressive chronic articular Rheumatism.*

This is the *rheumatic gout,* or *nodular rheumatism* of authors ; the *primary asthenic gout,* of Landré-Beauvais ; *the nodosities of the joints,* of Haygarth.

This form is the most serious ; it involves deplorable disability. Although affecting in preference the small joints, it also attacks the large ones ; often it is the cause of muscular retractions and other complications.

Two forms may be distinguished. Sometimes *primary,* sometimes *secondary* to the acute form (a rare occurrence), this affection may be either mild or severe. It is not always limited to the joints, and may be accompanied by visceral affections, which are sometimes like those of acute rheumatism (and occasionally are dependent on it), and sometimes peculiar to chronic rheumatism ; in this latter category *ophthalmia* and *albuminous nephritis* must be placed.

The local changes are those of the dry form of arthritis, which are, however, common to all sorts of chronic rheumatism except certain secondary modifications.

2. *Partial chronic articular Rheumatism.*

In this type the affected joints are few in number ; sometimes there is but one affected. The articular changes are the same as in the preceding form, but of much greater severity, as we see in the case of *morbus coxæ senilis.* The foreign bodies which occasionally develop in the joints, often reach an exceptional size in these cases.

On the contrary, visceral or non-articular affections are here uncommon ; they may, however, occur. It is especially in the mild form of the disease that they are met with ; in some of these patients we find certain forms of asthma and of cutaneous affections coming on.

It is quite otherwise in the severe form which scarcely admits of the viscera being affected, and in which the whole disease seems concentrated on the affected joint. In some exceptional cases, however, albuminuria has been noticed to come on.

3. *Heberden's Rheumatism.*

Heberden's *nodosities* (*digitorum nodi*) constitute the least grave type of this disease. It is especially in this form that a critical discussion will be necessary. When we are dealing with nodular rheumatism it is generally recognised that it differs from gout, at least in certain of its characteristics. The same cannot be said of the form I am now pointing out. Nobody, you may say, doubts that these lesions are placed in close and rightful relationship with gout. I am obliged to hold a diametrically opposite opinion. I intend to describe quite specially that form of arthritis which so commonly attacks the *second joint of the fingers*, and which deforms them in so singular a manner. No doubt these lesions have attracted the notice of many observers, but they have not yet been studied with all the care they merit. Morbid anatomy will soon make us recognise that, beyond their special seat, this form of joint-disease differs in nothing from those which constituted the two preceding forms; but we shall have occasion after a while to justify clinically the separation of this particular type.

For the present I shall content myself with pointing out that in the most ordinary case one meets merely with nodes on the phalanges, almost always indolent nodes, without other complication. Sometimes, however, several other joints, some of which are among the most important ones, become affected at the same time; lastly, the joint lesion may be accompanied by muscular or neuralgic pains, which affect sometimes the sciatic, sometimes the trifacial, sometimes other nerve trunks.

Among the visceral affections connected with this variety we may notice particularly *asthma* and *migraine*.

III. We will now consider the anatomical characters of chronic rheumatism.

When we tried to trace the history of gout, we all along came upon one fundamental fact, which determines all the symptomatic modifications of that disease, I mean the alteration of the blood which consists in its containing an excess of uric acid. We do not find for our guidance in the study of chronic rheumatism any character of such general importance; and although it is probable that in rheumatism, as in gout, a special modification of the liquids of the body does exist, this hypothesis is still far from being demonstrated.

We must therefore fall back upon a searching examination of the local lesions; we shall pursue these researches from the double point of view of clinical observation and morbid anatomy, insisting especially, however, on this latter aspect of the question, at least for the present.

Pathological anatomy enables us in the first place to demonstrate the *unity* of this disease; for the various forms which it may assume differ most in their clinical characters, and so far as the local changes are concerned, present a common type, modified by some differences of secondary importance. It enables us, in the second place, to connect the chronic form of articular rheumatism with the acute or subacute form; it enables us, lastly, to establish a radical distinction between this disease and the other diatheses which share with it the peculiarity of localisation in the joints; such for example as gout, scrofula, and syphilis.

We need not go far back in history to discover the first works relating to our subject.

The physicians of antiquity, as I have already pointed out to you, appear to have confounded articular rheumatism with gout, and the question has arisen whether the former of these two affections is not one peculiar to modern times. In this matter archeology comes to the aid of medicine, and the excavations at Pompeii have taught us that chronic rheumatism was already existent in the first century of the Christian era. Delle Chiaje, in a work called "Osteologia Pompeiana," has figured articular lesions which are identical with those which we find in the plates of Adams's classical work. There can be no doubt, therefore, on this point; yet chronic rheumatism has only been recognised as a special kind of disease since the works of Sydenham and Musgrave appeared; and the first monographs devoted to the study of this disease date from the commencement of this century; we may mention that of Landré-Beauvais (year viii.), of Haygarth (1809), and of Chomel (1813). It was a little later that the fundamental characters of chronic rheumatic arthritis were made clear; in France, Lobstein (1832) perceived that in this affection the bones are particularly fragile; that the destruction of the articular cartilages is followed by eburnation; and that at the margin of the articulating surfaces bony vegetations grow.

About the same period, an Irish physician named Colles observed that this inflammation differs from others by a perfectly special character; he said that two very opposite processes take place at the same time, namely, absorption of the original bone and of its cartilage of incrustation, and formation of fresh bone.

But it is especially to Adams,* contemporary and fellow-countryman of Colles, that we owe the best studies on this subject (1839—1857). As to naked-eye examination his description has left very little to be desired; still, special mention is due to the works of Deville and Broca on *dry arthritis* (1850). They have completed in certain respects the descriptions given by Adams. In our days, histological studies have thrown a clear light on this question.

In Germany, Leis, H. Meyer,† and Otto Weber,‡ have taught us in what way each tissue is modified when under the influence of chronic rheumatism, and have thus given the rationale of several phenomena which would otherwise have remained inexplicable.

In France these results have been confirmed and extended by Ranvier, Cornil, and Vergely.§

It is through the help of this literature, and relying on the studies I have myself made, that I shall give you a description of the morbid processes characteristic of chronic articular rheumatism.

A. *Concise Account of the Essential Characters of Chronic Rheumatic Arthritis.*

The affection which we are about to study affects the whole of

---

* *A Treatise on Rheumatic Gout,* by R. Adams, M.D. London, 1857.
† Müller's *Archiv,* 1849.   ‡ Virchow's *Archiv,* Jan., 1858, p. 74.
§ Ranvier, *Thèses de Paris,* 1865.—Cornil, Translation of Niemeyer's *Internal Pathologie,* vol. ii., p. 556.—Vergely, *Thèses de Paris,* 1856.

the constituent parts of the joint, but it attacks first of all the synovial membrane and the cartilages; these may be affected simultaneously or in succession. The synovial membrane becomes extremely vascular; the original synovial fringes increase in size and new villous appendages are formed; lastly, foreign bodies may develop either at the expense of the fringes themselves or in the substance of the synovial membrane.

At the same time a modification of the synovial fluid takes place; at the beginning the secretion of the fluid is increased, and this, according to Adams, is a constant phenomenon. Later on the synovia may undergo various changes, but it never contains *pus* unless there are special complications. The destruction of the cartilage goes on in a manner already known to William Hunter, and ably studied by Redfern;* it is known as the "velvety change." At first the cartilage is found to divide into fibrillæ; then these fibrillæ themselves disappear, and the cartilage is destroyed.

Let us see now what the changes are that are going on at the same period in the osseous tissue. We find, first, eburnation of the articular surface, either at the expense of the deep portion of the cartilage or of the original bone; at the same time there is a growth of bony vegetations, generally situated at the edge of the cartilage. These osteophytes have at first a cartilaginous structure; then they become impregnated with calcareous salts, and end by ossifying.

A third alteration, the importance of which is at least equal to that of the preceding lesions, is the thinning of the osseous tissue at the ends of the bones. At the outset there occurs an evident increase of vascularity below the eburnated layer, and newly formed marrow substance takes origin at this spot; next, the bone thins, and is transformed into a kind of fatty marrow below this point.

Such are the essential facts which it is well to state just now. There are no doubt many other changes, but as they are not common to all the forms of articular rheumatism, we shall study them at the proper time and place.

I shall now take up each of the facts which I have just pointed out, in order to study it more thoroughly by help of those means of investigation which we possess to-day.

* *Edinburgh Monthly Journal*, 1849.

B. *Histological Study.*

1. *Alterations in the synovial membrane.* Up to a certain point they consist in a mere exaggeration of the tendencies which, in a rudimentary state, exist under the normal conditions. You know that the synovial membrane is edged by fringes, and these latter have appendages.* You will find that in a morbid state these little prolongations increase in number, and appear intensely vascular.

In the normal state, cartilage cells exist in these synovial fringes (Kölliker). These cartilaginous nodules may become the starting points of the pedunculated foreign bodies which we have already mentioned. According to Ranvier, proliferation of the cells first occurs, and then formation of true cartilage; calcification follows, and, lastly, real ossification takes place with formation of bone corpuscles.

In the substance of the synovial membrane *sessile* foreign bodies may be formed, and these pass through exactly the same stages as the pedunculated ones.

2. *Alterations in the cartilage.* Concerning changes in the joint-cartilage we meet with two principal facts : the first is the *proliferation* of the cartilage cells and the formation of secondary capsules; the second is the *segmentation* of the ground substance. It divides into fibrillæ which become free at their extremities bordering the articular cavity.

This morbid process must be studied both at the surface of the cartilage and in its substance.

At the surface, the segmentation has the effect of opening a passage for the capsules, which burst in the articular cavity and empty their contents into it. They are often found there together with the *débris* of epithelial cells (Rindfleisch, O. Weber) ; at other times they undergo colloid change.

As to the fibrillæ of ground substance, they undergo mucous degeneration and are transformed into mucin (Rindfleisch), which is found in abundance in the synovial fluid.

At other times these altered portions of cartilage become gradually worn away by the friction of the articular surfaces ; at length they fall off and leave the surface of the bone bare.

* Kölliker, *Elements of Human Histology.*

In the deep portions, the proliferation of the cells ends in the formation of a new layer of bone. The mother-capsules become infiltrated with calcareous salts, and communicate with the superficial medullary spaces ; the cells which they contain become embryonic medullary cells, and at their expense the new bony tissue is formed.

It is thus that eburnation of the surface takes place. There is a sort of sclerosis of the bone, accompanied by increased vascularity of the deep parts. There now occurs a singular phenomenon, which recalls in certain points the facts observed by geologists with regard to the action of glaciers on the rocks. The eburnated surfaces present striæ—grooves which vary in depth and follow the direction of the articular movements, thus giving evidence of the imperfect reparative action which opposes the wear occasioned by friction.

The articular cartilage, as you know, is covered at its margin by the synovial membrane. When the joint is invaded by rheumatism, this arrangement, according to Ranvier, hinders the passage of the capsules into the cavity of the joint and their rupture there. They would then continue proliferating at this point and thus determine the formation of those enlargements, at first cartilaginous, then osseous, which are met with in this situation.

Thus Ranvier refers all the new bony formations, which develop under these circumstances, to proliferation of the cells of the articular cartilage. However, the periosteum probably takes some part in the process ; moreover there may occur a simultaneous ossification of the capsules of the joints, the ligaments, tendons, and muscles. As to the interarticular ligaments and fibro-cartilages, &c., they wear away and disappear in a manner analogous to that in which the articular cartilage is destroyed, but which has not yet been sufficiently studied.

Such, gentlemen, are the most general facts that I had to mention to you, but numerous modifications of these occur, according to the clinical form of rheumatism in question, and according to some special circumstances dependent on the actual conditions of the disease. Thus the changes met with in a joint kept at absolute rest, differ from those which accompany a more or less complete maintenance of articular movement. We have hitherto considered the subject on this latter hypothesis. We shall now study the modifications which occur when the joint is motionless.

In such a case, says Adams, eburnation is no longer observed, but there occurs a new growth of connective tissue at the expense of the synovial membrane. The cartilage may participate in this, according to Forster; sometimes it is the ground substance which undergoes this transformation ; sometimes, on the contrary, the cartilage cells assume the appearance of connective tissue corpuscles. However much truth there be in this theory, we find an embryonic tissue forming which unites the bones one to another, and which becomes vascular at a certain stage of growth ; then ankylosis occurs, sometimes fibrous, sometimes bony. This last event is very rare ; it only occurs in very small joints.

Prolonged repose has also the effect of inducing extreme atrophy and friability of the osseous tissue; the nodes and vegetations may disappear. This atrophic process, which is common in the general form of rheumatism, also occurs, though rarely, in *morbus coxæ senilis* (Adams).

C. *Modifications corresponding to the chief forms of chronic articular rheumatism.*

The description which I have just given applies chiefly to general rheumatism, and to the rheumatism of Heberden. Here the lesions of the dry form of arthritis are found in a rudimentary state ; but in partial arthritis they undergo enormous development and become almost unrecognisable. One finds an extreme degree of wasting and eburnation of the cartilages and bones, and consequent deformity of the ends of the bones. Lastly, in this form atrophy of the bones reaches its extreme development. Formerly these lesions were explained by osteo-malacia, or senile rickets (Malgaigne, Hattier).

In the joints, which, for imperfectly understood reasons, admit of the presence of foreign bodies, we find these growing in great numbers; this occurs, for example, in the shoulder and knee, but the case is quite otherwise in regard to the hip and finger joints. There occur besides considerable thickenings of the fibrous capsules, and ossification of ligaments and tendons. Let us note, however, that these differences cannot justify a radical distinction ; in partial rheumatism there may be several joints in which the changes only reach a much inferior degree of severity, and in general rheumatism some of the diseased joints may present lesions quite as pronounced as in partial rheumatism ; this occurs, for example, in the vertebral column.

To bring this study to an end we have still to compare chronic rheumatism with the other chronic joint-diseases from an anatomical point of view. But before entering on this subject I wish to point out to you the analogies which connect the chronic form of rheumatism with the acute.

LECTURE XII.

COMPARISON OF CHRONIC ARTICULAR RHEUMATISM AND THE OTHER
CHRONIC JOINT DISEASES FROM AN ANATOMICAL POINT OF VIEW.

SUMMARY.—Analogy between the lesions of chronic articular rheumatism and those of acute articular rheumatism.—Alterations of the joints in acute and subacute articular rheumatism.—Sometimes absent, sometimes manifest.—Arthritis with exudation.—The inflammation is not superficial.—The cartilages and bones may participate in it.—Lesion of the synovial membrane.—Lesions of the articular cartilages.—Lesions of the bones.—Nature of the fluid secreted into the synovial cavity.—Analogy between these lesions and those of chronic rheumatism.

Characters which distinguish *arthritis deformans* from the other joint affections.—Arthritis through prolonged repose.—Strumous arthritis.—Syphilitic disease of joints.—Gouty disease of joints.

The lesions of chronic rheumatism have not a specific character.—They may result from other than rheumatic influences.—In that case they are almost always monarticular.—Chronic rheumatism is generally polyarticular.

GENTLEMEN,—We are now in a position to compare, from the point of view of pathological anatomy, chronic articular rheumatism with the other slowly developing joint diseases.

But before undertaking this comparison, it is absolutely necessary to make clear the points of resemblance between the alterations in chronic articular rheumatism and those in acute articular rheumatism. We shall soon perceive that the lesions of the chronic form are only, so to speak, the higher expression of the lesions of the acute form ; they correspond to a more advanced phase of the morbid action. The analogy which I am indicating is not evident at first sight, especially if the comparison is made between extreme cases—if, for example, one brings together a transient acute attack and *morbus coxæ senilis ;* but it becomes most manifest, on the contrary, if one chooses as the terms of comparison those subacute cases, which, from the clinical as well as from the anatomical stand-point, constitute a transition between the acute and chronic forms of articular rheumatism.

I. *Changes in the Joints in Acute and Subacute Rheumatism.*

In the scholastic language of ancient medicine, the term *subacute* was applied to diseases the duration of which exceeded twenty-one days—the extreme limit of acute diseases properly so called—and might continue up to forty days. Pathological facts do not admit of such arbitrary divisions, and under the name *subacute articular rheumatism* we shall speak of a disease, the development of which is no doubt less rapid than that of acute articular rheumatism, but which also differs from it in other respects, though without being radically distinct. But we must also admit that this subacute form is already approaching chronic articular rheumatism in certain of its characteristics.

Thus, in this form of the disease the articular affection is less transient ; the fever is less intense, and resembles hectic fever ; the small joints are often affected, and sometimes in great numbers. You know that the contrary occurs in acute articular rheumatism. Moreover, the visceral affections, or at least some of them (endocarditis, pericarditis), are less frequently observed.

Such are the essential characters of subacute articular rheumatism. Later on I shall have some fresh considerations to offer you on this subject. At present I shall mention the lesions that are observed in the joints in acute and subacute articular rheumatism.

Interminable discussions took place at one time with regard to the lesions of acute articular rheumatism. May this affection end in suppuration or not ? Some maintained that articular rheumatism leaves no trace in the joints ; others declared that it is the cause of the most serious articular lesions, and may lead to purulent arthritis.

At the present day the question is decided, and a more rational appreciation of the facts has had the effect of proving that there was considerable exaggeration on both sides.

It is true that occasionally rheumatic inflammation of the joints may leave behind it no appreciable change (Grisolle, Macleod, Fuller), and that in certain cases, on the contrary, it may lead to purulent arthritis (Bouillaud). But facts of this kind are very exceptional, and in the immense majority of cases, what one meets with are the signs of arthritis with sero-fibrinous exudation ; the synovial membrane is red and injected, and its cavity contains a serous fluid, in which float fibrinous flakes.

It was thought for a long time that the inflammation in this case is quite superficial, and that the synovial membrane is alone affected (synovitis); but it has now been shown that the cartilages, and even the bones, may take part in these changes.

The lesions of the synovial membrane need not detain us long. We meet with : 1st, more or less injection of the synovial fringes which normally exist; 2nd, a varicose dilatation of their vessels (Lebert).

The changes in the cartilage are of much greater importance; we owe our knowledge of them to the interesting work of Ollivier and Ranvier.

It had already been noticed (Garrod) that the articular cartilage sometimes presents a certain degree of opacity, and loses the polish, blue tint, and consistence which characterise it in the healthy state. Ollivier and Ranvier have further shown that there are often changes appreciable to the naked eye; there are local swellings of the cartilage which give it a mammillated aspect, and sometimes even actual erosions. But even in cases where there is no change appreciable by the naked eye, the microscope reveals very manifest and probably constant lesions.

At an early stage the most superficial cell-spaces become globular; the contained cell divides and gives origin to one or two secondary cells.

Things may stop at this point, and it is easy to understand that in such a case the histological elements may return to the normal state; but at a more advanced stage there occurs a segmentation of the ground substance in a horizontal direction; a kind of velvety condition is produced, characterised by grooves which penetrate more or less deeply into the tissue. In the interior of these newly-formed grooves, the capsules burst and there empty their contained cells; the latter then mingle with the synovial fluid, and there undergo the mucous transformation. In this, you see, there are great analogies with what takes place in cases of *arthritis deformans.*

But the changes presented by the osseous surfaces make the analogy still more striking; they seem in certain cases to take part in the inflammatory action. According to Gurlt,* the medullary tissue of the ends of the bones undergoes a great increase of vascularity, with proliferation of its corpuscles.

* Forster, *Handbuch der path. Anat.,* p. 1000.

Hasse* and Kussmaul† have also referred to lesions of the bones and periosteum in acute articular rheumatism.

I have still a word to say on the nature of the fluid contained in the synovial cavity. It sometimes has an acid reaction, and holds albumin and mucin in solution ; we find floating in it fibrinous flakes, lumps of hardened mucus, and globular corpuscles, some of which are cartilage cells and epithelioid cells which have undergone fatty degeneration, whilst others much resemble the cells of pus ; sometimes, indeed, real pus cells are found. But it may be stated that, in general, this last element is not predominant save in exceptional cases in which the rheumatism is consecutive or symptomatic, or where a rheumatic inflammation is combined with the purulent diathesis.   If we try to interpret these phenomena, we may say, in brief, that the fibrin and pus cells are dependent on acute synovitis, whilst the mucin is produced by the transformation of the epithelioid cells and the ground substance of the cartilage.

These alterations, which offer incontestable analogies with those of chronic articular rheumatism, become still more like them in the subacute form.   Thus, in a case in which the rheumatism had lasted about two months, I found a thickening of the synovial membrane with very marked villous outgrowths ; erosions and a well-marked velvety condition were found at several spots.

In a patient who died on the twenty-fifth day, after showing cerebral symptoms, Bonnet had previously found analogous changes.‡   These lesions are met with as mere vestiges in patients who have succumbed to organic affections of the heart, after several previous attacks of acute articular rheumatism. There is an imperceptible transition between these cases and those in which, as a consequence of the persistence or constant return of the rheumatic affection, the disease has become decidedly chronic.   The lesions are then more severe ; synovial villous outgrowths are developed, foreign bodies begin to be formed, the articular surfaces begin to undergo eburnation, and osseous vegetations grow round the joints ; lastly, the osseous tissue becomes friable near the ends of the bones.

In this way it has been successfully proved from the anatomical

---

* Hasse, *Zeitschrift für rat. Med.*, vol. v., pp. 192—212.

† Kussmaul, *Arch. für physiol. Heilkunde*, vol. xi., 1852.

‡ Bonnet, *Traité des maladies des articulations*, Paris, 1845, vol. i., p. 329.

stand-point, that there is a close connection between the various forms of articular rheumatism. They are in no way distinct affections ; they are varieties of one and the same species of disease.

II. *Changes in the Joints in certain Affections not Rheumatic.*

One word now on the characters which distinguish *arthritis deformans* from the other chronic joint-diseases.

1. *Arthritis through prolonged disuse.* In an early phase, according to Teissier and Bonnet,* arthritis through prolonged repose gives rise to the following lesions : a sero-sanguineous secretion into the joint takes place ; even liquid blood is occasionally found there. The synovial membrane is injected and ecchymosed ; indeed, there is said to be sometimes ulceration of the cartilages.

But in a more advanced phase I have been able to determine the existence on the articular cartilage of central ulcerations with edges sharply cut as with a punch, and also of peripheral ulcerations. There are no osseous nodules and no fibrous ankylosis, but a very marked thinning of the osseous tissue takes place. But the essential characteristic of this affection of the joints is the existence of a layer of connective tissue which covers the articular cartilage in its whole extent ; this membrane may be readily detached from the subjacent surface, and one then comes upon the cartilage, the cells of which have undergone fatty degeneration *in situ*. This membrane is often penetrated by vascular ingrowths, which sometimes penetrate towards the central parts ; it is probable that the cases of vascularisation of cartilage mentioned by certain authors may be explained in this way. I have been able to demonstrate these lesions in patients long the victims of hemiplegia or paraplegia, especially in parts which remain uncovered, when an articular deformity exists.

You know that some of these changes are found associated with those of *arthritis deformans* in cases in which the joints are condemned to absolute disuse. It must be admitted that this is an important question, but as yet little studied and demanding fresh researches.

* Teissier, *Mémoire sur les effets de l'immobilité longtemps prolongée des articulations.* Lyon, 1844.—Bonnet, op. cit., vol. i.

2. *Scrofulous or fungous arthritis.* The researches of Ranvier show that *arthritis fungosa* is very different from dry arthritis, even when we only consider the elementary lesions. This is shown by a study of the lesions which characterise this disease. As to the bones and cartilage, in *arthritis deformans*, there is proliferation of the cellular elements; in *arthritis fungosa*, on the contrary, these elements die and undergo fatty degeneration, which can be seen in the bones and in the cells of the cartilage. Moreover, at a more advanced period of the disease the distinction becomes exceedingly evident: fungous arthritis gives rise to vegetations from bone and synovial membrane, with destruction and absorption of cartilage; then caries and necrosis of the bone follow; and, lastly, we find peripheral abscesses forming around the diseased joint.

There are analogies, however, between these two affections. In certain cases of scrofulous arthritis there is an active proliferation of the elements of the cartilage; but this is a secondary phenomenon. Sometimes, also, osseous stalactites are formed, but these are very vascular (Billroth); and they differ markedly from the large stalactites with rounded edges, like drops of tallow in form, and generally but little vascular, which characterise *arthritis deformans.* Thus the anatomical lesions of these two affections differ from one another, but there exist mixed cases in which they may be found together.

3. Let us pass now to *syphilitic* disease of joints. It is extremely probable that under this head rheumatism, either acute or chronic, occurring in syphilitic patients, has more than once been described, for these two diatheses are far from mutually excluding each other. However, certain clinical peculiarities, and the decisive influence of specific treatment in certain cases in which the supposed rheumatism has been long protracted, have led some physicians, among whom we may mention Babington, Boyer, and Lancereaux,* to think that there are really special forms of joint-disease, arising directly from venereal infection.

Lancereaux, to whom we owe a thorough investigation of this question, has endeavoured to give a careful description of the articular lesions of syphilis. He distinguishes two forms of them: 1st, *secondary* manifestations, which present the cha-

* Lancereaux, *Traité de la Syphilis,* 1866, p. 22.

racters of acute or subacute articular rheumatism ; 2nd, *tertiary* manifestations, which resemble some forms of chronic rheumatism ; these latter are the only forms which it has been possible to study anatomically. The morbid process commences in the subsynovial connective tissue and in the fibrous tissue, and it is characterised by the formation of new growths which in texture and external appearance exactly recall gummatous tumours.

In the cases observed by Lancereaux there was no alteration of the synovial membrane, but the articular cartilages were eroded.

4. *Gouty disease of the joints.* The lesions of *arthritis deformans* have sufficient resemblance to those of gout to be often readily confounded with them at the bedside ; but anatomically this is no longer the case. Not the least trace of a deposit of sodium urate is ever found either in the articular affections of rheumatism or in the other articular affections which I have just mentioned.

The uratic infiltration of the cartilage is, then, the essential character of articular gout ; further, no other constant lesion of the cartilage exists. There is no segmentation of the ground substance, nor proliferation of cells, so that if the two alterations are met with together, it is evidently from the simultaneous occurrence of the two diseases ; they never become transformed in such a way as to run into each other.*

We may regard the articular lesions of gout as the result of the presence of a foreign body in the substance of the tissues ; whilst the lesions of rheumatism, on the contrary, depend on real changes of the histological elements. Moreover, when a fragment of cartilage, raised from the surface of a joint attacked with gout, is treated by acetic acid, we see the crystals of sodium urate, with which the cells are infiltrated, dissolve, and the latter then resume their normal aspect.

I think we have demonstrated : 1st, the unity of the various clinical forms of chronic articular rheumatism, so far as morbid anatomy goes ; 2nd, the existence of an incontestable connection between the changes of acute rheumatism and those of partial or chronic rheumatic arthritis ; 3rd, the existence of a marked distinction, still from the anatomical point of view, between the

* Charcot and Cornil, Contributions á l'étude des alterations anatomiques de la goutte, *Mémoires de la Société de Biologie*, 1864.

affection we are now considering and the other articular affections of constitutional origin.

Gentlemen, in the course of this account, one question must have often occurred to your minds. Have the lesions I have been describing a specific character ? In other words, are they exclusively peculiar to the rheumatic diathesis ?

To speak only of what relates to chronic articular rheumatism, we have been led, even from a purely anatomical point of view, to admit that there are marked distinctions between the articular lesions determined by it and those which result from gout, scrofula, and syphilis.

It is important, however, to recognise that the elementary lesions, which, as a whole, constitute *arthritis deformans,* may also be met with in cases in which a rheumatic influence cannot be assumed. Thus in fungous arthritis proliferation of the capsules and segmentation of the ground substance of the cartilage may occur here and there under the influence of the inflammatory process, which at a certain stage lays hold of the different tissues. The rarefaction and condensation of the osseous tissue at the ends of the bones, the formation of osteophytes and bony nodules at the margin of the articular cartilages, are met with, as you know, in affections other than rheumatism. So that it is the simultaneous occurrence of these changes in different parts of the joints in the manner which I have already indicated, and the degree to which these lesions may proceed without becoming complicated by suppuration, which constitute in my view the *anatomical characteristics* of the disease.

At this point we are led to inquire whether an irritation completely different from the internal cause which determines rheumatism—a cut or blow, for example—may set up the various changes of *arthritis deformans* in a joint.

It is certain, gentlemen, that under these conditions we may meet with all the lesions which I have just described. But in such a case they are almost always limited to a single joint; and even here are we not justified in assuming the intervention of a latent influence determining the character of the local lesion ? Recall what happens in this respect in patients attacked with gout.

It always happens that when the articular affections are multiple (and this is commonly the case) they are spontaneously developed, and seem by this double characteristic to point to a general predisposition of the system.

In such a case it is the influence of *rheumatism* which must be invoked, for in the present state of science we are acquainted with no other diathetic state to which such effects can be attributed.

LECTURE XIII.

ACUTE ARTICULAR RHEUMATISM, CONSIDERED ESPECIALLY IN ITS
RELATIONSHIP WITH CHRONIC ARTICULAR RHEUMATISM AND
GOUT.

SUMMARY.—Concise description of acute and subacute articular rheumatism.—Its
analogy to chronic rheumatism ; differences which distinguish it from gout.—
Acute rheumatism ; subacute rheumatism.

Multiple arthritis.—Pain.—Swelling.—Redness.—Temperature.—Duration.—
Versatility of the affection.

General condition in rheumatism.—Fever.—Irregular progress of the disease.
—Relationship between the intensity of the febrile action and the number of
joints affected.—Pulse.—Secretions.—Saliva.—Urine.—Profound anæmia.

Comparison of acute articular rheumatism, gout, and subacute articular
rheumatism.—The pathology of the blood in acute and subacute articular
rheumatism.

GENTLEMEN,—I have no intention of giving you a complete
description of acute articular rheumatism. This study can only
be made with good result in the ordinary hospitals. Nothing is
rarer, in fact, in old people than the acute form of articular
rheumatism ; nothing, on the contrary, is commoner in them
than the chronic form of this disease : I have already proved
this fact to you.

We cannot, however, completely ignore the history of acute
rheumatism. For I am desirous of maintaining in the domain
of clinical medicine the comparison which I have already
made, so far as anatomy goes, between these two affections ;
and, in taking up this new stand-point, I shall once more
establish that there are not merely analogies between them, but
that in certain respects they are really identical. I want to
accomplish the demonstration of the theory which I hold ;
namely, that there are not two fundamentally distinct diseases to
be dealt with, as certain authors fancy, but only two different
manifestations of one and the same diathetic state ; and you will
readily perceive the striking features of resemblance which unite
them, in spite of the diversities in the symptomatic expression of
the disease, which result from the slow or rapid reaction of the
organism.

Contrariwise, we shall arrive at just the opposite conclusion in reference to the connection between rheumatism and gout; I shall enable you to perceive that, though certain phenomena may sometimes make these two diseases resemble each other, this is only the case in quite exceptional circumstances; and also that, thanks to the rules of diagnosis which I shall soon lay down, these two diseases may nearly always be accurately distinguished in practice.

I shall, therefore, give you a concise description of acute rheumatism, laying stress only on characters which are essential.

I. *Description of Acute Articular Rheumatism.*

Here again we meet with the two forms, the existence of which I have already mentioned : on the one hand acute articular rheumatism—rheumatic fever of English authors ; and on the other subacute articular rheumatism (Garrod, Copland), or capsular rheumatism (Macleod). The latter is a transitional form, as I have already stated, and its characters we shall presently study. At present we shall consider rheumatic fever.

The usually multiple articular lesions with which we are already acquainted from an anatomical point of view, and which we shall soon study in their clinical bearings, are far from being the sole constituents of acute rheumatism. There is associated with them a general reaction, which expresses itself in a very characteristic general condition, and a very marked change in the state [*crase*] of the blood (increase in the amount of fibrin and diminution in the number of red disks), as well as by the frequent, we might say habitual, coexistence of certain visceral affections. Endocarditis and pericarditis, for example, are among the fundamental events of acute rheumatism ; and this character is one great reason which induces us to regard this affection as a general disease, or at least one with no definite seat, and not as a mere group of articular inflammations more or less independent of one another.

We arrive at the same conclusion by studying the development of the disease, and the etiological conditions which may give rise to it, among which, as you know, heredity plays an important part.

Such, gentlemen, are the most general characters of rheumatic fever. But we must now enter upon some further particulars in reference to each of the points which we have mentioned.

A. *Articular Affections in Acute Rheumatism.*

The characteristics of these local lesions are already known to you ; I shall therefore confine myself to making clear the analogies and differences which connect them with, or distinguish them from, the articular lesions of gout. We shall study them separately at first, and then contemplate them as a whole.

1. *Pain.* It occurs especially at night; its intensity is less than in gout, but it is accompanied by muscular cramps as in the latter affection.

2. *Swelling.* It takes place specially in joints near the surface : it may be situated in the neighbouring connective tissue, or result from distension of the synovial cavity by a serous or sero-fibrinous secretion. Contrary to what happens in gout, it is accompanied by no local œdema which preserves the impress of the finger ; Garrod, however, has seen this symptom occur occasionally in cachectic patients. There is no desquamation when the swelling goes down.

3. *Redness.* It presents an erysipelatous appearance. It is less pronounced than in gout, and no ecchymoses are to be seen ; moreover, the veins are less prominent.

4. *Temperature.* According to Bouillaud and Neumann[*] there is sometimes a difference of one degree (C.) between the diseased spot and the surrounding parts which do not share in the heat resulting from the morbid action.

5. *Duration.* According to Budd each joint is inflamed for about from three to fifteen days.[†]

Let us now consider these articular affections in their mutual relations.

Generally several joints are attacked at the same time. Primary monarticular rheumatism probably does not exist; if it is secondary, the rheumatism is localised in a single joint. However, we will admit that rheumatism may be partial, that is to say, localised in a few joints, as opposed to that which is general or polyarticular. You know that in acute gout it is rare to find the affection general from the first.

---

[*] Neumann, *Ergebniss und Studien aus der medicinischen Klinik zu Bonn*, Leipzig, 1860, p. 33.

[†] Tweedie's *Library of Medicine*, art. "Rheumatism," vol. v., p. 191.

As to the mode of invasion, there are characters which distinguish rheumatism from gout very accurately. According to the researches of Prof. Monneret,* if rheumatism is monarticular, it hardly ever affects the great toe ; moreover, the disease attacks simultaneously the upper and lower limbs. In the majority of cases the knee, the wrist, and the instep are the seats of election. It is but rarely that the little joints are attacked, except in subacute rheumatism.

The tibio-tarsal joint is most frequently the first attacked, according to Budd and Prof. Monneret.

We often see rheumatic arthritis develop symmetrically on the two sides, but too much importance must not be attached to this phenomenon, which is common to nearly all the diathetic affections of joints.

Sometimes the sudden disappearance of the articular symptoms coincides with the sudden development of a visceral affection. But this is rather the exception than the rule ; at any rate there is no experimental proof of a *retrocession* of the disease, provoked by external influences, as we have seen to be the case in gout.

Lastly, one of the most characteristic clinical features of this affection is its excessive versatility, which allows it to leap from one joint to another, and to change its locality many times in the course of the disease.

B. *The general state in Acute Articular Rheumatism.*

The essential phenomenon here is *fever ;* for the febrile reaction, marked by a more or less pronounced elevation of the general temperature, is never completely wanting in the course of acute articular rheumatism.

The heat of the central parts may exceed 40° C., but it generally remains between 39° C. and 40° C. (102·2° F. and 104° F.) according to Wunderlich, Hardy, and Sydney Ringer.†

The febrile action assumes the continued type, with exacerbations and remissions which are generally very pronounced. The thermometric curves are very irregular, and, according to Wunderlich, cannot furnish any precise data relative to the pro-

---

* Monneret, *Thèse de concours pour le professorat,* 1851, p. 51.

† Aitken, *Science and Practice of Medicine,* vol. ii.—Russell Reynolds, *A System of Medicine,* vol. i., p. 896.

gress of the disease; however, the maximum of temperature is oftenest observed during the day, and the minimum at night.*

In brief, this affection proceeds in accordance with no regular type; its course has no definite cycle; there are no phases succeeding one another at definite periods, as in pneumonia and the eruptive fevers; we do not find any violent rigor marking its onset, and the disease generally becomes established by a gradual increase in the severity of the symptoms; an imperceptible transition conducts us from its initial period to its acme and its decline. The termination does not come about abruptly or by rapid defervescence; it takes place slowly and progressively, save in certain exceptional cases in which the temperature falls below the normal level.† Lastly, relapses are here rather the rule than the exception.

There remains one question to discuss, which has received various answers from authors. Is the fever dependent on the arthritis? is it, on the contrary, independent of any local lesion?

It is certain that the fever sometimes persists when all arthritis has disappeared; but in such a case it is almost always kept up by some latent visceral affection, for example endocarditis or pericarditis.

The fever may also precede the articular symptoms; but here again it is often (we do not say always) caused by one of those visceral lesions which sometimes precede the articular manifestations of rheumatism.

It is true that the febrile action is often of great intensity when the number of diseased joints is inconsiderable. There is therefore some unknown element which eludes us, and which seems almost to justify the opinion of Graves, Todd, and Fuller, according to whom the fever in rheumatism is *primary* and not *consecutive*.

We have contemplated rheumatic fever as a whole. Let us now proceed to study the details, and consider the accessory phenomena of the febrile state.

The *pulse*, the frequency of which according to Louis‡ does

---

* Wunderlich, *Pathol. und Therap.*, vol. iv., p. 621.

† Hardy, *Thèses de Paris*, 1859.

‡ Louis, *Recherches anatomiques, pathologiques, et therapeutiques sur la fièvre typhoïde*, 1841, vol. i., p. 433.

not exceed 90 or 100 beats per minute, offers special characters which are not met with to the same degree in other febrile maladies. According to Monneret, Todd, and Fuller,* the artery feels voluminous, as in certain cases of anæmia. The sphygmographic tracings explain this particular sensation wonderfully; they denote an enormous amplitude ;† a tolerably pronounced dicrotism, in fact a marked resemblance to the pulse of aortic incompetency. Of course if a cardiac affection supervenes, these characters are greatly modified.

The *secretions* in acute rheumatism deserve special attention. I shall put first in importance the *sweat*, which is generally remarkably abundant and of extreme acidity, especially in the neighbourhood of the affected joints.‡ There are sudamina containing fluid which is distinctly acid in reaction ; and this character of rheumatic sweat long resists alkaline treatment even in large doses. No doubt the sour odour exhaled from rheumatic patients is to be attributed to this acid secretion. But we cannot say exactly what the chemical principle is which determines this reaction ; it has been attributed to lactic acid, but without sufficient proof. Simon has proved that in the course of acute articular rheumatism acetic acid exists in sweat, which is not the case, according to him, in the normal state ; but Schottin has made it clear that, even in a state of health, sweat contains not only acetic acid but also butyric and formic acids.§

The *saliva* is acid in acute rheumatism according to Fuller ;‖ moreover, all the fluids of the system are, according to this author, remarkable for decided acidity ; and the serum secreted into the pericardium and the joints offers the same reaction. I have sometimes noticed this last phenomenon, but only in some exceptional cases ; it occurs besides in gout. Let us add further, that the intra-articular fluid, though sometimes acid, is also sometimes alkaline.

The state of the *urine* must engage our special attention, for we shall find in this respect a marked difference between rheumatism and gout. On inspection it appears high-coloured and

---

* Monneret, loc. cit., p. 53.
† Marey, *Physiologie médicale de la circulation du sang*, p. 545.
‡ Williams, *Principles of Medicine*, 3rd ed., London, 1856, p. 194.
§ Donders, *Physiologie*, vol. i., p. 450.
‖ Fuller, op. cit., p. 517.

scanty; on cooling it furnishes abundant uratic deposits of a brick-red colour.

Analysis discloses a notable diminution of the watery constituent, which is explained by the profuse perspiration, and also an increase of the chief solids. A particularly large proportion of urea and colouring matter is found; this last phenomenon is probably connected with a more considerable destruction of blood disks than occurs in any other inflammatory disease.

The proportion of uric acid is increased : it is found in the proportion of ·85 gram p. litre, according to Parkes;* ·75 gram, according to Garrod. This is another contrast with gout.

The proportion of chlorides is diminished, but less so than in pneumonia. Lastly, the urine is very acid ; nothing, however, shows that this depends on the presence of an excess of lactic acid.

The last characteristic of the general state in acute rheumatism to be referred to, is the profound anæmia which develops a few days after the onset, even in cases in which recourse has not been had to the antiphlogistic method. There is no doubt an analogous condition in inflammatory diseases, owing to the destruction of blood corpuscles, but it is much less in degree. Todd, O'Ferral, and Fuller in England ; Canstatt in Germany ; Monneret and Piorry in France, have laid much stress on this point. It happens quite differently in acute gout, and we cannot help seeing in this one more difference between them.

II. *Comparison between Acute Rheumatism, Gout, and Subacute Rheumatism.*

After this concise account of acute articular rheumatism we are in a position to bring into prominence the differences and analogies which it presents in relation to gout and subacute rheumatism.

1. With regard to *acute gout* we find but one analogy to point out; this is the irregular and paroxysmal course of the disease. In everything else we find only differences.

Thus in gout the temperature is less elevated (as far as can be stated in the present state of science), the fever is less intense ;

* Parkes, *On Urine*, London, 1860, p. 286.

it seems completely dependent on the number of joints affected, and only reaches a really high point when the gout is general.

The pulse has not the special feature which we found it present in rheumatism.

The perspiration is less profuse and has not the acidity which I pointed out in rheumatic sweat.

The state of the urine differs from that which I have shown to be present in rheumatism, although the external appearance may be the same ; for when we proceed to analyse the urine in gout, far from finding an increase of uric acid, we find rather a diminution of it.

Lastly, in acute gout anæmia never becomes pronounced from the commencement.

2. *Subacute* articular rheumatism still presents us with the characters of the acute state; but the febrile action is less intense, as well as the phenomena accompanying it; the anæmia, however, is quite as pronounced ; on the other hand, the articular affections are more persistent, a character contrasting with the extreme mobility of the local symptoms in the acute form. Lastly, there is a difference between these two forms of the disease in regard to duration ; according to Macleod this is from six weeks to two months in subacute rheumatism; in acute rheumatism it has been variously estimated, but is always much less than that which I have just mentioned; thus it lasts from one to two weeks according to Prof. Bouillaud, about three weeks according to Legroux, four weeks according to Chomel and Requin ; according to Lebert it varies with the treatment employed, and may last as long as from four to five weeks.

III. *Pathology of the Blood in Acute and Subacute Articular Rheumatism.*

The composition of the blood in articular rheumatism differs considerably from that which is found in acute gout, and that no doubt is one of the most important differences which distinguish these two diseases.

You know that the blood-clot in acute rheumatism is firm and retracted, and that it resembles the buffy clot of pleurisy *as an egg resembles an egg*, to quote Sydenham's rather familiar expression.

M

The researches of Nasse, Simon, Andral and Gavarret, Becquerel, and Rodier, have shown us the reason of this phenomenon ; they have found that there is a considerable increase in the proportion of fibrin, which may rise to 7 or 8 p. mil. instead of 3 p. mil., which is the normal amount. There is at the same time a considerable increase in the proportion of red disks. In this respect the composition of the blood in acute articular rheumatism may be taken as the type of inflammatory blood, and differs essentially from its composition in gout.

I must add that in rheumatism the blood-serum is alkaline, the proportion of urea is normal, and no excess of uric acid is met with. It would be impossible to exaggerate the importance of this fact, which is now beyond dispute.

But in acute articular rheumatism does not the blood possess some special characters which belong to it alone ? Does it not contain some pathological product, some substance foreign to its normal constitution, which would explain why acute articular rheumatism differs in so many respects from ordinary inflammatory diseases, which, however, induce modifications of the same kind in the composition of the blood ?

Numerous analogies argue in favour of this hypothesis, but as yet they are based on no positive fact.

In the last century, Van Swieten, Baynard,[*] and several other physicians supposed rheumatism to depend upon a peculiar acidity of the blood, and a retention of the acids and salts which the kidneys ought to eliminate. Recently an hypothesis has been formulated in England more in harmony with the facts of modern chemistry. It is supposed that lactic acid, a normal product of the disintegration of fibrous tissues, is formed in excess, and gives rise to all the phenomena which I have just described. This opinion has been supported by Prout, Williams, Todd, and Fuller ; but it rests on no solid foundation. Richardson, however, having injected lactic acid into the veins of dogs, found articular lesions and affections of the heart in these animals. But his experiments have been repeated in Germany, and it has been shown that, in the canine species, cardiac affections are exceedingly frequent apart from any artificial intervention. It seems clearly shown, then, that the endocardial lesions existed beforehand ; and as to the articular lesions, it

* Baynard, Phil. Trans. (abridged), vol. iii., p. 265.

must be remembered that the joints are affected in a great many different forms of poisoning.

One circumstance deserves mention before terminating this rapid description. *Inopexia*—the excessive coagulability of fibrin independently of its excessive amount—occurs to an extreme degree in acute articular rheumatism : hence the great frequency of thromboses in the blood-vessels and of fibrinous vegetations in the heart.

On the contrary, in several grave cases, a quite different condition has been observed. At the autopsy the blood is then found liquid and black ;* it does not redden on contact with the air, and it is especially under these circumstances that the fluid exuded into the serous cavities has a very acid reaction, as I have several times found to be the case.

Remember, lastly, that in certain patients rheumatism appears associated with the hemorrhagic diathesis.

To sum up ; I think we have proved that articular rheumatism, in all the varied forms which it may assume, constitutes one and the same morbid species, essentially distinct from gout. Acute rheumatism, chronic rheumatism, and subacute rheumatism, which forms a transition between the two extreme types, are at bottom only one and the same disease. We have tried to prove this by studying the articular lesions and the general characters of the malady ; we shall find a fresh proof of it in a study of the *visceral lesions*, a consideration of which we shall now enter upon.

* Vogel, Virchow's *Handbuch der spec. Pathologie und Therapie*, vol. i., p. 479.

M 2

LECTURE XIV.

VISCERAL AFFECTIONS IN ACUTE AND CHRONIC ARTICULAR RHEUMATISM.

SUMMARY.—Comparison between the visceral affections of gout and those of acute or chronic rheumatism.—Late development of visceral lesions in gout; early development of these affections in acute rheumatism.—These lesions only appear at a later period in chronic rheumatism.—Difference in the nature of the visceral lesions in rheumatism and gout.—Affections of the heart in rheumatism.—Rheumatic pericarditis.—Rheumatic endocarditis.—Modifications made in our knowledge of this disease by the progress of modern histology.—Structure of the lining membrane of the heart.—Inflammatory lesions of the endocardium.—They occur principally on the valves.—Description of this morbid process.—Swelling of the endocardium; vascularisation of this membrane.—Consequences of this pathological state.—Capillary embolism.—Disturbances of the circulation.—Typhoid state.—Chronic stage of the disease.—Multiple affections, the result of these lesions.—Ischæmia; local gangrene.—Ecchymotic spots.—Cerebral softening.—Deposits of fibrin in spleen, liver, kidneys.—Various complications of acute articular rheumatism.—The cardiac lesions may occur also in subacute and chronic rheumatism.—Lesions of the respiratory system.—Pleurisy, pneumonia, pulmonary congestion.—Asthma, emphysema.—Pulmonary phthisis.—Lesions of the urinary system.—Nephritis.—Albuminuria.—Cystitis.—Lesions of the nervous system.—Cerebral affections.—Affections of the cord.—Various other non-articular lesions.—Muscular pains.—Neuralgia.—Disorders of the visual organs.—Cutaneous affections : eczema ; psoriasis ; prurigo ; lichen, etc.

GENTLEMEN, — The non-articular affections in rheumatism will occupy our attention to-day. We shall first endeavour to compare them with the changes caused by gout in our internal organs; we shall then have to inquire whether the visceral lesions of acute rheumatism are also to be found with the same characters in the chronic forms of the disease.

During the course of attacks of acute gout purely functional troubles are long the only indication of the viscera being implicated; these leave behind them no material modifications; and it is only when the incessant return of the attacks begins to give a chronic form to the disease, that we find permanent alterations appearing, which day by day become more serious.

In articular rheumatism it may be said that events take an almost opposite course. Indeed, one of the chief characters of this affection (at least in its acute form) is the development from the beginning of certain visceral lesions (endocarditis, pericarditis, etc.), which often appear directly after the first attack, and scarcely wait until the disease has passed through its initial stage. It is here no longer a question of mere functional disturbances, but of permanent lesions which modify the structure of the organs, and almost always leave behind them indelible traces of their existence.

Primarily chronic rheumatism differs in this respect from the acute form. The existence of these visceral lesions in the chronic form is so rare as to have been called in question by several authors ; and it may be stated that the more tendency the disease has to assume a chronic form, the rarer is it to see such lesions develop during its course.

Another fact which it is important to make clear is that the visceral affections of rheumatism do not present any but the roughest analogy to those of gout ; they are at bottom essentially different lesions.

Thus the cardiac disorders which may supervene in gout are purely functional in their origin, and affect the muscular substance when they give rise to permanent lesions ; fatty degeneration is what we then observe.

In acute rheumatism, on the contrary, the cardiac affection appears in the form of inflammatory lesions, affecting the endocardium and pericardium, and only secondarily attacking the muscular tissue of the organ. The structural changes which these lesions so often leave behind them are the consequence of this inflammatory action. It is a fact that in nearly half the cases of permanent lesions of the auriculo-ventricular valves, these originate in acute articular rheumatism.

We shall dwell more especially in the course of this study on these cardiac affections, which form almost an integral part of acute articular rheumatism. They may be regarded as one of the characteristic features of the disease ; their frequency indeed is here so great that when we find acute endocarditis or pericarditis coexisting with an articular affection which is in other respects ill-defined, we are usually justified in referring this group of phenomena to rheumatism.

Therefore to these cardiac lesions, a knowledge of which is of such great importance, we shall chiefly devote our attention. The other visceral affections of rheumatism have less interest from our special point of view ; we shall, however, say a few words about them.

I. *Endocarditis and Pericarditis in Acute Articular Rheumatism.*

Rheumatic pericarditis is an affection which has long been known ; we may truly say that all the features of its history are now familiar to us. We know that there is an inflammation of the serous membrane covering the heart, and that this inflammation generally causes the secretion of a sero-fibrinous exudation, which in some exceptional cases may assume a hemorrhagic or purulent character.

I shall mention further on the group of symptoms which indicate its existence, and the peculiar circumstances in which it arises.

Our knowledge of endocarditis, on the other hand, has been remarkably modified by the progress of histological studies, and the endocarditis of rheumatism has been a large sharer in this change.

Not long ago the endocardium was considered to be a serous membrane, and it was supposed that its lesions would be found to present the characters of serous inflammations. You may know that in his *polypous carditis*, Kreysig had spoken of the secretion of plastic lymph as one of the chief characteristics of the disease, and you may know also that in his very remarkable studies on endocarditis, Prof. Bouillaud long insisted on the bright red colour which the lining membrane of the heart presents.

We now know that this view was wanting in exactitude in certain respects. The structure of the endocardium is not the same as that of serous membranes, and it cannot become inflamed in the same manner. But it is exaggeration in an opposite direction to deny that endocarditis occurs. The attempt has been made to refer all the lesions of this disease to simple fibrinous deposits (Simon). This is the excessive development of an idea once put forward by Laennec.

There is a certain amount of truth in both opinions. Endocarditis does occur, the lining membrane of the heart may become inflamed ; but here there could be no question of plastic exudation. On the other hand, the formation of clots in the interior of the cardiac cavities plays an important part in this disease ; but this phenomenon is always secondary and can never claim the first place.

Let us first examine the structure of the lining membrane of the heart; we shall then be in a better position to understand the alterations of which it may become the seat.

The endocardium is essentially composed of a very thin layer of connective tissue, containing some elastic fibres, and covered by pavement epithelium. According to Luschka the endocardium is a continuation of all the coats of the vessels ; but according to most authors it is continuous only with their lining-membrane.

The endocardium has no vessels of its own ; but on account of its slight thickness, the subjacent capillaries of the cardiac wall are in very close relation to it. It is quite different in the situation of the valves. Here the lining-membrane is thicker ; some vessels, according to Luschka, are to be found between the two layers of the mitral valve ; but in the sigmoid valves they never exist in the normal state.

Now it is precisely on the valves, that is, on the thickest part of the endocardium, and that most distant from the vessels, where the inflammatory lesions are usually situated ; they commence, moreover, on the external surface.

In what, then, does the morbid process consist ?

In the acute state, the morbid action commences by the swelling of the diseased part; little pimples form, made up of the pre-existent elements, the size of which is perceptibly increased, and of a new growth of nuclei and embryonic cells ; the whole pimple is soaked with a liquid, which has a reaction like that of mucus. This is the first stage of the disease.

In the second stage the pimples have sometimes acquired a permanent organisation : at other times their extremities are ulcerated, the consequence of a granular degeneration, which must not be confounded with the fatty change. These little ulcers have vertical margins.

Later on the swollen spot becomes covered with a layer of fibrin, differing in thickness according to the case. You know that a tendency to the coagulation of fibrin is an habitual result of rheumatism, as well as of the puerperal state and certain peculiar cachexias.

The vegetations on the valvular endocardium, then, are a

consequence of inflammation of the tissues themselves, and of the consecutive deposit of a fibrinous layer.

But while this action is going on, the vessels are undergoing a new development. In the mitral valve, where they existed before, they become more apparent; in the sigmoid valves they are formed anew; or at least the neighbouring capillaries send prolongations into the non-vascular parts, as happens in the cornea when it is inflamed ; and thus it is that vascular networks are to be found round the lesions which have invaded the orifices of the heart.*

The results of this pathological state it is important to study. Let us first see what are its immediate consequences.

Sometimes matters remain the same ; there are then no disturbances of circulation. Sometimes the fibrinous deposit softens, breaks into detritus, and gives origin to capillary emboli. This is an essentially clinical aspect of the question, and a quite new one, although the contrary has been stated. Sometimes, lastly, the ulceration goes on deepening; then perforations form in the valves, and give rise to the most varied circulatory troubles ; the meeting of several openings may lead to a detachment of a fragment of the valve and give rise to a more or less bulky embolon. Do not forget that valvular aneurisms are sometimes formed, and these may occur either in the sigmoid or the mitral.

In some cases, as a result of unknown causes, the process is different : pus may form—a rare event ; but more often we find that deleterious substances have been formed, which then proceed to infect the mass of the blood, thus giving rise to typhoid symptoms. This is usually spoken of as ulcerative endocarditis ; but speaking correctly, the ulcerative form of endocarditis is not necessarily accompanied by septicæmia.

The ulterior consequences of endocarditis are met with in the chronic stage of the disease. The inflammatory action goes on, while changing its character; the whole valve becomes indurated, and this causes it to become puckered up, and, as a consequence, incompetence results ; at other times adhesions are formed between the diseased valve and the circumference of the orifice, a condition which gives rise sometimes to incompetence, sometimes, on the contrary, to obstruction.

* Ball, *Du rhumatisme viscéral, Thèse de concours pour l'aggrégation,* 1866, p. 28.

Sometimes compensatory changes occur, as has been well shown by Jacks. The shortening of one of the sigmoid valves, for example, leaves a gap, which is sometimes found filled up by the lengthening of the two others ; and the mechanical part of the affection may be cured in this way. I have myself met with evident examples of this in the cadaver.

Such are the elementary lesions of endocarditis. We shall not dwell in this place on their appearance to the naked eye. You know that they occupy in preference the left side of the heart, and the auriculo-ventricular orifice ; that on the mitral valve they affect especially the auricular surface and the neighbouring parts ; and that on the sigmoid valves they readily assume the form of a wreath of vegetations. But what it is now of importance to make clear is that there often exist no disturbances of the circulation. Often there is only a formation of mere pimples, which during life give rise to no appreciable functional trouble, and are only recognised at the autopsy.* This is the case much more frequently than is supposed; and by taking account of these rudimentary lesions we increase very largely the number of times in which affections of the heart and rheumatism coexist. It is especially in the chronic form that it is important to take account of this point, as we shall see later on.

But I first wish to say a word about those multiple affections which originate in endocarditis ; this is one of the most curious aspects of the question, and one of the most recent conquests of science.

At the present day we know that moveable bodies may become detached from the diseased orifices, either at the expense of the fibrinous deposits, or of the valves themselves ; and that, dropped into the current of the circulation, they proceed to set up various symptoms at a distance.

We must here distinguish between the phenomena caused by the displacement of bulky concretions, and those which result from the transportation of almost molecular fragments.

1. The emboli that are strictly *arterial* may obstruct the circulation in vessels of the first order ; the femoral and even the external iliac have been noticed to become suddenly impervious to the blood-current, on account of the presence of an immense clot from the heart.

* Charcot, *Comptes rendus de la Société de Biologie*, 3e série, 1862, vol. iii., p. 269.

When the arteries of the limbs are thus obliterated, a disturbance of the circulation is caused, which usually ends in gangrene. Watson, Tufnell, and several other authors, have reported examples of this in rheumatic endocarditis.*

2. *Capillary* embolism, which is infinitely more frequent, may affect almost any organ and give rise to the most varied lesions.

A. When the capillaries of the skin are obliterated we find more or less considerable ecchymotic spots produced.

B. When the encephalic vessels are affected, softening, sometimes red, sometimes white, ensues, and this is one of the commonest causes of hemiplegia in people who have not yet reached old age. When the obliterated artery is one of considerable calibre, there sometimes occurs instantaneous hemiplegia; consequent softening almost always takes place. An extremely remarkable case of this kind was reported by Kirkes.

We sometimes find that similar symptoms arise, although the chief arteries of the brain are found quite permeable after death. At first we notice the appearance of all the symptoms of softening, which follow their ordinary course; but after death no lesion is discovered in the chief vascular channels. There are two explanations of this anomalous condition. Actual obliteration of vessels of considerable calibre may have taken place; but the clot becoming absorbed, the artery has become permeable again, although the consequent softening has been persistent. On the other hand, we may suppose that very small vessels having been obliterated, a cerebral affection arose, without any obstacle existing in the main channels of the encephalic circulation.

I have myself witnessed a case of this kind. The patient, a woman, was first admitted into a ward of Trousseau's, and this eminent clinicist supposed that there was a cerebral embolism, consequent on a valvular lesion of the heart. This woman afterwards dying under my care at the Salpêtrière, I demonstrated at the autopsy that there had been a former endocarditis, with vegetations on the mitral valve, but I found no obliteration of the arteries at the base.† Cases of this kind may be explained by absorption of the thrombus; this is sometimes complete at

* Watson, *Principles and Practice of Physic*, vol. ii., p. 314, 4th ed.—Tufnell, *Dublin Quarterly Journal*, vol. xv., p. 371.—Goodfellow, *Trans. of the Med. Chir. Soc. of London*, vol. xxviii., 2nd series, 1862.

† Trousseau, *Clinique méd. de l'Hôtel-Dieu*, vol. ii., p. 587.—Bouchard, *Comptes rendus de la Soc. de Biol.*, 1864, p. 111.

the time of the autopsy, but in other cases one still finds vestiges of the obstructing clot, thus enabling one in some degree to determine the nature of the case.

Lesions of this kind are so frequent as a sequence of rheumatic heart disease, that Lancereaux in his thesis attributes more than half the pathological incidents he has collected to this cause.*

C. The spleen very often becomes the seat of capillary embolism, which gives rise to wedge-shaped infarcts, with the apex directed towards the hilus, thus corresponding with the well-known mode of distribution of the splenic vessels.

I have myself had the opportunity of observing an interesting case in which this lesion occurred as the sequel to a rheumatic affection of the heart. The patient was a man of 24, who was affected with articular rheumatism, at first acute, then chronic. During life he had a rough double murmur at the apex. He often complained of acute pain in the region of the spleen, and this organ had acquired considerable size; the man died with the usual symptoms of heart disease.

At the autopsy fibrinous vegetations were found on the mitral and sigmoid valves, as well as two fibrinous deposits in the spleen, one of which was of considerable size, the other a little smaller.

D. The kidneys may also be affected with similar lesions. Rayer, without knowing their origin, has described them very well under the name of *rheumatic nephritis*. Figs. 2, 5, 6, 7, of plate F in the Atlas of the " Traité des Maladies des reins " are examples of rheumatic nephritis in patients suffering from heart disease.

Capillary emboli in the kidney give rise to morbid changes which have been very well described in the thesis of Dr. Herrmann.† They chiefly consist of fatty degeneration which develops round the injured spot, and this is after a while followed by a depressed cicatrix.

E. The liver itself is not free from these occurrences; but they only happen rarely in this situation.

F. To these lesions, dependent on arterial or capillary emboli, those septicæmic phenomena must be added, which sometimes

---

* *De la thrombose et de l'embolie cérébrales* (Thèses de Paris, 1862).

† *Des lésions viscérales suites d'embolie* (Thèse de Strasbourg, 1854).

appear as a sequence of rheumatic heart disease. Then we see the phenomena of the *typhoid state*, of *grave icterus*, and of *symptomatic intermittent fever* supervening and becoming associated with the symptoms of acute articular rheumatism.*

II. *Endocarditis and Pericarditis in Subacute and Chronic Articular Rheumatism.*

Gentlemen, after having thus traced the history of endocarditis and pericarditis in acute rheumatism, I shall try to prove to you that these complications are not exclusively peculiar to this form of the disease.

In the first place, they are met with pretty frequently in subacute rheumatism, in spite of the celebrated law of Prof. Bouillaud—a rigorous, tyrannical law, if I may so express myself.

No doubt endocarditis and pericarditis are more frequent in acute polyarticular rheumatism. Valleix, Latham, Bamberger, and Fuller agree in this matter with the learned French clinicist.

Cardiac complications, however, are met with pretty often where the affected joints are few, and where the febrile action is not intense. West has shown this in the case of children; Walshe, Ormerod, and Garrod in adults. If I may here mention my own experience, I have seen several cases of subacute rheumatism, in which an autopsy has been made, accompanied by affections of the heart. One of these cases is recorded in Dr. Ball's thesis.†

But the thing is to prove that these lesions may occur in really chronic rheumatism, in nodular rheumatism.

1. It must be remembered that rheumatic *endocarditis* is an affection very often latent during life, but it almost always leaves traces behind it which are recognisable after death. So we must not always expect to meet with manifest murmurs in patients attacked with chronic rheumatism; but morbid anatomy enables us to demonstrate in this matter a relationship between the

---

* When the right side of the heart is the starting-point of migratory clots, pulmonary embolism may occur and sometimes determine almost immediate death. A case of this kind has been reported by Goddard-Rogers. It was one of acute articular rheumatism with endocarditis, in which the patient was suddenly seized on the fifteenth day with a fit of orthopnœa, ending in death after ten minutes. At the autopsy the pulmonary artery was found obliterated by a bulky clot from the right ventricle. *Lancet*, p. 19, 1865.

† *Du rhumatisme viscéral*, p. 61.

acute and chronic forms of articular rheumatism, proving once again that it is one and the same disease, in spite of the diversity of its morbid manifestations.

Cardiac lesions are found pretty frequently in nodular rheumatism. A case of this kind was mentioned by Romberg in 1846.* Two others are to be found recorded in Trastour's thesis and in my own, out of a total of 41 observations. Since this time, attention having been aroused on this point, cases have multiplied. Some years ago in a clinical lecture Beau showed in a young girl the coexistence of nodular arthritis and aortic stenosis ;† and Dr. Ollivier has observed in the clinic of Prof. Grisolle the case of a man, 23 years of age, in whom the characteristic deformities of nodular rheumatism were present, and in whom the signs of a lesion of the aortic valves were found to exist.

There has generally been in these cases at a former period an attack of acute rheumatism ; but I have collected a considerable number of cases in which endocarditis has developed in chronic rheumatics without the disease having ever assumed an acute form. Two of these are recorded in Dr. Ball's thesis.‡

The first case was that of a woman of 60, a concierge, whose right hand presented the characteristic deformities of chronic rheumatism. She attributed this disease to the dampness of the room in which she had long lived.

When first admitted into the infirmary for right hemiplegia she showed at first no sign of heart disease, and returned to her sleeping-room after treatment for two months.

But on entering the infirmary a second time she showed evident signs of heart disease. The symptoms of this affection becoming rapidly aggravated, death was not long delayed.

At the autopsy was found *general adhesion of the pericardium to the heart, this condition being evidently of recent origin,* for the pericardium could be easily detached from the subjacent tissues. The heart had acquired an enormous size ; *vegetations arranged in wreaths were found on the aortic valves and on the mitral, the ventricular surface of which presented very remarkable vascularity.*

---

* *Klinische Ergebnisse,* Berlin, 1846. An analogous case had been already mentioned by Todd in 1843.

† *Gazette des Hôpitaux,* 19th July, 1864.   ‡ Op. cit., p. 121, et seq.

In the second case, the patient, a woman of 84, died in the infirmary of the Salpêtrière of cancer of the liver and stomach. In her case the lesions of dry arthritis were found in the shoulders, elbows, and knees. The heart was flabby, large, and loaded with fat. *On the aortic valves there were manifest traces of former endocarditis.*

It seems, therefore, evident to me, considering the cases which I have just related, that one may meet with organic lesions of the heart in the case of primarily chronic rheumatism.

2. *Pericarditis* probably occurs frequently in chronic rheumatism, for in nine autopsies which I performed in 1863 with Dr. Cornil,* I met with it four times. We have, moreover, at the present time a case of this kind under observation, and Dr. Mauriac has observed a very remarkable example at the *Hospice des Ménages.*

Here is the analysis of this interesting case.

In a woman, 71 years of age, long a sufferer from chronic articular rheumatism and pulmonary catarrh, rather intense dyspnœa suddenly appeared, with marked pain on the right side. Percussion disclosed slight increase of precordial dulness, and on auscultation a rough and grating pericardial friction sound was heard over the whole lower half of the sternum, where it masked the normal sounds of the heart. Under the influence of appropriate treatment, the patient recovered at the end of six weeks, after suffering from inflammatory symptoms in the joints already diseased.

This may be compared with another observation made by Martel at the hospital of St. Eugénie in Dr. Barthez' clinic. In a child of ten, attacked with chronic articular rheumatism, it was noticed that pericarditis appeared, characterised by friction sounds in the precordial region. This affection, however, did not last long. The rheumatism had undergone an exacerbation during the time that the pericarditis occurred. This child afterwards presented in a very high degree the characteristic lesions of nodular rheumatism.

Since the time when my attention was directed to this point, I have several times seen the appearance of pericarditis coincide with exacerbation of the joint affection in patients attacked with

* Cornil, *Mémoire sur les coïncidences pathologiques du rhumatisme articulaire chronique; Mem. de la Soc. de Biol.,* vol. iv., 4th series, 1865.

chronic rheumatism. The cases which I have just related are therefore in perfect harmony with my own observations.

To sum up; endocarditis and pericarditis undoubtedly occur in some cases of chronic articular rheumatism ; these affections present the same characters as in acute rheumatism. They appear especially when there is an exacerbation of the disease, and when there is some approach to the acute state. But these affections are generally less grave in character when they appear in the course of chronic rheumatism.

III. Other Non-articular Affections in Chronic Rheumatism.

Cardiac affections are not the only visceral manifestations of the rheumatic diathesis. It is important to remark here that the other ordinary complications of acute articular rheumatism are met with more rarely than the preceding ones in chronic rheumatism. But we shall soon perceive that, on the contrary, this latter form of the disease is compatible with certain complications almost completely unknown in acute articular rheumatism.

We shall pass in review one by one the chief functional systems of the body in reference to this point.

RESPIRATORY SYSTEM. *Pleurisy* is found in subacute and chronic rheumatism, but it is much less common than in the acute form.

Acute pneumonia is a frequent complication of acute rheumatism ; I have never met with it in the chronic form. I have certainly observed some cases of chronic pneumonia in rheumatics, but they have been cachectic patients.

Pulmonary congestion in rheumatism, a very formidable event, exposing the patients to almost immediate death, may be met with in chronic or subacute rheumatism. Dr. Ball has reported a very remarkable case of this kind in his thesis.*

Certain chest affections occur especially in the chronic and ill-defined forms of articular rheumatism. *Asthma* followed by *emphysema* is as common in this disease as in gout. Twice I have myself seen this complication present at the Salpêtrière.

The first case was that of a woman, sixty years old, who for twenty-five years had followed the occupation of laundress.

* Op. cit., p. 61.

The asthma dated from ten years back. At the commencement the attacks were infrequent and nocturnal; at the time when she was under our observation, they were so near together, so confluent, that the patient passed most of the day and night sitting up in bed, and breathing with great difficulty.

Sibilant rhonchi could generally be heard even from a distance. Auscultation showed great feebleness of the vesicular breath-sounds over the whole of both lungs. Expectoration was scanty.

This woman had never had general acute articular rheumatism, but on several occasions for seventeen years she had had arthritic pains accompanied by swelling of the joints. The articulations chiefly affected were the knees and shoulders, and the metacarpo-phalangeal joint of the right index-finger. There were no characteristic deformities, but the knees were the seat of well-marked creaking.*

The second case was that of a woman of 70, who, having long inhabited a very damp dwelling, seems to have had an attack of acute rheumatism; she remained in bed for six weeks, and two months after getting up could only walk with crutches. From that period there had been from time to time lumbago and transient articular pains. When 40 years of age she had a fresh attack of subacute articular rheumatism. A last attack of the same kind occurred four years before her admission into the hospital.

The menopause took place at 55, and it was not long after this period that she began to feel oppression in breathing. At the commencement of the pulmonary affection she was unable to lie down in bed for about two months. The attacks, always very lengthy, were at first tolerably far apart; then they came so closely after one another that after about three years the oppression was always present; it became much more intense during its course.

When the thoracic affection had reached this intensity the articular pains became slighter and more transient. There was no deformity of the joints, but creaking in the knees was very evident.

After a pretty long residence in the infirmary this woman at last died after considerable œdema of the lower limbs had appeared.

* Op. cit., p. 129.

The autopsy determined the presence of:

1. Hypertrophy of the *right* ventricle, without valvular lesions, and with no trace of old or recent pericarditis;

2. Articular lesions, almost exactly the same as those of acute rheumatism, but with no synovial secretion into the joint, and with a much more velvety condition of the ends of the bones;

3. In the lungs, pronounced congestion and evident hyperæmia of the bronchial mucous membrane; these tubes contained a considerable quantity of greenish and tenacious mucus.

This woman's son has long been asthmatic.*

It is clear that in this interesting case there was articular rheumatism, at first acute, then subacute, and finally chronic. The occurrence of asthma in this patient along with articular symptoms is a fact of capital importance from our present point of view.

You know that the occurrence of *laryngitis* in association with acute rheumatism has long been noticed. Garrod has also described a peculiar form of chronic laryngitis in nodular rheumatism.

Has *pulmonary phthisis* any connection with chronic rheumatism? This point is still doubtful, and we shall discuss it farther on.

URINARY ORGANS. In acute rheumatism there is a special form of *nephritis* which I have recently mentioned [embolic]. In gout morbid changes in the kidney are almost the rule. In chronic rheumatism *albuminous nephritis* is pretty common in advanced periods, to judge by the researches which Cornil and I carried out on this subject. These lesions, moreover, are always met with in patients who are profoundly cachectic.

Affections of the *bladder* are not very common in acute rheumatism. You must not confound with vesical gout that burning sensation which rheumatic patients experience on micturition, and which depends on the extreme concentration of the urine.

In chronic rheumatism, on the other hand, *cystitis* is pretty frequent, especially in patients long confined to bed.

NERVOUS SYSTEM. A. *Cerebral affections.* I have shown you the great analogies between disease of the brain in rheumatism and the cerebral symptoms of gout. *Rheumatic insanity,*

* This case is reported in Ball's thesis, but incompletely.

N

described by Burrows, Mesnet, and Griesinger, is pretty often found associated with the subacute forms of rheumatism.

Symptoms of this kind in chronic rheumatism have been pointed out by Fuller and by Vidal. But these occurrences are not common.

Migraine, so common between the attacks of gout, also occurs in chronic rheumatism.*

B. *Affections of the cord.* Chorea, the connection of which with acute rheumatism has been so often demonstrated, does not seem to occur in chronic rheumatism; at least I have never met with it in this affection.

But several diseases dependent on the spinal cord are met with in the chronic form of rheumatism.

Paralysis agitans, or at least *tremors,* may be associated with partial or general chronic rheumatism.

I have seen several cases of *locomotor ataxy* accompany dry arthritis and nodosities of joints. But as we now know that the articular symptoms of ataxic patients appear from the onset of the disease, it becomes extremely difficult to make out exactly the part which rheumatism plays.†

As to paraplegia, it is rarely associated with acute or subacute rheumatism, and great care must be taken not to confound the *articular pains* of spinal affections with rheumatism affecting the joints; for lesions of the spinal cord sometimes give rise to painful swelling of the joints, as Mitchell, Morehouse, Remak, and several other observers have noticed.

We have now to mention certain lesions, which, though not occurring in internal viscera, are nevertheless found away from the joints. We have seen that gout sometimes causes non-articular affections that are not visceral; the same thing happens in the acute and chronic forms of rheumatism.

Thus the *muscular pains* of gout, followed by cramps and retraction of the muscles (Guilbert), may also be found in acute rheumatism; but they are much more often found in chronic rheumatism.

Sciatic and trifacial neuralgia, which occur both in gout and rheumatism, belong especially to the subacute and slight forms of these two diseases. They may also be found in

---

* Consult on this point the thesis of Dr. Malherbe, Paris, 1866, p. 45.

† Charcot, *Archives de physiologie,* 1868, p. 162.

Heberden's rheumatism. Dr. Bastien has told me of a case of this kind.

The visual organs may be affected both in gout and rheumatism. I have already spoken of gouty *iritis* and *sclerotitis*. Ocular affections in acute rheumatism are uncommon ; but it is quite otherwise in subacute rheumatism (Garrod, Fuller) and chronic rheumatism (Cornil). It is generally a case of *iritis*, but obstinate *conjunctivitis* may also occur. Evident alternation is often observed between the ocular phenomena and the affection of the joints.

Lastly, *cutaneous affections*, so well known in gout and acute rheumatism, are also met with in chronic rheumatism. They are not common in the severe form of this disease, and are especially found in partial chronic rheumatism. Bazin pointed out, besides, that the cutaneous affections are most lasting and obstinate when the articular symptoms are least pronounced.

I have frequently found in chronic rheumatics the skin affections described by Bazin : *eczema, nummular psoriasis, lichen, arthritic prurigo*.

Lastly, I have seen *erysipelas* associated with nodular rheumatism.

At our next meeting we shall begin to study the symptomatology of chronic rheumatism.

LECTURE XV.

SYMPTOMATOLOGY OF PROGRESSIVE CHRONIC ARTICULAR RHEUMATISM.

SUMMARY.—Three fundamental types of chronic articular rheumatism.—They form in reality one and the same disease.—Progressive chronic articular rheumatism or nodular rheumatism.—Often confounded with gout, from which it differs essentially.—It specially affects the small joints.

Joint symptoms dependent on nodular rheumatism.—They often resemble those of acute rheumatism to begin with.—Spasmodic retraction of muscles.—Abnormal attitudes.—Permanent disorders.—Pain.—Creaking.—Deformity of bones.—Joints which are specially affected.—The hands are almost always first attacked.—Symmetrical invasion.—Mode of sequence of the articular inflammations.—General from the commencement in young subjects; progressive course in the old.—Consequent deformities of the limbs.—Two chief types; their varieties.

Course of the disease.—Secondary changes.—Atrophic form; œdematous form.—Loss of movement.

Deformity of lower limbs.—Of the vertebral column.—Deviation of the head.—General invasion of all the joints.

Mode of production of these lesions.—Various opinions.—Spasmodic contraction.—Accessory causes.

General symptoms.—Pathology of the blood.—General reaction.—Rapid evolution.—Slow evolution.

GENTLEMEN,—Hitherto we have regarded rheumatism from one point of view. The morbid anatomy of this affection has so far been the object of our studies; but it is time for us to reach the clinical stand-point, and for me to place before you the external symptoms which reveal the presence of this disease.

We have already dwelt on the need of recognising three fundamental types in the anatomy of the disease; it seems equally necessary to make this distinction in regard to the symptomatology. As you already know, we have to deal with nodular rheumatism, or progressive chronic articular rheumatism, partial chronic articular rheumatism, and Heberden's rheumatism.

These are not, however, three distinct diseases, but three specialised forms of one and the same disease. But it is no less indispensable to distinguish them, for the nature and relationship of the symptoms, the prognosis, and even the treatment, differ in each of these three types of chronic rheumatism.

We shall devote this lecture to the study of *progressive chronic articular rheumatism.*

From a medical point of view, nodular rheumatism is the most interesting of the three types which I have just pointed out. Often confounded with gout, it has sometimes been spoken of as *rheumatic gout* [*rheumatisme goutteux*]. I have already shown that a complete distinction must be made between them. Rheumatism must never be confounded with gout ; but all the varieties of articular rheumatism form part of one and the same pathological family, and must have a place to themselves.

Nodular rheumatism is to the other forms of chronic rheumatism what general acute rheumatism is to subacute or partial rheumatism. It affects especially the small joints, particularly those of the hands. It is a disease which too often shows itself beyond the resources of art, and which gives rise to deplorable infirmities.

I shall have in the first place to describe the articular symptoms which result from this disease, and then the symptoms dependent on the general condition of the system.

I. *Articular symptoms.* In the first stage, the articular symptoms, if we disregard their locality, differ in no way from those of acute and subacute rheumatism. You find in the affected joints the pain, redness, swelling, and heat which also characterise the acute disease ; only the symptoms are of less intensity and infinitely less changeable in their seat. Observe, also, that there is no œdema or desquamation, as in gout.

But a new phenomenón often becomes associated with this group of symptoms, even from the beginning, a phenomenon which in the acute form does not occur to nearly the same extent. I refer to spasmodic retraction of the muscles, which gives rise to peculiar and often permanent malpositions of the affected limbs.

In the second stage permanent lesions are produced. The enlargement has taken hold of the soft parts, producing sometimes hydarthrus, sometimes thickening of the synovial membrane and subsynovial tissue ; it has also spread to the hard structures, and it is then that we find foreign bodies developed, rarely in certain joints, more commonly in others ; bony nodes,

which deform the ends of the bones; and, lastly, partial dislocations of the articular extremities.

Pain, either spontaneous or when provoked, becomes permanently established at this time; it may affect the joint itself,
the shaft of the bones, or the neighbouring muscles in the form
of painful cramps.

You may now make out creaking, due to eburnation of the
osseous surfaces, provided the joint still retains some mobility;
but often also the rigidity, resulting from fibrous ankylosis, and
from retraction of the fibrous structures, makes itself perceptible
at this time. And you then notice the appearance of deformity
of the bones according to certain laws, certain rules, which we
shall study later on.

Let us see now which are the joints chiefly affected. We
have remarked that the small joints are the locality usually
chosen by the disease. The larger joints do not begin until
afterwards; and even when the invasion is general, the shoulder
and the hip are often respected. But we must here add that
the upper limbs are almost always the first to be attacked; it is
quite different in gout, in which the upper limbs are generally
only secondarily affected.

The mode of invasion of nodular rheumatism is somewhat
peculiar in character. Symmetry is here the rule, as Budd
pointed out; this observation has been confirmed by Romberg,
and I have myself verified its truth. You know that in gout
such a rule is by no means strictly followed. But note that in
some exceptional cases chronic rheumatism is asymmetrical,
and the rarity of the occurrence induces me to point it out.
In this case we see one side of the body only attacked at first,
and then at a later period the articular symptoms become general.

There is a no less marked distinction between gout and
nodular rheumatism with regard to the regions first affected.
In gout it is the great toe; in nodular rheumatism it is usually
the metacarpo-phalangeal joints of the index and middle fingers
which are first attacked; and this happens on both sides at
once, conformably to the law of symmetry which I have just
enunciated. Do not forget, however, that onset in a large joint
is much more common here than in gout, and that this fact
alone may often aid us in diagnosis. Here are some statistics
on this point.

Origin in—

1. Hands and feet only, small joints .... 25 times
  „ „ great toe .... 4 „
2. Hands and feet at the same time as a large joint.... 7 „
3. First a large joint; then the fingers...................... 9 „

Let us now inquire into the manner in which the joints succeed one another in becoming inflamed in nodular rheumatism. Usually the arthritis spreads from periphery to centre : the fingers are first affected; then the elbow; then the shoulder. But this regular succession is hardly ever found except in cases in which the disease develops slowly. In young patients, from 16 to 20, we often find, on the contrary, that the affection is general from the first; in subjects of greater age, from 40 to 60, it follows the progressive course I have just indicated. In the former case the development of the disease is rapid ; in the second, its course is slow. There is, however, no absolute rule in this respect, for often at the period of the menopause one sees the symptoms come on abruptly, and the affection assume from the first the appearance of an acute disease.

We have still to mention the deformities of the limbs which are the result of this morbid action. They are particularly pronounced in young patients, when there are spasmodic pains and well-marked retraction of the muscles. They are not due in these cases to actual deformity of the joints themselves, but to malpositions, resulting from changes of relative position between different parts of the limb.

These deformities are almost always the same ; they are in accordance with definite laws. Those of the upper limb may be referred to two chief types, with derivative secondary forms.

In both forms the hand is more or less decidedly pronated ; this is a character common to them all, but they differ in many other respects. I will give a concise account of them.

First type. This is the form most often met with. It is characterised by—

1. Flexion of the ungual phalanx on the second to an obtuse, right, or even acute, angle.

2. Extension of the second phalanx on the first.

3. Flexion of the first phalanx on the metacarpal bone.

4. Flexion, to a less obtuse angle, of the metacarpals and carpus on the bones of the fore-arm.

5. In a great many of the cases, inclination of all the fingers

towards the ulnar border of the hand, and a deviation in the opposite direction of the second phalanges on the first. The former of these two lesions is often one of the first deformities which mark the onset of the disease.

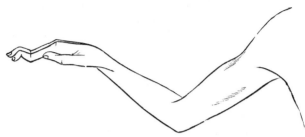

Fig. 1. FIRST TYPE.

There are two variations from this type. In the first, most of the characters which I have described are retained ; but the first and second phalanges are in the same axis, and form a single column.

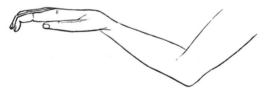

Fig. 2. FIRST VARIETY OF THE FIRST TYPE.

In the second there is no flexion of the ungual on the second phalanx, and the backs of the fingers appear excavated beyond the prominent heads of the metacarpal bones.

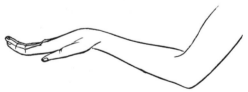

Fig. 3. SECOND VARIETY OF THE FIRST TYPE.

Second type. It is characterised by—

1. Extension of the ungual phalanx on the second.
2. Flexion of the second phalanx on the first.
3. Extension of the first phalanx on the metacarpal bone.

4. More or less marked flexion of the carpus on the bones of the forearm.

5. In some cases deviation of all the fingers towards the ulnar border of the hand.

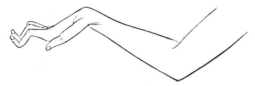

Fig. 4. SECOND TYPE.

This type, like the former, may present two variations.

In the first, there is flexion of all the segments of the hand on one another, so as to appear rolled up.

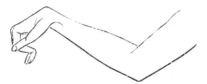

Fig. 5. FIRST VARIETY OF THE SECOND TYPE.

In the second the same characters are found, but there is besides extension of the second phalanx on the first.

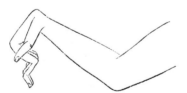

Fig. 6. SECOND VARIETY OF THE SECOND TYPE.

Hitherto we have only considered malpositions of the fingers ; but what about the thumb ?

Here, as elsewhere, the metacarpo-phalangeal joint is the one specially affected. The first phalanx of the thumb is usually in a flexed position, but occasionally it is extended.

The other joints of the upper limb take some share in these deformities.

Thus flexion of the elbow joint is more or less decided, sometimes extreme; extension is impossible. The forearm is pronated. There is more or less complete flexion of the carpus and metacarpus on the forearm, with projection of the ulna and radius. Lastly, the shoulder joint may be rigid and the upper limb fixed to the chest.

Let us now notice in what manner and in what order of succession the joints of the upper limb are attacked. Two groups of cases are found :—

A. In young patients the course of the disease is rapid, and the spasmodic contraction of the muscles being very pronounced, the deformities are very well-marked. The ends of the bones project in consequence of the partial dislocations which have taken place.

Thus in the hand, in the second type, considerable projection of the bones of the forearm behind the carpus takes place; subluxation of the first phalanges forwards and outwards on the heads of the metacarpals, which form a considerable prominence on the back of the hand; slight forward subluxation of the second phalanges on the first, the heads of the latter projecting on the posterior aspect of the fingers. Lastly, on account of the extreme flexion of the third phalanges on the second, the little condyles of the latter project backward.

It must be noted that the bony vegetations at the margin of the phalangeal joints do not always surround the ends of the bones; they are sometimes nodular, sometimes in the form of more or less elongated needles; in any case these osteophytes contribute little to the articular deformities.

Lastly, in the form which we are studying, there is more complete immobility, and hence greater rigidity of the ligaments and fibrous structures; fibrous ankylosis soon occurs, and there is rapid wasting of the parts. The term *nodular rheumatism* is scarcely applicable to cases of this kind

B. In older patients, the evolution of the disease is less rapid, and mobility of joints is in part retained. Thus the malpositions are less pronounced, while the size of the ends of the bones and of the osseous stalactites is greater.

There is, in fact, a certain contrast between the extent of the malpositions and the size of the osteophytes, as well as the extent of the deformity resulting from the latter.

When the disease has been protracted for a certain time, we

find morbid changes occurring which are a result of this state of things. Atrophy of the bones, atrophy of the muscles, and wasting of the soft parts are the usual symptoms in such a case.

But two quite opposite forms may be here distinguished. In the *atrophic* form (Vidal), induration of the skin, a sort of scleroderma, develops; the cutaneous covering is cold, pale, smooth, polished, and will not wrinkle.

In the other form we find the limb becoming *œdematous,* a condition simulating elephantiasis; this swelling is often accompanied by inflammatory symptoms; these occurrences are met with especially in the lower limbs.

However, the muscles of the upper limbs always undergo in the long run some amount of atrophy and fatty degeneration, as a consequence of the immobility of the parts.

The immediate consequence of these morbid changes is that the patients find they have lost the power of movement in the upper limbs, and are not able to do for themselves. It is at this stage that ingenious inventions appear upon the scene, such as those long forks, the size and form of which vary according to the degree of the patient's infirmity, but the object of which is always to enable them to lift food to the mouth by means of the more or less restricted movements which they have retained.

Notice in reference to this point, that the deformities of the right hand, which the patients still make use of, are not of so regular a type as those of the left hand, which is usually condemned to absolute immobility.

We shall now study the articular lesions which may occur in other parts of the skeleton.

The lower limbs are sometimes unaffected at a time when the hands have undergone very well-marked morbid changes. This state of things, however, is rare, and in general the lower limbs are symmetrically deformed and malposed, and become incapable of performing their usual movements.

The hip-joint usually retains its mobility, but this is not the case with the knees. Usually one finds the thigh flexed on the body, as well as flexion of the leg on the thigh. The chief deformities thence resulting are the following :—

The lower end of the femur projects in front of the head of the tibia.

The internal condyle of the femur becomes prominent.

The patella, thrown outward, rests on the outer condyle.

The head of the fibula projects externally.

It is rare, however, to meet with complete ankylosis of the knee-joint ; but osteophytes almost always develop there, and foreign bodies may be found in great abundance.

In the tibio-tarsal joint, on the contrary, ankylosis occurs very frequently. The foot may be kept abducted, and then rests on its inner edge in such a way as to simulate talipes valgus. It may, on the contrary, be in a position of adduction, giving rise to talipes equino-varus.

The big toe is turned outward, so as to cover the other digits.

Important deformities may also appear in connection with the cervical vertebræ. In several cases which I have myself observed at the Salpêtrière, I have seen the head inclined forward, and bent on the sternum ; the chin almost touched the chest. The movements of the head were much restricted, and gave rise to creaking sounds. In most of these patients the neck was widened posteriorly.

In the same manner most of the other joints may be attacked in the same individual, in cases of general chronic rheumatism ; and then the unfortunate patients are obliged to remain in bed for the rest of their lives. One sometimes finds them living more than twenty years in this dreadful condition.

But we have still to study the *mode of production* of these malpositions. Some physicians attribute them to an intentional arrangement (Beau) designed to lessen the intensity of the pain. According to Trastour they result from the attitude instinctively assumed by the patients.

For my part I am of a diametrically opposite opinion. In the majority of cases these deformities are the result of muscular contractions, spasmodic—almost convulsive. They are caused by a kind of reflex action, the starting-point of which is in the affected joints.

I will not dwell long on this subject. The arguments which I formerly enunciated, strengthened by those of M. Crocq, seem to me to have clearly demonstrated that the thing really happens in this way.

To this end we may adduce :

1. The actual form of the malpositions ; they are evidently attitudes forced upon the patient.

2. The resistance with which the patients oppose these spasmodic contractions, and which, though powerless to prevent them, is enough to prove that they are involuntary.

3. The general aspect of the malpositions, which exactly accords with the notion of muscular spasm; the deviations, in fact, form a group even when the joints involved are not all diseased.

4. Lastly, the presence of these same deformities in cases in which the joints are in no way affected; we can then only refer them to spasmodic contraction of the muscles. Thus in paralysis agitans, in congenital atrophy of the brain, in atrophy of the interosseous muscles, you may sometimes see the limbs assume shapes which are in every way like those observed in chronic rheumatism.

It would, however, be impossible to deny the existence of causes which are accessory to this fundamental cause of rheumatic deformities. The weight of the limbs, the more or less decided laxity of the ligaments, contribute in greater or less measure to the production of these malpositions; but these various conditions are insufficient to give rise to such effects without the co-operation of muscular contractions. Do we not see in some cases of hydrarthrosis extreme laxity of the ligaments of the knee, although no consequent deformities are produced? The limb remains, on the contrary, in a completely flaccid state.

The deformities which we have just described are not, as we have seen, exclusively peculiar to rheumatism. But the morbid changes in the joints, the creaking, the swelling of the joints, the fibrous ankylosis and consequent rigidity of the joints, and the symmetry of the lesions, distinguish the effects of chronic rheumatism from those which are produced by paralysis agitans and various other maladies. Gout, however, gives rise to the same spasmodic contractions, and the same malpositions. Guilbert laid stress on these muscular contractions in his *Traité de la Goutte*. But the presence of tophi, which usually accompany this kind of deformity in the gouty, is a really specific character. In rheumatism, we sometimes find that nodosities pierce the overlying skin; but the denuded portion is bone, and not a tophaceous deposit as in gout.

General symptoms : course of the disease. A. Examination of the state of the blood and the chemical study of the secretions have up to the present time given only negative results.

Musgrave says that the blood forms a buffy clot; this is decidedly the case in the acute forms. Uric acid has never been found in it. I have myself examined the blood in thirty-five cases of chronic articular rheumatism, but I have never found the least trace of this substance.

In a case reported by Böcker, chemical analysis gave very interesting results. This case is quoted as one of gout, but it would really be one of nodular rheumatism, for the ends of the bones were enlarged, a circumstance which does not happen in gout. The blood and the urine were examined, and in the latter a notable decrease of the normal proportion of phosphate of calcium was found; in the blood, on the other hand, there was four times as much calcic phosphate as in the normal state. The quantity of uric acid does not seem to have been increased; at least the author does not mention this point.

B. With regard to the general reaction and the course of the symptoms we may recognise two essentially distinct forms.

In chronic articular rheumatism of *rapid* evolution, we generally have to do with young subjects of from 16 to 30, or with women in a pregnant or puerperal condition; moral emotions and the action of sharp cold may also exert a certain influence.

In such cases we find a great many joints attacked at the same time. The muscular contractions are more pronounced; the pain is very intense; redness and swelling are pretty decided, and the disease is less variable than in the other type.

The general symptoms are those of acute or subacute articular rheumatism; there is marked elevation of the temperature, evident acceleration of the pulse, and profuse sweats. It is especially in affections of this kind that we meet with cardiac affections.

We might suppose that in these cases, the rheumatism, at first acute, has ultimately assumed a chronic form; this opinion, maintained by various authors, may be true in certain cases. Dr. Ball has shown me a patient in whom the metacarpo-phalangeal joints were affected during an attack of acute rheumatism; the result was a deviation of the fingers towards the ulnar border of the hand, and the man, who has now recovered, still retains this characteristic deformity of nodular rheumatism.

I fancy, however, that most frequently it is really chronic

rheumatism from the beginning, but that its course presents some of the characters of the acute state.

After a time the fever changes to a remittent type resembling hectic fever; after a while a series of exacerbations appears, each followed by a long interval of remission.

In cases of this kind the disease does not generally continue so long. After two, three, or four years, the joints almost entirely cease to be painful, and things remain as they are. Sometimes, indeed, deformities which have been produced, disappear. I have myself observed cases of this kind, but unfortunately they are very rare. Thus there was a woman attacked at first with subacute rheumatism of febrile type, affecting the shoulders and the metacarpo-phalangeal joints; spasmodic contraction of the fingers appeared three months after the onset of the disease; the consequent deformity lasted a whole year; then the patient recovered.

In chronic rheumatism of *slow* evolution, we generally have to do with older patients, people of from 40 to 60; one often meets with this affection about the period of the menopause. This form has been described by Geist* as senile gout. It is here especially that Haygarth's nodosities of the joints are met with.

The joints are attacked successively one by one; it is especially in these cases that you may study the mode of invasion of the disease. The pain is less acute; there is less redness, often indeed there is none. The *malpositions* caused by muscular contractions are less marked; on the contrary, the *deformities* of each joint are more decided.

As to the general condition, there is rarely any febrile reaction; only from time to time a slight touch of pyrexia is observed. Lastly, the prognosis is on the whole less grave than in the preceding case.

We have compared the two extreme forms in order to bring out their analogies and differences, but between these two points there is a number of intermediate conditions which make a gradual transition between them. Note also that in spite of the rule which we have enunciated, cases are met with in young people which behave like those occurring in old age: the converse is equally true.

* *Klinik der Greisenkrankheiten.* Erlangen, 1860.

LECTURE XVI.

SYMPTOMATOLOGY OF PARTIAL CHRONIC RHEUMATISM AND HEBERDEN'S NODOSITIES.

SUMMARY.—Partial chronic rheumatism.—Various names it has received.—Does not differ essentially from nodular rheumatism.—Its peculiar characters.—Small number of joints affected.—The large joints are the oftenest attacked.—Insidious onset; primarily chronic form.—Articular deformities.—Diathetic manifestations. —Cutaneous affections.—Visceral lesions.

Mode of development.—Sometimes follows acute rheumatism.—May be chronic from the beginning.—Sometimes becomes general.

Articular symptoms.—Deformities.—Pain.—Absence of tenderness to touch. —Creaking.

Prognosis relatively favourable.—More or less complete abolition of movement.—Spasmodic contraction of muscles not common.—Extreme rigidity of the joint.

Heberden's nodosities.—Independent of gout.—Situated at the joints between the ungual and the second phalanges.—Lesions those of dry arthritis.—The other joints of the hand often affected, but to a less degree. This affection depends on the rheumatic diathesis.—It may, though rarely, coexist with gout.

GENTLEMEN,—We shall complete our description of the symptoms of chronic rheumatism, by studying two important forms of this disease which follow nodular rheumatism in the classification which we have adopted. These are *partial chronic rheumatism*, and *Heberden's nodosities*.

Partial chronic rheumatism, which we shall first consider, has received a great many different names from different authors. When it occurs in the hip it is called *Morbus coxæ senilis;* when it occurs somewhere else, the names *senile arthritis* and *dry arthritis* have been given to it. It is the malady which produces the best characterised deformities; it is *Arthritis deformans*.

This disease does not differ fundamentally from the preceding; but it is distinguished by some peculiar symptoms. I have already mentioned some of them; and shall now remind you of the most characteristic differences which distinguish these two forms of the same affection.

1. The joints attacked are few in number, in comparison with the number affected in general rheumatism.

2. The large joints, even those which are only very exceptionally attacked in the preceding form, are those most frequently affected in this.

3. The primarily chronic form is here the rule. The onset is usually insidious; pain is not a prominent symptom; the affected limbs usually retain their power of movement, at least up to a certain point. But, on the contrary, considerable deformities are often produced in the neighbourhood of the joints on account of the luxuriant growth of osteophytes; sometimes also sufficient swelling of the joint is met with to contribute to the deformity (*Hypertrophic form* of Adams).

This disease has been specially studied with regard to its external pathology; attention has been specially directed to those cases in which the affection is localised in a single joint. Indeed the diagnosis may then offer great difficulties; for this form of rheumatism may simulate a dislocation, a fracture, and still more closely white swelling. These are questions which have especially attracted the attention of surgeons; nevertheless the study of this disease has a great interest for the physician; in fact it is almost always a diathetic affection, and may often be accompanied by cutaneous manifestations * and visceral lesions (asthma, heart-disease), the meaning of which is shown by the very fact of their coexisting with chronic joint affections.

We must observe also that the localisation of the disease in a single joint, the latent onset of the affection, the luxuriance of the new osteophytic growths, are characters which are exceptional rather than habitual, and which are particularly striking on account of their singularity. The articular disorders of partial chronic rheumatism very frequently appear with all these characters, much less-marked certainly, but perfectly appreciable. This fact is of great clinical importance, for the satisfactorily demonstrated existence of these articular lesions may be a readily appreciable indication of the rheumatic diathesis; and it is especially from this point of view that they interest us.

I shall not attempt, gentlemen, to give you a regular description of this form of rheumatism; it belongs especially, as I said, to the domain of surgery, on which I do not wish to trespass. I cannot, however, forbear to make you acquainted with those features of the affection which are most interesting to us from our present point of view.

A. Partial chronic rheumatism appears sometimes to follow

* See Colombel, *Recherches sur l'arthrite sèche.* Thèses de Paris, 1852.

acute articular rheumatism, of which it may then be regarded as the sequel.

Adams, who has devoted special study to this question, recognises this mode of development of the morbid phenomena. Under such circumstances it is one of the forms of nodular rheumatism that we have to deal with. Two cases may arise : either the rheumatism degenerates into white swelling, or it assumes the characters of *arthritis deformans*. The latter is what usually happens, and there is nothing which need surprise us in this transition, for we know that acute rheumatism presents, in germ, the lesions of the chronic form.

B. The onset of *arthritis deformans* may be acute although the rheumatism is originally partial in its distribution.* Adams and Colombel† have reported examples of this, and I have myself observed some cases at the Salpêtrière. Thus, in a woman of 53, there were at the commencement a few joints acutely inflamed, together with fever and muscular spasms; then the disease progressed in the form of dry arthritis ; at last symmetrically disposed pain appeared in the hands, and the affection was seen to pass into nodular rheumatism.

C. On the other hand, the onset of the disease may, as we have seen, be slow and insidious, the symptoms at first remaining localised in a single joint ; but the real nature of the affection is made clear in the long run, by one or several more joints becoming inflamed, or by the appearance of some of the non-articular manifestations which associate themselves with rheumatism. There is now at the Salpêtrière a woman of 46, who, after having first suffered from dry inflammation of the hip-joint, was attacked subsequently with a similar affection of the knees. In another woman, 63 years of age, there was at first dry arthritis of the right hip, then of the left hip; then painful swelling of the left knee with creaking; and, lastly, Heberden's nodosities appeared.

D. Lastly, one meets with a good many cases in which the rheumatism, after having been limited for a longer or shorter time to a few joints, then becomes general. One may meet with the two converse transformations ; sometimes it is partial rheumatism which becomes general; sometimes, on the contrary, in general rheumatism the affection in one joint is seen to pre-

* Op. cit., pp. 44 and 301, obs. xvii.   † Op. cit., p. 71, obs. v.

dominate, and in this joint the lesions of *arthritis deformans* at last appear. Adams has reported several examples of this occurrence.

He quotes, among others, the case of Dr. Percival, a very distinguished physician, who died in 1839, at the age of 82, having long been a sufferer from this disease. In 1818 he had had pretty sharp pains in the hands and wrists, accompanied by slight swelling. Two years later slight pain appeared in the right hip-joint, and little by little walking became extremely difficult. The limb became shortened, and remained in a state of external rotation; movement of it was accompanied by very manifest creaking, and it was only at rest when the legs were crossed; he could not change this attitude without experiencing a painful sensation. Five years before his death analogous symptoms appeared in the left hip. Dr. Percival died of an affection of the bladder, and conformably to his last desires, the autopsy was performed by Dr. Colles, and the specimens presented to the Pathological Society of Dublin. The joints presented the best characterised type of senile disease of the articulations; the ends of the bones were flattened and eburnated, as well as the two cotyloid cavities. The ligamentum teres had completely disappeared. The neck of the femur was shortened; the head of the left femur was red and hyperæmic, and numerous bony formations covered the fibrous capsule.

In a lady of 60, a sufferer from nodular rheumatism for twenty-five years, the disease became at last localised in the knees, which were ankylosed at a right angle, and presented the classical characters of dry arthritis.

But whatever the origin of partial rheumatism, when it has once become chronic it is rather an infirmity than a disease,—barring the visceral lesions which may become associated with it. However, it must not be forgotten that acute exacerbations sometimes occur. Then the articular affection, long painless, at length gives rise to acute suffering; the skin reddens, and an evident aggravation of the chronic symptoms is observed.

The purely articular symptoms, when the disease is thoroughly established, are the following :—

1. There is more or less pronounced deformity of the joint; there are bony projections, foreign bodies, swelling.

2. The patient feels spontaneous pain, not intense, and dis-

appearing when he walks, but which in the end becomes more marked.

3. Pain on touch or percussion is absent, or nearly so, which distinguishes this form of joint disease from those of less benignant nature.

4. There is always more or less pronounced creaking.

This affiction does not threaten life, when it is free from any complication, but it abolishes more or less completely the motility of the affected parts. However, the patients continue to walk, though not without difficulty. It is in such cases that, when we examine the joint at the autopsy, we notice grooves on the eburnated portion of the articular surfaces.

Spasmodic contraction of the muscles is very rare in this form, except at the onset, but there is sometimes extreme laxity of the ligaments; or perhaps, as one often finds in the hip, extreme rigidity of the joint, resulting from deformity of the heads of the bones or of the concavities which receive them.

Heberden's Nodosities. We shall now proceed to consider Heberden's nodosities, a special form of chronic rheumatism which has not yet been sufficiently described, and which is hardly mentioned by authors. Most physicians unhesitatingly class it with gout.

When it is a question of *nodular rheumatism,* physicians readily admit that it differs from gout in certain of its characters ; but as to Heberden's nodosities, doubt, say they, is no longer allowable ; it is really gout that is before us.

For my part I am of an entirely opposite opinion, and I speak of this form of rheumatism as the *nodosities of Heberden* because this author was the first who felt the necessity of distinguishing these lesions from gout.

He asks in his Commentaries : What is the nature of those small hard nodules, about the size of a pea, so often met with on the fingers, usually a little above their extremities, near the joints ? *They have no connection with gout,* he adds.

These little nodosities, as Heberden pointed out, are situated close to the joints between the second and third phalanges. Generally the end of the finger is a little bent either to the right or left. There are two nodules at the level of the joint, and the joint itself seems wider than usual. There is rigidity but no creaking in the diseased articulation.

Usually the onset of this disease is very obscure; however, there are attacks of redness, heat, and temporary swelling of the soft parts. These are really exacerbations of the affection, which the patients often regard as paroxysms of gout.

The anatomical lesions in this miniature joint-disease have not yet been described. According to the numerous investigations which I have had the opportunity of making at the Salpêtrière, you will find here, as in the two other forms of chronic articular rheumatism, the morbid changes of dry arthritis. I have many times assured myself of this fact by dissection. The articular cartilages undergo the velvety change; then they disappear, and an eburnated osseous layer is found in their place. The articular surfaces enlarge in all directions, on account of the growth of osteophytes, which almost exactly reproduce in an exaggerated form their shape and normal contours. The pea-like enlargements, which, as Heberden said, are met with in the neighbourhood of the second phalangeal joint, are nothing but the osseous nodules, which exist normally on the head of the second phalanx at its dorsal aspect; only the size of these nodules is considerably increased by the growth of new layers of bone. There is no trace of sodium urate deposits, either in the substance of the articular cartilage or in the soft parts in the neighbourhood of the joints.

The other joints of the hand are generally affected, but to a much less degree. Contrary to what obtains in nodular rheumatism, the joints between the first and second phalanges especially, and nextly the metacarpo-phalangeal joints, present more or less decided lesions in such cases.

These nodosities are interesting ,to the observer because they reveal a constitutional state, which is none other than the *rheumatic diathesis*.

This affection, which is very frequent at the Salpêtrière, belongs especially to old age; however, it would not do to suppose that it is never met with in young people. On the contrary, we often discover it at less advanced periods of life, and this is a point which it is important to make clear. It is a hereditary disease, and may appear in several members of the same family. It presents evident affinities both with nodular rheumatism, and, especially, with partial rheumatism ; in fact you may often find it along with disease of the hip or knee.

It occasionally happens that in the same family some individuals have Heberden's nodosities, others general chronic rheumatism, and still others partial rheumatism ; a fresh proof of the affinity which unites these three forms of one and the same affection.

Heberden's rheumatism is often accompanied by asthma, migrain, neuralgia, especially of the sciatic nerve, and muscular rheumatism. These manifestations may alternate, moreover, with the exacerbations of this disease. It is not uncommon to meet with it in patients suffering from cancer of the breast, or of some other organ.

Lastly, these little nodosities may coexist with gout, as I have myself had a recent opportunity of proving. In this case the nodosities had preceded the gout by several years.

LECTURE XVII.

ETIOLOGY OF ARTICULAR RHEUMATISM.

SUMMARY.—Chief causes of articular rheumatism.—They are common to all forms of the disease.—Historical sketch.—Prominence of gout in the writings of the physicians of antiquity.—Nodular rheumatism, however, already existed.—Geographical distribution.—Acute articular rheumatism is a disease belonging especially to temperate climates.—It is unknown in the neighbourhood of the poles and the equator.—Chronic articular rheumatism abounds in temperate countries, but also exists in hot countries.—Heredity: its influence indisputable.—Statistics borrowed from various authors.—Age.—The classical age for acute rheumatism is from 15 to 30.—Chronic rheumatism is met with especially at two periods of life: from 20 to 30 and from 40 to 60.—Sex.—Men are more subject to acute articular rheumatism, women to nodular rheumatism.

External causes.—Damp cold.—Damp dwellings.—Destitution, bad food.—Traumatic causes.—Blows, falls, inflammations, whitlows.—Pathological causes.—Erysipelas, Angina, Scarlatina, Gonorrhœa.

Uterine functions.— Chlorosis. —Dysmenorrhœa.— Menopause.—Pregnancy.—Prolonged lactation.

Comparison between the etiology of rheumatism and that of gout.—These two affections are not identical, but there is a certain amount of affinity between them.

GENTLEMEN,—The study of the causes which determine articular rheumatism will furnish fresh proofs in support of the opinion which I have all along maintained.

In the domain of etiology, indeed, we shall see the different forms of this disease meet and mingle ; on the contrary, we shall see them becoming more distinct from gout ; and we shall demonstrate that the types I have hitherto been describing, apparently so different, have in reality a common origin.

It must not, however, be forgotten, that according to some observations that have been made, articular rheumatism may through inheritance create a predisposition to gout ; and the converse of this appears equally true.

I. *Historical and geographical account of the disease.* We have already found, while studying the history of gout, that articular rheumatism attracted very little attention from the physicians of antiquity, whose descriptions relate almost exclusively to gout ; moreover, they confounded this latter affection with rheumatism under the common title of *articulorum passio.* Baillou was the first author who pointed out that rheumatism is a separate disease ; and a proof that this distinction took some time to become established is to be found in the fact that it was not yet recognised in the first editions of Boerhaave.

The silence of the ancients has made some authors fancy that rheumatism did not exist before modern times. But the bones found in the excavations at Pompeii have supplied us with more positive information on this point than could be furnished by medical literature,—at least so far as chronic rheumatism goes ; in several cases the lesions characteristic of this disease have been found in the human relics. Precious facts about this subject are to be found in the *Osteologia Pompeiana* of Prof. Delle-Chiaje of Naples. The figures which accompany the text can leave no doubt in the reader's mind.

The *medical geography* of rheumatism is still to be worked out. Under the influence of preconceived ideas regrettable confusion has arisen about all the diseases which are dependent on cold as a cause ; and it is clear how difficult the task of criticism becomes when observations made in distant regions have to be compared.

It seems proved, however, that acute articular rheumatism is a disease which belongs especially to temperate climates ; it is unknown in the immediate neighbourhood of the poles and equator. However, the disease is met with pretty often in hot climates ; it is common in Egypt according to Pruner Bey, and in the East Indies according to Webb ; in this latter country it is often complicated with endocarditis and pericarditis.

At the Cape of Good Hope, in the land of the geranium, the English army gives a proportion of 57 rheumatic out of 1,000 invalids ; whilst in the rigorous climate of Nova Scotia, out of the same number of patients only 30 cases of rheumatism are met with.

As to chronic articular rheumatism we possess no precise information. It is certain at any rate that it abounds in temperate countries, in England, Ireland, France, Germany, and the whole of central Europe. But it seems to exist also in hot countries. In India Malcolmson has pointed out its occurrence among the Sepoys, and I have myself seen that it is frequent at Naples.

II. *Heredity.* The study of this question is of great interest in reference to the theory of rheumatism ; for hereditary affections are not accidental transient maladies, but are part of the very constitution of the individual; we see this distinctly in the case of gout.

The statistics of Chomel and Requin establish the frequency of hereditary transmission in this case; unfortunately these authors have mixed up rheumatism and gout. But Fuller, who takes account of the distinction, found hereditary transmission in 96 cases out of 300 of rheumatism, giving a proportion of 29 p.c.; for gout the proportion is 50 p.c.

As to chronic articular rheumatism fresh inquiries are necessary. Still, what we do know tends to prove that this affection is often handed down hereditarily, either from acute rheumatism, or directly from chronic rheumatism.

It is necessary, however, to make a distinction here between the three types which I have described.

In the case of *nodular rheumatism* there can be no doubt on this point. Out of 45 cases of this kind Trastour found the father and mother rheumatic 10 times, and 3 times that affected women had children already attacked with chronic rheumatism. I have myself observed an interesting case of this kind. There is now at the Salpêtrière a woman suffering from nodular rheumatism, whose daughter and grand-daughter are already experiencing pains in their small joints. There you see three generations successively attacked by the same affection.

As for *Heberden's rheumatism,* my own observations seem to me to have established its heredity; it very often runs in a family. Moreover, this is a point which Garrod had already made out.

Concerning *partial chronic rheumatism* the question is still under consideration, and I could not give an opinion on it.

III. *Age.* The classical period for *acute articular rheumatism* is from 15 to 30, but it is not uncommon in the very early years of life; you will meet with it in children of from 5 to 10; and according to West and most other authors, diseases of the heart occur more frequently in young rheumatic patients than in older subjects.

So that there is a distinction to be pointed out here between rheumatism and gout, which hardly ever appears before 20,— a fact which we have already remarked.

The acute form of rheumatism rarely presents itself after 50. Out of 199 cases, Macleod only found it develop once after 55 ; and Fuller, out of 289 cases, only seven times after 50.

I have myself observed two cases of this kind after 70 years of age. The first was a mild case of acute rheumatism, the second, very obstinate subacute rheumatism with febrile symptoms.

Trastour and I have shown that there are two periods of life during which people are peculiarly liable to suffer from attacks of *nodular rheumatism*. These are from 20 to 30, the period when development reaches completion ; and from 40 to 60, the date of the menopause. Haygarth then was in error when he associated chronic rheumatism almost exclusively with the menopause.

Nevertheless this disease may appear either before or after the periods which I have just mentioned. We have several observations which supply the proof of this statement.

Thus Laborde showed to the Société de Biologie a little boy of eight who presented all the characteristic deformities of nodular rheumatism ; the disease originated when he was four years old. I have already mentioned, when speaking of rheumatic pericarditis, the very remarkable case which Martel has reported from the clinic of Dr. Barthez. I have myself observed the following examples.

An invalid of the Salpêtrière, who had been brought up in a damp dwelling, was attacked with nodular rheumatism at the age of ten.

Another invalid at the same hospital, who had lived during her childhood in a damp room, was attacked at the age of sixteen.

Lastly, a man who had grown up in one of the abandoned quarries on the banks of the Loire, which are often used as dwellings, was attacked by nodular rheumatism at the age of twenty.

Partial rheumatism, and especially *arthritis deformans*, are usually met with in people of advanced age ; they are often met with in middle life, and it is only in quite young subjects that they are really exceptional. Moreover, some cases below thirty have been noticed.

As to *Heberden's nodosities*, we have seen that although they are especially common in old age, they may nevertheless appear in young people.

IV. *Sex.* Men are more subject than women to *acute articular rheumatism.* There is, however, no very decided difference between them.

Nodular rheumatism is incomparably more common in women than in men (Trastour, Vidal). To convince oneself of this one need but compare the inhabitants of the Bicêtre with the infirm women at the Salpêtrière.

Partial rheumatism is perhaps commoner in men; this is especially the case in *arthritis deformans.*

Heberden's nodosities seem to be more common in the female sex, but this point has not yet been well worked out.

V. *External causes.* 1. *Damp cold.* A sudden transient chill can only be regarded as an occasional and in no way specific cause of rheumatism. It will not do to imitate the mistake of Eisenmann, who has written a book called "*Erkaltungskrankheiten*" (*Diseases caused by chill*), in which rheumatism includes the whole of pathology, or nearly so.

It is certain, however, that in predisposed persons the power of cold in developing both acute articular rheumatism and rapidly-developing chronic rheumatism is great.

But I am far from disputing the influence of *prolonged sojourn in a damp dwelling.* On the contrary, I recognise that this is the most efficient cause both of acute articular rheumatism and especially of nodular rheumatism.

About three-quarters of the women attacked by this latter disease refer it to the prolonged influence of damp cold. When Beau affirms that this condition is a constant one, he doubtless exaggerates an indisputable truth, but it is certain that this cause does exist in the majority of cases.

Rooms on the ground floor, damp dark chambers, wet sheets, walls from which the paper is falling, these are the conditions we shall meet with in most cases where people are attacked by chronic rheumatism. Moreover, most of the patients have dwelt a long time in these miserable habitations; for four, six, eight, or even *ten years.* There are in the neighbourhood of Chantilly dwellings which are really like those of Cave Men; they are excavations underneath the ground in old abandoned quarries. Among the wretched people who have taken refuge there, are a large number, to judge from Beau's account, who suffer from nodular rheumatism. This is not surprising ; but it must not be forgotten that in many regions the people still live in subterranean dwellings, without seeming to experience much inconvenience. This is the case, for example, in certain provinces of the Russian empire, and notably in Georgia. You know that during the retreat of the Ten Thousand, the Greeks, having reached Armenia, found the inhabitants of the country living in excavations of this kind, and that in the midst of a glacial winter they got along very comfortably in these well-warmed pits.* Remember also that these are very cold countries, and the people only go into their burrows to escape the rigours of the climate. Now we have seen that excessive cold is not generally at all favourable to the development of rheumatism. But in temperate climates it is more difficult to avoid this consequence of living under such conditions.

And yet as a rule the disease does not declare itself at once ; there is usually an incubation period, during which only vague muscular pains are experienced. Often the articular symptoms do not appear until three or four years after their cause has ceased to operate.

2. The influence of *poverty* and bad food on the development of rheumatism cannot be disputed : the workhouse paupers of England and Ireland supply many instances of nodular rheumatism, a fact showing well that it is a disease occurring specially among the poorer classes, although the contrary opinion was maintained by Haygarth.

3. *Traumatic influences,* as in the case of gout, may determine both the onset of the disease and its primary locality.

There are several cases reported in which acute or chronic rheumatism has appeared after a blow, a fall, a boil, a whitlow, commencing in the joint nearest the injured spot.

A woman suffered from nodular rheumatism, originating in the right shoulder, which had been severely bruised at a former period.

In a butcher, already rheumatic, a boil developed in consequence of a puncture on the hand, and an attack of acute

* Xenophon, *Anabasis,* iv., 48.

rheumatism came on, commencing in the wrist near the chief seat of the phlegmonous inflammation.

In the case of a woman at the Salpêtrière, a whitlow which had appeared in one of her fingers marked the onset of nodular rheumatism, which commenced in the joints nearest the affected part.

Partial rheumatism often develops after a blow or a fall, and it is difficult to decide in such a case whether we have to do with a general affection or with a purely local disease resulting from external violence.

VI. The *pathological causes* often act like external influences. Acute articular rheumatism may be observed after a great many different diseases.

In an individual already rheumatic, facial erysipelas, caught during an epidemic of this affection, was the starting-point of acute rheumatism. This case must be distinguished from those in which the erysipelas is one of the manifestations of the rheumatic diathesis; for I might mention several cases of nodular rheumatism in which the attacks of erysipelas have alternated with the articular symptoms.

Some facts seem to show that there is a rheumatic angina, but it is very certain that an angina otherwise caused has often been the starting-point of an attack of acute articular rheumatism.

You know the connection there is between articular affections and scarlatina. Two classes of cases must be here distinguished. Sometimes the scarlatina determines the appearance of an articular affection which differs in nothing from acute rheumatism; sometimes, on the contrary, it is evidently a special form of arthritis, usually mild in nature, as Todd remarks, but sometimes assuming great gravity and becoming purulent, as Garrod pointed out. These latter cases alone deserve the name of scarlatinal arthritis; the former belong to acute articular rheumatism, scarlatina being merely the determining cause. The case of gonorrhœa is similar.

Does gonorrhœal rheumatism exist? This is a question which deserves our attention for a moment.

Usually when articular symptoms appear after a urethral affection, one sees a subacute form of arthritis arise, affecting

two or three joints and accompanied by iritis (Rollet) ; that is
the classical type of gonorrhœal arthritis.

But acute articular rheumatism with endocarditis may also be
found along with a simple clap. A case of this kind 'has been
observed by Brandes, and Prof. Lorain has told me of another.

Lastly, chronic rheumatism with deformity of the joints may
also appear in connection with this disease (Garrod, Lorain,
Broadhurst, Trousseau).*

How shall we interpret these facts ? Is there always here a
manifestation of rheumatism ? Certainly not. We know that
the articular symptoms following fevers are not always dependent
on this diathesis. The articular symptoms of morve, variola,
and purulent infection are evidently not rheumatic. It may be
then that there is a scarlatinal or gonorrhœal arthritis independent
of rheumatism ; I am even convinced that this is often the case.
But frequently the articular affection which originates under
these circumstances *is really rheumatism*, developing as a sequela
of affections which also in certain cases have the power of acting
directly on the joints on their own account.†

VII. *Uterine functions.* All authors have recognised the
influence exerted on the development of the different forms of
articular rheumatism by the functions of the female generative
organs. This is true not only for the acute form but also for the
chronic form of the disease.

The appearance of the catamenia, the menopause, pregnancy,
labour, the puerperal state, lactation, all these exert a potent
influence on the development of articular rheumatism in women.

On this point we must go into a few details.

Chlorosis is a condition from which the joint-symptoms of
rheumatism readily spring. Musgrave quotes several examples
of *arthritis ex chlorosi*, which were evidently cases of nodular
rheumatism. The good effects of preparations of iron have been
shown in several cases of this kind.

It is well known that the menopause is often marked by a
condition like the chlorosis of young girls, and it is also known
that chronic rheumatism often develops at this period of life.

* Garrod, *On Gout*, p. 545.—Broadhurst in *Reynolds's System*, vol. i., p. 920.—Trousseau,
Clin. méd. de l'Hôtel-Dieu, t. iii., p. 375.—Lorain's case verbally communicated.

† Refer on this point to the discussion at the Société médicale des hôpitaux, *Union
médicale*, 23rd Dec., 1866, and 5th March, 1867.

Pseudo-membranous *dysmenorrhœa* has been mentioned by Todd among the affections coexisting with nodular rheumatism. It is not perhaps uninteresting to point out in this connection that dysmenorrhœa is often accompanied by eruptions (erythema nodosum for example) which are sometimes met with in acute or subacute rheumatism. In persons already affected, an exacerbation of the pain has been observed to occur at each menstrual period. The sudden suppression of the courses consequent on strong emotion has sometimes been the starting-point of nodular rheumatism.

Pregnancy is also one of the causes of this affection. In a work which he has been good enough to send me, my colleague, M. Lorain, reports several cases of acute or subacute rheumatism occurring in pregnant women. In my thesis I have reported several examples of *nodular rheumatism* appearing under the same conditions ; Todd had already observed this coincidence. It is not uncommon to see individual joints affected during pregnancy, and then the disease become general after delivery. It is a fact that acute rheumatism itself has been observed in the course of pregnancy (Chomel and Requin, Todd). It must not, however, be forgotten that multiple purulent arthritis may appear in women during confinement. It is a mistake in my opinion to speak of these cases as puerperal rheumatism.

Another condition in which the different forms of rheumatism (especially subacute and chronic rheumatism) may often appear is lactation, especially when prolonged. (Lorain, Garrod.)*

It would be interesting to compare this etiology with that of gout, and to bring into prominence the differences between them; but time presses, and we must be content with a general glance.

It is true, speaking broadly, that the causes of gout are connected with comfort, excess, and good-cheer ; the causes of rheumatism, broadly speaking, and especially of chronic rheumatism, are rather poverty, damp cold, insufficient food, and weakening influences of every kind.

But the contrast becomes more striking still if we compare the affections which most frequently accompany rheumatism and those usually associated with gout. On the one hand we find

* On Gout, p. 568.

diabetes,* corpulence, gravel,† the affinity of which with gout I have already shown, and which are only rarely met with in rheumatism ; on the other hand scrofula,‡ phthisis, cancerous affections,§ which are common in chronic rheumatism, but rare in gout.

Thus there are many contrasts, from the point of view of causation, between these two diatheses, and yet in spite of the great differences which distinguish them, and which I have endeavoured to make clear, they present remarkable analogies, and have often been confounded ; even when we distinguish them, we are obliged to place them near together in any satisfactory classification of diseases.

It is, moreover, certain that a relationship which may show itself in various ways connects rheumatism with gout.

They are sometimes seen to coexist in the same individual who presents the lesions of gout and those of chronic articular rheumatism at the same time.

At other times acute articular rheumatism occurs during a patient's youth ; then at its favourite period gout comes on.‖ Some see in this a transformation, others a succession.

Again, the relationship may show itself through inheritance. Acute articular rheumatism is frequent in the children of gouty parents. (Heberden, Fuller, Todd.) The children of rheumatic individuals often become gouty. (Fuller.) Lastly, the hereditary

---

* Out of 225 cases of diabetes, acute articular rheumatism is noted twice only by Griesinger in his "Studies on Diabetes." I do not think diabetes has ever been observed as a complication of chronic rheumatism.

† I have seen uric acid gravel together with nodular rheumatism in a woman, but the blood, examined on several occasions, never contained an excess of uric acid.

‡ Scrofula very often figures among the antecedents of those who are suffering from progressive chronic rheumatism. It is very common to see these persons with specific scars on the neck. I might quote several cases of women who were affected with white swelling in youth, and who, in later life, have suffered from nodular rheumatism. In 119 cases of nodular rheumatism, Fuller (op. cit., p. 334) mentions 23 ($\frac{1}{5}$) in which the father, mother, and collateral relatives presented evident signs of pulmonary phthisis. This affection, I am sure, often carries off invalids who are suffering from nodular rheumatism, and in such cases it seems to me that the phthisis is remarkable for its slow development. In patients with acute rheumatism phthisis is rare (Wunderlich, Hamernjk). Still the coexistence of these two affections is possible ; M. Danjoy, who has called attention to this point, believes that the evolution of the disease is then retarded.

§ I have often been able to convince myself at the Salpêtrière that the coexistence of Heberden's nodosities, both with mammary and uterine cancer, is not exceptional.

‖ On this point see Baillou, t. iv., p. 415. Is it this which made Junker say, *Rheumatismus arthritidem ordine antecedit ?*

connection may show itself in collateral relatives. I have myself observed nodular rheumatism appear in a woman whose brother was gouty.

Do these relationships, apparently so intimate, prove the identity of these two affections? Certainly not; all the more must we admit that they have a common basis and background, that there is an *articular predisposition,* an *arthritic* state, from which both take their origin.

LECTURE XVIII.

TREATMENT OF GOUT AND CHRONIC ARTICULAR RHEUMATISM.

SUMMARY.—General considerations on the treatment of gout.—Treatment of the attacks.—Expectant treatment.—Remedies of charlatans.—Colchicum.—Advantages and drawbacks of this agent.—Rules to be followed in its employment.—Narcotics : henbane, opium.—Sulphate of quinin.—Iodide of potassium.—Tincture of guaiacum.—Local applications.—Leeches.—Blisters.—Moxæ.—Treatment of the constitutional state.—Alkalis.—Their various properties.—Soda, potash, lithia.—Action of these drugs.—Cases in which alkalis are contraindicated.—Mineral waters.—Tonics.—Treatment of the local affection, of the tophi and rigidity of joints.—Treatment of abnormal gout.—Dietetics.

Treatment of chronic articular rheumatism.—Unsatisfactory state of our knowledge in this direction.—Treatment of the acute exacerbations.—Opium, sulphate of quinin, blood-letting.—Alkalis.—Tincture of iodin.—Arsenic internally and externally —Tincture of guaiacum.—Iodide of potassium.—Iron, cod-liver oil.—Blisters, revulsives.—Mineral waters.—Impotence of our art in the majority of cases.

GENTLEMEN,—We enter to-day on the last part of our course. We have postponed the treatment of gout until the end of these lectures, so as to be able to compare it with that of chronic articular rheumatism. This is the subject which will occupy us to-day.

TREATMENT OF GOUT.

I. *General considerations.* Gout is a hereditary constitutional disease, primarily chronic, in spite of its acute manifestations.

But gout is sometimes also an acquired disease, sometimes through errors of diet, sometimes from other causes ; this is a kind of spontaneous generation.

One may hence conclude that hygienic influences here hold the first place, and therapeutic agents only the second. This, moreover, is what experience has long proved.

I do not affirm that the disease is radically incurable ; there are examples of spontaneous cure, but art has not yet managed to reproduce with certainty the methods of nature.

Still there are means by which the effects of the disease can be lessened and its paroxysms averted ; it is on these measures as a whole that the treatment of the constitutional state in the intervals between the attacks depends.

But we have a more humble though very useful mission to perform. The periodic manifestations, the paroxysms of gout, whether acute or chronic, are accompanied by extreme, almost insupportable, suffering. Can we remove these crises of pain, or at least diminish their intensity and shorten their duration? This is what constitutes the treatment of the gouty paroxysm. Let us first of all consider this part of the subject.

II. *Treatment of the fits of acute and chronic gout.* The treatment is here mainly palliative. Some physicians go so far as to forbid all measures of alleviation as dangerous and pernicious. This is the school of Sydenham, which regards things from a teleological point of view. "*Dolor acerrimum naturæ pharmacum,*" said the great master. "Gout is the best remedy for gout," said Mead. And Cullen said, "Patience and flannel."

The partisans of expectant treatment rest their views upon the slight efficacy of known remedies, upon the danger of their application, and especially upon the relief experienced by the patient after the attack. But it may be replied to their arguments, that for instructed men to abstain from action is to open the door to quacks. If the physician holds aloof from the gouty patient, charlatans get hold of him. They arrive with means of relief whose effect is almost instantaneous, and which, though sometimes giving rise to grave incidents, are often without any real danger. Such are Reynolds' elixir, liqueur de Laville, the wine of Anduran, the pills of Lartigue, etc.

Now it seems clearly proved that these pretended specifics owe their efficacy for the most part to the presence of *colchicum.* It is then the business of the physician to study attentively the therapeutic properties of this redoubtable agent, which sometimes gives immense relief to the patient and does no harm, but sometimes causes serious symptoms which may lead to death. Nobody, however, not even its most inveterate enemy, contests its power. It causes the gouty inflammation and the terrible pain which accompanies it, to disappear as if by enchantment. Its action in this respect is almost like that of cinchona in intermittent fevers, and this is another differential character distinguishing gout from articular rheumatism. In the acute form of this latter disease, Prof. Monneret had already demonstrated the uselessness of colchicum ; and in the different forms of chronic rheumatism I have been able to convince myself that this drug does no good.

Let us now see what it can do in gout. From the 6th century of the Christian era the ancients knew the advantages and drawbacks of colchicum. Alexander Trallianus tells us that in his time it was only given to people who were pressed with business and had no time to be ill. Demetrius Pepagomenus, who lived about 1200 A.D., calls it *Theriaca articulorum*.

But the colchicum of the ancients is not our colchicum. They made use of *colchicum variegatum* (*hermodactyle*), we employ *colchicum autumnale*.

Fallen into disuse, this drug was again brought forward by the effects of *Husson's cure*. Everard Home extolled colchicum, which had already been restored to honour by Störck, for affections other than gout. More lately its effects have been well studied by Wandt, Halford, Watson, and Garrod.

All parts of the plant are made use of, bulbs, seeds, and flowers. It is administered in extract, wine, and tincture. The wine made from the bulbs may be given in doses of $\mathfrak{m}$x to $\mathfrak{m}$xxx three or four times during the twenty-four hours ; the acetic extract is prescribed in doses of from ½ gr. to 2 grs.

One word on the physiological effects of this drug. In large doses it causes—

1. Phenomena of gastro-enteritis, more or less serious.

2. Marked depression of the circulatory system, with a tendency to algidity and slowing of the pulse.

3. Lastly, nervous symptoms and a peculiar delirium.

In small doses, it only gives rise to slight nausea and moderate depression of the circulation.

Now it is in small doses, or at least when well borne, that it acts favourably in gout; in administering it one must avoid exciting inflammatory action in the alimentary canal; moreover, its action seems the more efficacious the less the operative effects are decided.

Its specific action is shown by the disappearance of the gouty inflammation and of the pain which accompanies it; this takes place as though by enchantment in from eight to fourteen hours. It is far from possessing the same amount of influence on other inflammations, and the various forms of articular rheumatism, as I have already pointed out.

What, then, is its manner of action ? A question still unanswerable. Its effects have been attributed to the elimination of uric acid ; this opinion, supported by Chelius, Maclagan, and Gregory, has been disputed by Garrod, Böcker, and Hammond. The opinion of these latter observers is based upon careful analyses of the urine, which seem to leave no opening for criticism.

Its sedative action on the circulatory system has been invoked ; but this is not the secret, for it does not act in the same way in other inflammations.

Neither is it the effect of its purgative action ; for its specific virtue may be manifested when there is no evacuation of the intestines.

Nor can one refer to its narcotic power, for its effects are quite special to gout.

In whatever way caused, its efficacy is beyond question. But we must look at the reverse of the medal, and see what its dangers are.

It is undeniable that when it is imprudently administered, very serious symptoms may result. What are the rules that should guide us in its employment ?

1. As I have already shown, gout is a disease in which retrocession occurs. If, therefore, you suddenly stop the attack, visceral troubles may be caused ; but you need fear no danger of this kind when small doses are employed. Moreover, there is no need to administer colchicum immediately on the onset of the attack (Halford, Trousseau) ; several days may pass before beginning to use it. Again, its irritant action on the gastro-intestinal canal is to be dreaded, another reason for prescribing very small doses.

2. Not only must large doses be avoided, but it is important to suspend the use of the drug at times ; for in some individuals its effects seem to be cumulative. In that case one would be afraid of the sudden impression that might be made on the nervous system. I should be inclined to suppose that several cases in which gout has apparently retroceded under the influence of colchicum and caused death, are cases of poisoning by this substance (Potton).

3. The patient must not be habituated to the use of colchicum, for then he is obliged to take ever-increasing doses. There are colchicum-drinkers, just as there are opium-eaters and alcoholics (Todd). Under these conditions a more or less profound modification of the system is produced, and the gout under this influence may pass into the *atonic state*.

4. Colchicum ought not to be employed in asthenic gout, but it may be made use of in some of the paroxysms of chronic gout. It is sometimes accused of prolonging the attacks, but often, on the contrary, it seems to shorten their duration (Goupil, de Rennes).

5. The action of colchicum should be assisted by a suitable regimen (diet, repose in bed), and by adjuvants such as the alkalis which act on the excess of uric acid ; the preference must be given to the potassic and lithic salts. Lastly, purgatives are often employed with good result, but you must avoid mercurials, of which experience has shown the serious inconvenience.

There are cases where colchicum cannot be employed, but medicine is not thereby completely disarmed ; there are other measures to which recourse may beneficially be had.

Internally, during the acute attacks, narcotics may be given, especially henbane. Opium may also be prescribed, but it has the drawback of retarding the secretions, and this may impede the regular evolution of the disease. In certain individuals also it gives rise to effects quite out of proportion to the doses employed ; on several occasions I have seen these drugs cause alarming cerebral symptoms, and in cases of renal affection, even give rise to the phenomena of uræmia. You will have especially to dread symptoms of this kind when the gout is already of long-standing and the lesions of gouty kidney already well-marked. A remarkable case of this kind has been reported by Todd.

Sulphate of quinin may also be administered with some chance of success ; but its action is far from being so efficacious in gout as in acute rheumatism.

In exacerbations of the chronic state, sulphate of quinin is also useful. After the attacks, the more or less permanent pains of which the joints are often the seat may sometimes be successfully combatted by iodide of potassium and the ammoniated tincture of guaiacum.

Externally, during the attacks, various local applications may be employed. Cold water has often been applied to the affected joints, but nothing, as I have already shown, is more apt to cause retrocession.

Formerly leeches were prescribed *loco dolenti*. This treatment is now abandoned, for it has been found that the joints recovered their normal mobility with difficulty. Narcotics, on the contrary, and especially atropin, may with advantage be applied to the suffering articulation.

Blisters are often useful both in acute and subacute cases. A small blister, not bigger than a franc-piece, applied to the red and swollen joint often acts efficiently during a paroxysm (Todd, Cartwright). I have sometimes employed this treatment with good results.

Lastly, moxæ have sometimes been employed. For example, there was the Chancellor, William Temple, who used to apply them himself, every time he had an attack of gout.

III. *Treatment of the constitutional state.* The proper indication here would be not only to modify the state of the blood, but to prevent the formation of uric acid in excess. That would be the ideal treatment, but how realise it ? One can scarcely do anything in this direction but combat the dyspepsia, prevent the attacks, and restrict the patient to a suitable diet.

But when once uric acid is formed in the blood, one may meet the effects resulting from its presence in excess. Its excretion by the kidneys must be facilitated, and we have powerful remedies for this purpose ; deposits of sodium urate must be prevented from forming in the tissues ; and when these deposits already exist, an attempt must be made to dissolve them.

Empirical experience had brought to light a group of agents answering to these indications, long before uric acid had been discovered. These agents are the alkaline bodies. Under this head are included :—

1. The alkalis (soda, potash, lithia) and their carbonates. They have a marked action on the stomach in neutralising acidity.

2. The organic salts of alkaline bases (citrates, tartrates, etc.).

3. The phosphates of sodium and ammonium, which have an alkaline reaction and a special influence on the excretion of urine.

It would be a mistake to suppose that all the alkalis may be used indiscriminately. On this point the experiments of Claude

Bernard and Grandeau, repeated more recently by Guttmann,* should be remembered. These observers have shown that a gram of a potassium salt injected into the veins of a medium-sized dog is sufficient to kill it; twenty centigrams sufficed to kill a rabbit. To obtain the same results with a sodium salt, a dose at least three times as large was needful.

Let us see, therefore, what is the special action of each of these substances, and, to begin with the two bases most commonly employed, let us compare potassium and sodium.

The salts of potassium have a diuretic action, the reality of which has been well shown by Mitscherlich. That of the sodium salts is not so marked.

The action of potash in dissolving uric acid is much more energetic than that of soda. You know that urate of potassium is much more soluble than urate of sodium. And if you plunge a cartilage incrusted with sodic urate into a solution of potassic carbonate you will find that a rapid solvent action occurs; if, on the contrary, you plunge it into a solution of sodic carbonate you will obtain scarcely any appreciable result in the same space of time.

Thus potash, speaking a priori, should be more efficacious than soda; † this latter base is, however, useful to the gouty, in cases where there is a hepatic affection (Garrod).

But there exists a still little-known substance, lithia, which seems to surpass potash and soda in all respects.

This base, which was discovered in 1817 by Arfwedson, occurs in several mineral waters, at Carlsbad, Vals, Vichy, Baden-Baden, Weilbach, at which last place there is a new spring which has been called Natrolithionquelle, and which contains a large proportion of this substance.

Spectrum analysis has enabled Bunsen and Kirchoff to determine its presence in human milk and blood, so that it is a substance not foreign to the system; and if potash exists in the corpuscles, and soda in the serum, lithia occurs also, though in small quantity, in the nutrient liquid of the body.

This new agent answers all the indications I have spoken of. Its diuretic action is very decided; it makes the urine very alkaline, and speedily dissolves uric acid. In this respect it is

* Berlin. Klin. Woch., 1865.

† Previous to the publication of Garrod's treatise, Dr. Galtier-Bossière had already directed attention to the more intense solvent action of potash, as compared with soda, in the treatment of gout. (De la Goutte, Thèse de Paris, 1859, p. 112.)

very superior to potash, for lithic urate is the most soluble of all the urates.

Garrod bases his views on the following experiment: into three solutions, the first containing 5 centigrams of lithic carbonate; the second, 5 centigrams of potassic carbonate; the third, 5 centigrams of sodic carbonate, to 30 grams of water, throw fragments of the same cartilage impregnated with sodium urate. At the end of forty-eight hours the lithic solution has accomplished complete solution ; the potassic has exerted a very slight action ; the sodic has had no effect at all.

Urate of lithium is, therefore, the most soluble of all the urates.

What will be the mode of action of the alkalis on the blood in gout ? They have no power to lessen the formation of uric acid ; neither can they dissolve it, as has been maintained, for it exists as urate of sodium. But by rendering the tissues alkaline, they may hinder the formation of deposits ; moreover, the carbonates of lithium and potassium would dissolve the deposits already formed, which carbonate of sodium could not do. However, their influence would be useless, had they not at the same time a diuretic action.

That is what theory says ; let us now consult therapeutic experimentation.

The alkalis, especially potash and lithia, administered in small doses and much diluted, for the action of water is very efficacious, and especially administered for a long period of time, have a remarkable action on gout. They defer its paroxysms, they sometimes dissolve and remove the deposits already formed, and give more mobility to the joints.

Carbonate of lithium is administered in doses of 4 or 5 grains during the twenty-four hours. I have myself prescribed a dose of more than 6 grains without producing any unpleasant effect on the stomach.

Stricker[*] has succeeded in causing the tophaceous deposits to disappear in a woman, by giving her an artificial imitation of the waters of Weilbach, according to the following formula :—

Water charged with carbonic acid .... 1 pint.
Bicarbonate of sodium .... 4 grains.
Carbonate of lithium .... 1½ grains.
This quantity represents the daily dose.

[*] Virchow's *Archiv.*, Bd. xxxv.

Schutzenberger has recommended the employment of water charged with protoxide of nitrogen, and containing a gram of lithia per litre (8½ grains to the pint).

By prescribing alkalis according to this method, the system is enabled to tolerate them for several months. No serious inconvenience is caused if the doses we have indicated are kept to.

It is necessary also to be acquainted with the cases in which the alkaline treatment is applicable. It is formally contra-indicated—

1. In persons of advanced age ;
2. In those whose kidneys, being more or less altered, have no longer any power of elimination ;
3. In individuals whose peculiar idiosyncrasy prevents them from bearing alkalis well.

It is not perhaps without use to mention here that the dangers from saturating the blood with alkalis have been much exaggerated, so far, at least, as sodium bicarbonate is concerned. My own experience is opposed to the generally received opinion on this subject. Many a time have I administered sodium bicarbonate to patients with chronic rheumatism in the apparently enormous dose of 20 to 30 grams in the twenty-four hours, sometimes for several months together; and I have never observed the supervention in such cases, either of profound anæmia, or *solution of the blood*, or multiple hemorrhages, which, from the generally received ideas, one might have anticipated. But I have not had the opportunity of directly studying the effects of large doses of potash, and I am quite ignorant of the consequences that might ensue.

We have still to say a few words about mineral waters in the treatment of gout; this will be the natural conclusion of the subject which has just occupied us.

Generally speaking, waters containing much saline matter hasten the attacks, and determine the crisis we want to avoid. Certainly, this is no absolute contraindication, but it is a fact that the physician must always bear in mind, so as not to be taken unawares by the effects of the treatment which he has recommended.

Waters in general are contraindicated in patients with organic affections of the heart and kidneys.

The alkaline springs (Vals, Vichy, Carlsbad, etc.) seem useful at the onset of the disease in robust persons, and especially in those whose livers are affected. But they cannot effect the solution of tophi, and they are not of much use in chronic gout unless dyspepsia exists.

The sulphurous saline (Aix-la-Chapelle) or simply saline (Wiesbaden) waters are suited to the torpid state, to atonic cases.

There are some waters with very little solid matter, which, to employ a favourite term in Germany, I may call *indifferent*, in which the real active principle is the water drunk in large quantity. We may place in this class, at least from our present point of view, Wildbad, Töplitz, Gastein, Bath, Buxton, and Contrexeville. They are often very useful in chronic gout. I have several times seen the waters of Contrexeville ordered in cases of long-standing gout with tophaceous deposits, and the results have seemed favourable.

Lastly, the ferruginous waters (Pyrmont, Schwalbach, Spa) may also be useful in cases where iron is indicated.

We will not go beyond this brief statement of the action of mineral waters in the treatment of gout. If one wanted to give a critical account of all that has been written on this subject, both by the declared partisans of the waters, and by their adversaries, one would easily fill a volume. I need only make the general remark that on both sides there has been much exaggeration.

Going on to *tonics* and *strengthening medicines*, I may point out that they have an indirect action upon gout by modifying the condition of the stomach and increasing the strength. They are very useful in the asthenic forms of gout.

Decoction of ash-leaves (*Fraxinus excelsior*) has been used with success ; its employment is recommended by Pouget and Peyraud. It is prepared as follows :—

Take of ash leaves .... 30 grams.
,,　　water .... 1 litre.

Boil for ten minutes. (About ½ ounce to the pint.)

Garrod has made use of this infusion with some success.

Cinchona and gentian (one of the active principles of *Portland powder*) is also used with benefit.

IV. *Treatment of the local affection, tophi, and rigidity of joints.* Gouty people should be enjoined to take exercise; it helps to remove rigidity, as Sydenham showed. In order to dissolve chalk-stones it has been recommended to bathe the part with potash or lithia; and if the concretions are small and superficial, the skin may be punctured to extract them, especially if they are semi-liquid. But generally when they are large, hard, and deep, all operation must be avoided; ulcers, healing with difficulty, are often the result of such concretions; moreover, it should not be forgotten that under the influence of the least prick, a bad form of erysipelas may come on in gouty persons with renal affections and especially with diabetes.

When spontaneous ulcers have formed, it is the rule to take great care of them.

V. *Treatment of irregular gout.* There is a general agreement in admitting that, when gout has retroceded, especially if to the stomach, recourse must be had to the application of revulsives to the joints; without disputing their good effects, I will point out that there are very few authentic observations adapted to establish the efficacy of this treatment in bringing back the gouty inflammation to the joints. Stimulants, cordials, brandy, are, however, often followed by readily appreciable effects; experience seems to have demonstrated their usefulness.

When we are dealing with *misplaced* gout (migraine, ophthalmia, etc.), colchicum in small doses is indicated, according to Watson, Holland, and some other authors. But this seems to me a subject which is still far from being cleared up.

VI. *Dietetics.* The gouty patient is recommended to take exercise; he should be abstemious in his feeding, but must not carry this too far, lest he should favour the development of atonic gout. You must rigorously forbid him strong beer, and wines rich in alcohol, but you may allow him the light beers, moselle, and bordeaux. He may travel; change of climate is often beneficial, according to the English physicians, who recommend India, Egypt, Malta, and other stations in hot countries; but this would in no way make an observance of dietetic rules unnecessary.

Lastly, one must regulate the mental hygiene, combat the irritability so natural to this class of patients, guard against melancholy, anxiety, and excess of intellectual work.

TREATMENT OF CHRONIC ARTICULAR RHEUMATISM.

The details into which we have been entering make it necessary for us to shorten the latter part of this lecture ; besides, I must say that the treatment of chronic articular rheumatism is still less efficacious than that of gout; we are even less advanced in this respect, and we have not even colchicum to combat the most urgent symptoms of the disease.

In cases in which there are any acute symptoms, the indications for treatment are nearly the same as in acute articular rheumatism. You may prescribe opium, sulphate of quinin, local abstraction of blood, etc., a treatment sometimes successful; but most frequently one is powerless to hinder the progressive course of the disease.

Large doses of alkaline medicines are here less efficacious, according to Garrod, than they are in acute articular rheumatism. This is, however, the treatment in which from my own experience I should have most confidence, and I combine quinin with them. This is of course a purely empirical mode of treatment. I have often prescribed 30 or 40 grams of the carbonate of sodium each day for several weeks with beneficial results. I have never seen symptoms of *solution of the blood* produced, as I remarked when speaking of gout ; on the contrary, patients have seemed to me inclined to gain in weight. By this treatment one at least succeeds in giving them some relief during the febrile exacerbations of the disease.

Tincture of iodin has been extolled by Prof. Lasègue for internal use. The dose was progressively increased from 8 or 10 drops a-day to 5 or 6 grams, taken during meals with a little *eau sucrée*, or better, Spanish wine, as vehicle. The treatment may be continued for several weeks, and if needful, several months. Under its influence none of the symptoms of iodin poisoning have ever been observed.*

Arsenic has been employed by Bardsley and Jenkinson, Begbie, Fuller, and Garrod in England ; by Beau and Guéneau

* *Arch. gén. de méd.*, 1856, vol. ii.

de Mussy in France.* It was especially in treating chronic rheumatism of the large joints that this drug was employed by Bardsley; but the other authors, whom I have just mentioned, employed it especially against nodular rheumatism. I have myself tried this plan of treatment at the Salpêtrière, and, like Garrod, I have sometimes seen arsenic cause great improvement, and at other times fail completely. But I think I can state that arsenic remains without effect, or is even injurious in very inveterate cases of nodular rheumatism, and when the disease has appeared at an advanced age.

One of the first effects of the administration of this drug is often to revive the pains, and to intensify them in the joints usually and most seriously affected. Sometimes, indeed, redness and swelling appear where they did not exist before, and one is obliged to suspend the treatment for a time. But generally a few days bring tolerance of the drug, and then the dose can be progressively increased. It is well, at least in my opinion, to give arsenic in the form of Fowler's solution in a two to six drop dose, and according to the English method, that is, shortly after meals.

In France, where arsenic is given internally, it has also been employed in the form of baths by Guéneau de Mussy and Beau. I made use of this method of treatment myself at the Hôpital Lariboisière, in 1861. M. Ducom, head-pharmacist of that establishment, was good enough to undertake the analysis of the urine of the patients whom I had put under arsenical treatment. In cases of internal administration we found that arsenic appeared in the urine after a short time. In the other class of cases the results were invariably negative. It seems, therefore, pretty clear that these two methods do not act on the system in the same manner, even admitting that they are both equally efficacious in combatting the disease, which I should be disposed to doubt.

There is another drug which I have used in cases of this kind with results analogous to those obtained by arsenic. This is the *ammoniated tincture of guaiacum*, which at first intensifies the local symptoms, and then markedly ameliorates them; the

* Bardsley, *Medical Reports*, London, 1807.—Kellie, *Edin. Med. and Surg. Journ.*, 1808, vol. iii.—J. Begbie (same journal), No. 35, May, 1858.—Fuller, *On Rheumatism*, 2nd ed., London, 1860.—Guéneau de Mussy, *Bull. de therapeutique*, vol. lxvii., 1864, p. 24.—Beau, *Gaz. des hôpitaux*, 19th July, 1864.

mobility of the joints returns occasionally after some time, and the patient experiences manifest relief.

Iodide of potassium has sometimes been prescribed with success against chronic rheumatism.

In chlorotic or debilitated subjects, iron and cod-liver oil may indirectly have a beneficial influence by modifying the general health.

The local measures most employed are blisters, painting with tincture of iodin, and the actual cautery. This last measure is especially useful in the partial form of chronic rheumatism.

As to the mineral waters, those of Mont-Dore, Lamalou l'Ancien, Vals, Néris, Plombières, have been recommended; most of these waters contain arsenic. Is it to this circumstance that the efficacy attributed to them is due?

We are far from having exhausted the long list of remedies that have been extolled against chronic rheumatism by various authors, or which I have myself made trial of. I have endeavoured to bring into prominence those therapeutic measures which seem to me endowed with the most real efficacy; but, it must be admitted, chronic rheumatism is an affection which in the majority of cases, not all the resources of medicine can succeed in curing.

LECTURE XIX.*

SUMMARY.—Importance of clinical thermometry in general.—Its application to the pathology of the aged.—Central algidity.—Normal temperature of old people.—Axillary and rectal thermometry.—Temperature of the aged in disease.—Extreme limits of the central temperature.—Febrile temperatures, low, moderate, and high.—Danger from high temperatures long maintained.—Rational explanation of the danger of this symptom.—Physiological experiments.—Danger from fall of temperature.

GENTLEMEN,—At our previous meetings I endeavoured to make clear to you the very remarkable characters which give to senile pathology a physiognomy of its own. I sought especially to bring into prominence by striking examples the aid obtainable by medicine from the methodic employment of the thermometer, —aid in diagnosis, prognosis, and treatment, when one has to take one's bearings amid the innumerable dangers which threaten the physician who practises among old people. To-day I intend to resume this study, adding some further particulars, which the form of my previous lectures was too concise to enable me to give you.

To-day it is no longer necessary to consume much eloquence in favour of the clinical use of the thermometer; the method has made its way and has spread almost everywhere. This was hardly the case when, in 1863, we applied it to every-day practice in this hospital; and perhaps there is still some need to show that it is a method not adapted exclusively for scientific researches.

Clinical thermometry is of course a physical method of exploration in the same sense as auscultation and percussion; only, whilst the latter are specially applicable to local lesions, the former deals with the fundamental symptom of the febrile state, of which it may be said to supply a measure.† What, then, is fever? To this question all the authors still reply by Galen's definition: *Calor præter naturam.* For, in point of fact, all the other symptoms of fever may be absent; the rise of animal temperature is the only invariable necessary fact.

Such is the law—a general law, from which old people them-

---

* The three next lectures, reported by Dr. Joffroy, are printed in the original as an Appendix, On the importance of thermometry in the treatment of the aged.—*Transl.*

† Wunderlich, *Verhalten der Eigenwärme in Krankheiten.* Leipzig, 1868.

selves do not escape. For, gentlemen, that isolation of the organs, that want of general reaction, which I pointed out to you in my former lectures, are only apparent. As in the infant and in the adult, fever, or at least elevation of the temperature of the body, occurs in old persons, and it often acquires in them an almost equal intensity ; only, in the latter more often than in the former, it may remain latent, that is to say, may not reveal itself by the external symptoms which usually accompany it. But we must know how, with the aid of the thermometer, to seek for the manifestation of it in the central regions of the body.

It is particularly when we are dealing with diseases in which the temperature rises above the normal that I can make evident to you how important is the use of the thermometer ; there are, however, especially in the old, a certain number of affections which give rise to the inverse phenomenon, causing a real lowering of the temperature. Now, this central algidity can only be certainly recognised with the help of the thermometer, which here, too, may be called on to render great services. This is a subject still little explored, but which, I hope, will nevertheless give me the opportunity of pointing out some important facts.

I.

Before entering into the detail of our subject we must establish some preliminary points.

A. *Normal temperature in the old.* You are not unaware that in old persons the respiratory function is diminished, a fact shown by the diminution in the quantity of carbonic acid exhaled, by the increase in the number of respirations, and by the decided reduction of the vital capacity of the lungs. It is admitted also that the nutritive actions of integration and disintegration are likewise diminished at this time of life ; but I am not aware that any decisive researches have been undertaken on this last point. However this may be, gentlemen, it is a remarkable fact that, in spite of these evidently unfavourable circumstances, *the temperature undergoes no appreciable modification with the progress of age ;* $37\cdot2^\circ$, $37\cdot5^\circ$, rarely 38° ($98\cdot9^\circ$, $99\cdot5^\circ$, $100\cdot4^\circ$ F.), in the rectum, and sometimes a little less,

Q

sometimes a little more than 1° (1·8° F.) below these figures in
the axilla,—such, according to the very numerous researches
which I have made on the subject, are the normal temperatures
in old age, up to the extreme limits of life.

De Haen formerly, and in these latter times Von Baerensprung,
have maintained that in very old people the temperature is higher
than that represented by the above figures.   I think this is only
the case in exceptional circumstances.   I showed at one of these
meetings, three years ago, a woman of more than a hundred,
who enjoyed excellent health ; her axillary temperature was
habitually 37·4° (99·3° F.), and her rectal temperature 38°
(100·4° F.).   Since then I have rarely met with this temperature
of 38° in normal health, even in individuals who have reached
the last limits of old age.

Thus, to sum up, the internal temperature is the same in the
aged as in the adult ; I will add that it presents in both cases
the same invariability, and that it only rises decidedly, though
temporarily, in a condition of disease.

How shall we explain the fact that in the old the normal temperature is found at least as high as in the adult, although in
old age the nutritive functions are evidently less active ?   No
doubt the chief cause is the state of the skin in the former, for
its blood-capillary network is notably less rich, and its secre-
tory activity is at the same time much less than in the adult ;
the aged probably produce less heat than do adults, but they
lose less, both from the skin and from pulmonary passages, and
thus compensation is established.

B. *Axillary and rectal thermometry in the aged.*   I could not
leave the subject which we have just considered without saying
a few words to you about the use of the axilla for the thermometer in old people, compared with the use of the natural
cavities, and especially of the rectum.   You will often hear me
speak of the rectal temperature, and it is in fact this natural
cavity that I always prefer for my thermometric explorations in
aged subjects.   I must point out to you the reasons which from
the commencement of my studies on this subject, that is, for
nearly seven years, have led me to this choice, which at first
sight might appear rather odd.

It is easy to prove, gentlemen, and every one admits, that the
temperature taken in the axilla is always below that indicated

by rectal observation. The axilla, so far as temperature goes, is like the surface of the body; the rectum represents the internal viscera. In the adult the difference in temperature between these two localities, besides being in general very slight, maintains almost always the same proportion. But this is not the case in old people, where the discrepancy is sometimes considerable (more than a degree [C.] for example), sometimes much less marked, according to the most varied circumstances. Thus in old age the internal temperature alone is constant; the axillary temperature is, on the contrary, extremely variable, like the outer skin, though to a less degree.

But it is especially in disease, and particularly in the febrile state, that the discrepancy between the central and the external temperature in old age most markedly shows itself. Here is a diagram relating to a case of lobar pneumonia in a woman of 65 ; you see that the curves for the rectal temperatures and those for the axillary temperatures, although nearly parallel in the greater part of their course, yet separate from one another at several points in the most irregular manner. You see, indeed, that on several occasions the oscillations presented by the two tracings are in opposite directions. Thus, on the morning of the fifth day of the disease, when the temperature in the armpit was only 37° (98·6° F.), that in the rectum rose to 40·2° (104·3° F.), a difference of more than three degrees. In the evening the two curves approached each other, and the difference was not more than a degree. On the sixth day there is a point where the two tracings almost touch each other ; but next day they are very decidedly separated again. In this patient there had been uncontrollable diarrhœa, and on several occasions symptoms of collapse indicated by very marked chilling of the skin. I shall have to return later to the signification of these symptoms of collapse, which it is common enough to observe during the acute diseases of old persons ; at present I will only point out that the striking disagreement which we find in this case, taken as an example, between the data supplied by the axillary and rectal tracings, is very often met with clinically in aged patients.

This is the chief reason which has led me to prefer in practice an observation in the rectum to one in the axilla ; there is another, very secondary doubtless, which would certainly not have determined my choice, but which is not devoid of all value. To obtain accurate information from an observation in the axilla, fifteen minutes at least are necessary, especially in the aged. After an average of five minutes, on the contrary, the mercurial column of a thermometer placed in the rectum ceases to oscillate. So that rectal thermometry, you see, has a marked advantage over the other mode of observation from its rapidity of execution, a point not to be despised in the practice of a large hospital.

I shall say nothing to you about the very natural repugnance which patients often show to this mode of exploration, for persuasion almost always succeeds in smoothing away this difficulty.

C. *The temperature of the body in old people in disease.*

1. *Extreme limits of the internal temperature above and below the normal.* In clinical thermometry, gentlemen, there are a certain number of fundamental facts, the reality of which has been many times verified, and which one might almost put forward as axioms. I will state some of these leading facts.

If the internal temperature at any period whatever of a malady, and in whatever disease, reaches 41·5° (106·7° F.), the danger is great. If it reaches 41·75° or 42° (107·1°, 107·6° F.), death is certain. These figures, given by Wunderlich with special reference to the pathology of the adult, have, I am sure, an equal significance in the old; but it may be said that in the latter the situation is already exceedingly critical at 41° C. (105·8° F.).

If the elevation of the central temperature above a certain point is enough by itself, and independently of concomitant circumstances, to give warning of very great danger, fall of temperature below the normal, when it reaches a certain point, 35° (95° F.) for example (I only guarantee this figure for the aged), also shows that the case is a very grave one.

You see, gentlemen, that there are almost constant limits which the temperature apparently cannot exceed without the existence of the patient being very much endangered. Temperatures which overstep these two limits are rare and exceptional, and they indicate with certainty a fatal termination.

You cannot help seeing already that thermometry furnishes

us, at least with regard to prognosis, with a sign of the highest importance, for *its signification* may be regarded as *absolute*. I shall have many opportunities of pointing out to you applications which are quite as remarkable.

2. *Low, moderate, and elevated febrile temperatures in the old.* Speaking generally, it may be said that in the old, as in the adult, a temperature a little above 38° (100·4° F.) corresponds to slight fever (subfebrile temperature) ; below 39·5° (103·1° F.), it is of moderate intensity ; between 39·5° and 40° (104° F.) it is intense ; above 40° it is very intense (*hyperpyrexia*).

These facts, like the preceding, are as applicable to old people as to adults, for in regard to the point which the temperature may reach, the former are in no way behind the latter. This is a point which I endeavoured to establish some time ago, and my later researches have only confirmed it.

But, gentlemen,—it is important you should note this,—when I establish an identity between the febrile temperatures of the adult and the aged, I am only speaking of healthy subjects, or rather of those who are free from any previous disease, or cachectic state, at the time when the fever appeared ; for it is certain that in previously debilitated persons, *whatever their age*, the temperature (even in the case of a disease which usually gives rise to intense fever) may not rise during the whole course of the affection above medium febrile temperatures—39°, 39·5° (102·2°, 103·1° F.), although the case is of the gravest and terminates in death. But I repeat, and this is a point of the highest importance in my opinion, this relative weakness of the thermic reaction is not a characteristic of senility.

In a woman of 75, feeble and cachectic, suffering from lobar pneumonia, the maxima at the height of the disease did not exceed 39·5° but once. In another case of pneumonia which came on in a woman of about 50, and hence relatively young, but suffering from very advanced uterine cancer, and profoundly cachectic, the maxima never reached 40° ; they stopped at 39·5°, or less. This patient, like the preceding one, succumbed *during defervescence*, which is the most frequent occurrence in cases of this kind. You see how these observations in subjects of very different age are nevertheless analogous in all respects.

Look now at the counterpart of this behaviour. The three

tracings which I now show you* relate to three patients, the
first of whom is a child of 3 (Ziemssen), the second a man of
38 (Wunderlich), the third a woman of 75 (Salpêtrière); all
three relate to lobar pneumonia; as you see, there are striking
analogies between them, and you would have great difficulty,
if you were not told beforehand, in distinguishing one from
another. Thus, when Wunderlich (*loc. cit.*) maintains that by
simple inspection of a thermometric tracing, the age of the
patient can be recognised, because in old age the maxima remain
at a relatively low point, the proposition does not appear to me
to be perfectly accurate. But, nevertheless, one could recognise
in this way whether it were the case of a robust subject, or, on
the contrary, of a previously debilitated individual.

3. *Danger of high temperatures maintained for several days
in the aged.* Here is now a third point : a hyperpyretic temperature, 40·5° (104·9° F.), may occur, and yet the case not be
serious, provided it only persists at this level for a very short
space of time, as in an attack of intermittent fever, for example,
or abortive pneumonia. But if such temperatures are maintained for several days together almost without interruption, as
occurs in a disease of continued type—lobar pneumonia, for
example—the case is very serious. What I state is founded on
the numerous observations which I have been able to make on
this subject in the case of the pneumonia of the aged ; but it
seems proved that the same thing holds at the other periods of
life. However this may be, death has supervened in most of
the cases of lobar pneumonia observed at the Salpêtrière, in
which during the course of the disease the maxima several times
exceeded 40·5° ; and, on the contrary, when they stopped at 40°
or under, recovery has been frequent.

Do not conclude from this that all the cases of pneumonia in
old age, when the temperature remains at a relatively low point,
are favourable. Far from this, you already know that a large
number, perhaps the majority, of *pneumonias of low temperature*,
as we generally call them, are remarkable for their fatality,
But this is a point to which we shall have to return several
times in the sequel.

* We have not thought it needful to insert these three tracings in the text.

II.

You have seen the thoroughly practical importance of the facts which have just been stated; but we are only acquainted with them so far as the result of a purely empirical study without theoretical pre-considerations. The interest you already feel in them would certainly be still greater if we were able to penetrate their physiological rationale. Wherefore these narrow limits traced on the scale of the thermometer, which cannot be reached without life being very seriously endangered, and beyond which there is no longer any hope of saving the patient? Why is it that when the temperature rises to a point much within these limits, but remains thus for several days without decided remissions, does it tell us that the case is grave, no matter what the name of the disease?

Such are the questions which will have occurred to your minds. We cannot in the present state of science give them a definite, accurate answer; but we may hope at least, depending on physiology and experimental pathology, to recognise in what direction the solution may be found.

Let us make it clear in the first place that this disturbance of the whole economy, which is called fever, is a danger in itself when it is intense, independently of the cause which produced it. A patient is attacked with pneumonia; the respiratory functions are not more disturbed than is usual in such a case; there are no complications, and yet the patient succumbs in an intensely febrile state. The autopsy is performed, and reveals the existence of a lobar hepatisation which auscultation had recognised during life, but which has remained limited to so small an extent of a pulmonary lobe, that it is impossible to admit that the local lesion accounts in this case for the fatal issue. It will be enough· for me to have quoted this example, for, thanks to the progress of morbid anatomy, we can no longer believe with Hoffmann that the autopsy always discloses a gross organic lesion in some organ, which accounts for death. We must then look to the general state—that kind of general state which we call fever; but what element of this general disturbance of the system is to be specially blamed?

This leads us to a digression.

The febrile state, with its crowd of symptoms, some fundamental and essential, others accessory—elevation of temperature, acceleration of pulse, nervous disturbance, and the rest—is the result of phenomena that are very complex, but which may be referred to a few principal heads.

The starting-point seems to be a rapid metamorphosis, or rather an exaggerated combustion, of blood and tissues, which goes on almost everywhere throughout the organism, and which has been set up by a morbid poison or some other cause.

The elevation of the internal temperature is one of the perceptible results of the intimate chemical processes which constitute this exaggerated combustion.

The products of this combustion, the organic ashes, *urea and extractives*, accumulate in the blood and circulate with it. Sooner or later they must necessarily be got rid of by the natural emunctories, for the organism has no room for them.

Moreover, in cases of fever with local affection, certain disturbances resulting from the abnormal functioning of the affected organ are superadded to the general disorder giving rise to the fever. Thus in double pneumonia and capillary bronchitis, oxygenation of blood being seriously impeded, there may be *anoxæmia* with accumulation of carbonic acid in the blood; or if it is a case of acute parenchymatous hepatitis (acute yellow atrophy of the liver), then in consequence of the rapid destruction of the secreting elements of the organ, the materials destined to form bile will be retained in the blood, and there will be *acholia*.

But I don't want to enter into details; I will restrict myself to the most general facts.

Whence then comes the danger of fever?

The rapid consumption of the tissues, manifesting itself by more or less marked emaciation, by diminution of body-weight, and by prostration of strength, cannot be regarded as the chief element at any rate, except in diseases of chronic development. It could not take a leading part in a fever of rapid course like that determined by the lobar pneumonia which we took just now as an example.

The presence in the system of organic *débris*, the products of the febrile combustion, is also no doubt a serious danger in cases where excretion of these products is badly performed. Here, in fact, are the conditions of *auto-toxæmia*, for these products in certain doses are for the most part deleterious. But this self-poisoning, like the cholæmia and anoxæmia which we spoke of just now, can only occur in certain peculiar cases to which I shall allude presently. It is indicated, moreover, by special symptoms, which do not necessarily accompany the febrile state, even when most intense. The elevation of the temperature is still to be considered. Might it be that the organs and tissues, exposed for a time to these extreme temperatures to which your attention has been directed, would undergo at a certain point such profound modifications of their material condition as to render their functional activity impossible? According to this hypothesis the elevation of temperature in fever would be not only a resultant, a symptom; it would be the cause of disturbances sometimes sufficiently serious to lead to death.

The laity, who know scarcely anything of fever but the febrile heat, admit without difficulty " that an intense fever may carry off the patient." This popular opinion, gentlemen, must not be treated with too much disdain; for it has been to a certain extent embraced by masters in our art—Sydenham, Boerhaave, Van Swieten. In our own days it has been taken up again, and, as it were, restored to youth by several worthy authors— Liebermeister* in Germany, and Richardson in England; and the arguments which these physicians have put forward in its favour appear to me worthy to be taken into serious consideration.†

The most solid of these arguments are those furnished by experiment. You are aware that in man, as in animals, the central temperature can be artificially raised, and consequently a condition at any rate very analogous to the febrile state produced. The disturbances caused when the temperature of the body has been thus raised to a certain level above the normal recall the symptoms of fever: thus the pulse quickens, the respiratory movements grow more rapid; inexpressible malaise comes on, with headache, various nervous disturbances, at first excitement, then great prostration of strength; and when, in the case of animals, the experiment is pushed very far, coma supervenes, then general resolution, and soon death.

* *Ueber die Wirkung der febrilen Temperatursteigerung. Deutches Archiv*, Band i., 1866.—Niemeyer, *Spec. Pathol.*, 7th ed., 1868.

† *Med. Times*, May, 1869.

True, it is known from the celebrated experiments of Blagden and Dobson that men may be exposed to very elevated temperatures, even for a longish time, without any very remarkable disturbance of their condition being caused ; thus Richardson has recently borne without inconvenience a bath of hot air at a temperature of 212° F. for nearly twenty minutes. But this is only possible on the express condition that during the experiment the *internal temperature shall not rise above a certain point*, not far above the normal. In such a case, as you are aware, the pulmonary surface and the skin lose an enormous amount of heat, thus maintaining the equilibrium ; moreover, such experiments are only possible in dry air. They are extremely perilous if use is made of a bath of water raised to from 40° to 44° (104° to 111·2° F.), or indeed of damp air, even when the temperature does not rise above 40° or 45° ; for then the temperature of the body has been found to rise to 39°, 40°, even 41° (102·2°, 104°, 105·8° F.), as in a case observed by Bartels, and at the same time serious symptoms have almost immediately appeared, and have caused some apprehension of an unfortunate issue.

It is, moreover, under very similar conditions that one meets with the formidable accident, so well known to the physicians of the English army in India under the name of *sun-stroke*, *heat-stroke*, and which is even observed in our own climate when an army is on the march in hot damp weather ; the poor men affected by sun-stroke are sometimes almost literally thunder-struck, and cases of this kind are reported where the central temperature had risen at the moment of death to 44° C. (111·2° F.).

But let us come back to the experiments, and consider the case where experimentation is pushed to the last limits. Of course we are here dealing with animals. Now, gentlemen, death always occurs in such a case when the internal temperature has exceeded the normal for the animal experimented on by 4° or 5° C. (about 45° C. (113° F.) for mammals), and it occurs quite suddenly. So there is, you see, for each species of animal a fatal figure not to be reached without death ensuing.

This recalls what we just now found to occur in man in a state of disease. You have not forgotten that at about 42° in the adult (that is, when the normal has been exceeded by about

5°), and a little below this in the aged, death is certain, necessary; thence it becomes at least very probable that in this latter case, as in the case of the animals submitted to experiment, the extreme elevation of the central temperature has been the main cause of the fatal termination.

But what is the mechanism of death in these cases? The experiments of Claude Bernard * and Calliburcès, repeated by Panum, prove that it is especially the heart that suffers; at first excited in its action, it ceases to beat at about 45°. The organ presents no gross lesions; but its tissue has undergone profound modifications, for muscular rigidity like that of the cadaver has been caused, and the return of its movements under the influence of excitants, even for a time, has become thenceforth impossible.

The blood also presents marked changes in its constitution; sometimes it is very fluid, sometimes, on the contrary, coagulated; according to Richardson the former condition occurs when death has been very rapid; the latter, on the other hand, when it has occurred a longer time after the commencement of the experiment.

This is the place to remind you that in cases of disease observed in man where death has come on rapidly after a considerable rise of temperature, the blood has been found sometimes in a state of extreme fluidity, sometimes, on the contrary, coagulated in the cardiac cavities. Boerhaave supposed that coagulation of blood in the vessels is one cause of death in fever, and quite recently Weikart has tried to prove that this is to be regarded as the cause of death when the temperature rises to about 42° (107·6° F.).

The preceding facts all relate to cases in which death supervenes after extreme elevation of the internal temperature. As to those in which the febrile heat is maintained at a lower, though still very high, point for a considerable period, we can no longer rely upon the facts of experimental physiology, experimentation having never been directed to this particular subject. But certain facts may be mentioned which tend to show that here again elevation of temperature may give rise to serious symptoms and be itself a cause of danger.

* See the recent researches of Bernard on the influence of heat on animals, *Revue scientifique*, 19th year, 1871, No. 8.

First, notice that, as Liebermeister pointed out, the majority of febrile affections of whatever nature, in which the temperature remains for a considerable time more or less permanently at an elevated point, have an almost constant character in common. It is this, that after death certain organs present changes of their tissue which have sometimes been spoken of as *steatose*. The liver, the voluntary muscles, the kidneys, and above all the heart, undergo this morbid change. I shall only particularise here the more or less marked softening which we may find in this organ in typhoid fever (Louis), and according to Stokes in typhus. With these lesions symptoms of cardiac weakness, of asystole, are usually associated during life. Will it do to refer these changes, those of the heart especially, and the disorders consequent upon them, to the persistence of high temperature? One would be inclined to admit this, judging by the way in which extreme temperatures act on the tissue of the heart.

Moreover, we know that the extreme acceleration of the pulse, which in cases of this kind is a most inauspicious sign, is, up to a certain point, proportional to the rise of temperature.

But here is a rather more direct argument; it is drawn from the indisputable advantages of what is called antipyretic treatment, applied to acute diseases with high temperature. Now, what is the most striking effect, at once the most constant and the best established, of the different modes of applying this treatment? It is, more or less markedly and for a longer or shorter time, to lower the internal temperature, even at the height of the febrile process. This is how digitalis and veratria act in pneumonia, and sulphate of quinin in acute rheumatism; this also is the mode of action of prolonged and often repeated cool baths, employed latterly in Germany with so much enthusiasm in the treatment of typhoid fever, and which seem to have given results really worthy of attention (Brand, Jurgensen, Liebermeister, Gerhardt).

After what precedes, I think I may offer you this conclusion, *that the elevation of the internal temperature is in itself a danger*, not as a rigorously demonstrated truth, but as a very probable hypothesis.

But, for a moment, let us leave fever and rise of temperature on one side; let us consider briefly the movement of the thermometer in the opposite direction : in other words, let us try to see why the lowering of the temperature to a certain point below the normal level is almost necessarily followed by death. Has the chilling of the interior of the body in a case of this kind an action upon the organs and tissues, capable of diminishing the energy of the organic processes necessary to the maintenance of life? It can hardly be questioned, gentlemen, that this is really the case.

If an animal is exposed under certain conditions to the action of a low temperature, to complete inanition, to poisoning by substances such as opium, ammonia, hydrocyanic acid; if its body is covered with an impermeable coating, as in the experiments of Fourcault and Edenhuizen, the central temperature always sinks, and at the same time the respiratory movements grow feeble, the absorption of oxygen and exhalation of carbonic acid diminish.* If the experiment is pushed very far, the temperature sinks to a certain point, beyond which death occurs. Now, what happens in these very varied circumstances ? It may be said that the animal *dies of cold*. It dies of cold, for artificial warming always postpones the fatal termination, or even allows a complete return to life, under favourable conditions.

Thus, gentlemen, both theory and experiment indicate that heat and cold of body, reaching a certain point, are matters of the first importance, which it is necessary to take into consideration, not only to guide our prognosis in a given case of disease, but also to regulate the administration of therapeutic agents.

But I perceive rather late that the digression into which I have entered has led me a long way, and it is time to return from it to senile pathology.

It is not enough to have recognised the fact that in old age the rise or fall of internal temperature to a certain level has the same meaning as at other periods of life; we must now show that in the course of certain diseases, oscillations of temperature carefully recorded from day to day, from hour to hour, in the form of graphic tracings, have constant and characteristic types for each of these diseases in old age, as I have shown them to have in adult life; for the diagnosis of febrile diseases by

* Valentin, *Arch. für physiol. Heilk.*, 1858, p. 433.

temperature, of which so much has been said just lately, is based on this very circumstance. You will recognise, as I have done, that these specific types undergo no notable modifications in old age. They remain in the aged what they were in the adult, at least in their essential characters. In the next lecture I shall endeavour to establish this assertion on fresh data. This will afford us an opportunity of reviewing from our special point of view the affections which give rise to fever in the aged.

LECTURE XX.

SUMMARY.—Thermic characters of febrile diseases in old people.—Febrile diseases of continued type.—Febrile diseases of remittent type.—Febrile diseases of intermittent type. Rapid rise of the central temperature at the time of death in certain diseases of the nervous centres.—Tetanus.—Epi'epsy.—Hysteria.—Hemorrhage and cerebral softening.—Epileptiform and apoplectiform attacks.

GENTLEMEN,—In closing our last meeting, I told you that the fundamental characters of the thermometric curves are not notably modified by age. Let me justify this assertion by taking some examples from the *typical* febrile diseases that are met with in the old. These diseases may be arranged in three groups, according as the type of fever is continued, remittent, or intermittent.

§ I. *Thermic characters of the typical febrile diseases in old age.*

1. *Febrile diseases of continued type.* They are much less numerous than in the adult; the eruptive fevers are absent; but I have occasionally observed variola at the Salpêtrière ; in most of the cases that I have seen, it has assumed the hemorrhagic form with collapse. In these cases the patients usually presented a remarkable lowering of the central temperature, a *real algidity*, well worthy of your attention, and of which I intend to treat in the next lecture.

The chief malady in this group is *lobar* pneumonia, which, spite of the statement to the contrary of several authors, is observed in the aged more frequently than broncho-pneumonia.

a. The disease generally commences with a rigor (it is a mistake to say that the aged do not shiver much). At the same time the extremities grow cold. This *pyrogenetic* period is marked by a *sudden rise* of the thermometric tracing; by the second day the temperature will have risen to 40°, for example (104° F.). This character is alone sufficient to distinguish the affection from those of the following group, in which the rise is slow and progressive.

b. When the disease is established, the temperature, having reached a certain level, remains almost stationary for some days. I must, however, mention the diurnal variations, which take place within tolerably narrow limits, and do not exceed a degree (C.). In this part of its course the curve sometimes shows a progressive tendency to rise, and then the case is serious; sometimes a tendency to sink, occasionally indicating a favourable issue, but only if the rest of the symptoms do not become aggravated.

The regular course of the curve may be modified by various circumstances; at present I will only mention to you the modifications resulting from the employment of drugs.

c. The third period will give a different kind of curve, according as the issue is to be favourable or fatal.

In the former case you will observe a period of favourable defervescence, sometimes preceded by a temporary exacerbation of all the symptoms, and a sudden rise of the curve. This corresponds to what the ancients spoke of as *perturbatio critica*. This aggravation of the symptoms is of short duration in cases which are about to end in recovery; it does not last more than a few hours. Then defervescence takes place, usually in a very rapid manner; the curve descends without a break, thus recalling, though the direction is reversed, the sudden change of temperature which marked the onset. In this rapid fall you may not unfrequently notice *subnormal* temperatures, accompanied by the symptoms of *collapse*, to which we shall return anon. But soon the curve rises again to the normal level, and remains there permanently. Convalescence has begun in spite of the persistence of the local symptoms.

It is generally after the commencement of defervescence that the critical phenomena, of which the ancients thought so much, may be observed. Thermometry here shows itself superior to the old method of observation, since the final lowering of temperature precedes the appearance of the critical phenomena. Observe, by the way, that these phenomena are less frequent in the aged than in the adult. Very rarely they consist of epistaxis or sweats; generally they show themselves as diarrhœa, or more often by the passing of abundant or turbid urine.

When the issue of the case is to be fatal, a sudden rise of temperature is often observed, which I have noticed to go on increasing even after death. This is much the most common case in the adult. It is also what occurs in old people who have been in good health, whilst in those who are feeble, death most frequently comes on during defervescence. In this bad kind of defervescence the temperature does not generally descend so low as in the auspicious form of defervescence. We shall see in the next lecture by what characters we may make out whether the end is, or is not, to be favourable, in a case where defervescence is occurring towards the close of lobar pneumonia.

2. *Febrile diseases of remittent type.* Lobular or catarrhal pneumonia here takes the first place ; it is, however, as I have said, much less common in the aged than has been maintained.

In the period of invasion, the rise of temperature is slow and jerky. When the disease is fully established, the diurnal oscillations are considerable, and generally exceed a degree centigrade ; lastly, no critical phenomena are observed at the time of defervescence.

As to typhoid fever and acute catarrhal phthisis, which are among the most important forms of this group in the adult, they are almost completely absent in the old.

3. *Febrile diseases of intermittent type.* At the Salpêtrière marsh fever is very rare, and I am not sure that I have ever observed it. But, on the other hand, we frequently meet in this hospital with intermittent fevers which are symptomatic of affections of the urinary passages or biliary canals. These symptomatic fevers may be distinguished from the paludal intermittent fevers by means of certain symptoms, and considering their frequency, they seem to me to fully merit the attention which I shall devote to them in some of our next meetings.*

§ II. *On the rapid and considerable rise of central temperature which comes on at the time of death in certain diseases of the nervous centres.*

Hitherto I have only had the febrile diseases in view ; but in the course of other diseases one may notice at a certain period the sudden occurrence of an enormous rise of the internal temperature. Allow me to stop a few moments, in order that we may study this phenomenon, which is still little understood, but

* The recent thesis of Dr. Magnin contains the substance of these lectures, *De quelques accidents de la lithiase biliaire.* Paris, 1869.

is well worthy of your attention, if only on account of its importance in prognosis.

Profound coma, sometimes, but rarely, preceded by delirium ; very great acceleration of the pulse; contracted pupils; occasionally tonic or clonic convulsions ; rapid development of sores on the buttocks ; these are the symptoms which usually accompany this rise of internal temperature. It rapidly reaches 41°, 42°, sometimes more (105·8°, 107·6° F.) ; it may rise still further in the moments which follow death.

It is to be inquired whether, in cases of this kind, the ordinary process of fever must be called in to explain the production of these high temperatures. Wunderlich says, rather vaguely however, that in these cases "the products of tissue-metamorphosis do not appear in the urine in excess." In two cases of tetanus observed in the horse, Senator says he has only found a small proportion of urea in the urine.*

What is certain is, that in all these cases the nervous system is profoundly affected. It is diseases such as *tetanus* (traumatic or non-traumatic) and *epilepsy* of essential nature which give us the type of this final rise of temperature.

These two diseases are associated with tonic convulsions, and it is generally after repeated fits that the rise of temperature takes place ; nevertheless, we cannot assume the muscular contraction as the cause of this considerable increase of heat; for in ordinary cases, whether of tetanus or epilepsy, the most intense convulsions only produce a comparatively slight increase of temperature (A. Monti, *Beiträge zur Thermometrie des Tetanus. Centralblatt*, 1869, No. 44). It is then rare for the thermometer to reach 39° (102·2° F.). On the other hand, in cases where this very marked elevation is noticed, the convulsions have sometimes ceased for a long time, and have given place to more or less profound coma. Some cases of *hysteria*, or at least of *hysteriform affections*, with or without convulsions, have also been mentioned as ending in death, and exhibiting this final elevation of temperature.

A general fact is that in none of the cases in question does one find, either in the nervous centres or the viscera, any recent

* Quite recently, in a case of tetanus in man with rise of central temperature and ending in death, Senator found the excretion of urea below the normal. (Virchow's *Archiv*, Oct., 1869.)

structural change capable of accounting for the final symptoms and the rise of temperature. You are aware that in *general paralysis* of the insane attacks are pretty frequently observed, which are sometimes apoplectiform and accompanied by more or less persistent paralysis, sometimes epileptiform and followed by coma. The researches of Westphal have shown that a quarter of an hour or an hour after these attacks the temperature rises to about 39°, whether or no there have been convulsions. It sinks rapidly if the case is a favourable one; but if death is to ensue, it remains high, or even rises farther. At the autopsy you do not find any other lesions than those of diffuse periencephalitis. In some cases, however, the existence of pulmonary indurations of recent formation has been noted, but in the majority nothing has turned up to explain the closing symptoms.

I should not have mentioned these facts, gentlemen, which belong to mental pathology, did they not find their analogies in the affections which belong more particularly to the domain of senile pathology. We have, indeed, in our wards a great number of patients affected for considerable periods with hemiplegia, which has followed hemorrhage or softening of the brain. Now, it is not uncommon in these cases to notice the appearance of a condition which is marked by attacks sometimes of apoplectiform, sometimes of epileptiform, character, and recurring at varying intervals. There is the greatest analogy, with regard both to form and consequences, between these attacks and the corresponding symptoms of paralysis of the insane. Death may occur during the attacks or after them, as in diffuse periencephalitis, and in such cases a rapid and very marked rise of the central temperature is observed. Now, however much care is devoted to the autopsy, it is impossible to discover, either in the nervous centres or the viscera, any *recent* lesion of a kind to explain the grave symptoms which have led to death. You find only the old lesions (hemorrhagic or softened patches) on which the hemiplegia depended, and the secondary degenerations of crus, pons, and cord, which result from the morbid changes in the hemispheres. I think it will be useful to show you as examples two diagrams relating to cases of this kind.*

The first refers to a woman of 32 years of age, affected with

* It has not been thought needful to reproduce these diagrams.— *Transl.*

incomplete hemiplegia of the right side, dating from infancy,
with atrophy and shortening of the paralysed limbs, as generally
happens in such a case. She was subject to epileptic attacks.
After a more violent fit than usual she was brought to the
infirmary. The rectal temperature was 38° (100·4° F.) on the
day of admission. The fits ran into one another, and recurred
about a hundred times a day; between them was more or less
profound coma ; sores formed rapidly on the buttocks, and the
patient died on the sixth day.

The central temperature rose each day, reaching 42·2° (108° F.)
on the day of death. At the autopsy were found a considerable depression of the encephalon on the left side, an
extensive yellow patch, and atrophy of the whole hemisphere on
this side. There was no recent lesion either in the nervous
centres or in the viscera.

The second case is that of a woman aged 61, with right
hemiplegia due to a cerebral hemorrhage two years before. This
woman had already had several epileptiform attacks, generally
quite slight. One day a violent and prolonged epileptiform fit
came on, and was followed by an apoplectiform condition. Two
hours after the onset the rectal temperature was 38·6° (101·5° F.);
five hours later it rose to 40° (104° F.). Next day, *although the
convulsions had ceased*, the temperature was 41°, and the day
after, the day of death, it reached 42·5° (108·5° F.). At
the autopsy two yellowish foci were found, one in the corpus
striatum, the other in the substance of a convolution. But there
was no recent lesion capable of explaining the symptoms.

Presently I shall make clear to you the clinical usefulness of
the thermometer in cases of this kind; I shall show you that the
results which it gives may furnish indications of great value, not
only in prognosis but also in diagnosis. But I have not yet
concluded the list of affections of the nervous centres, in which
high temperatures are met with at death. I proceed to affections
in which there are recent lesions, beginning with those of a
traumatic nature.

Since Brodie's celebrated case, a considerable number of
analogous observations have been published (quite lately by
Fischer, Naunyn, and Quincke). This was a case in which the
spinal cord was crushed on account of a dislocation of the 5th
and 6th cervical vertebræ, and in which a temperature of

43·7° (110·7°) was observed. In a lecture given in England some years ago, Brown-Séquard had already collected some of these cases, and their analysis led him to this important conclusion, that elevation of temperature indicates a grave central lesion, whilst if the cord is simply irritated, the body is found to cool. Lately Dr. Fischer has made the same distinction.

It is not only lesions of the cord, moreover, that may have these consequences. Billroth has seen death follow rapidly after a fracture of the skull without external wound ; the internal temperature had risen to 40·9° (105·6°).

We meet with the same thing in severe non-traumatic lesions of the encephalon, caused by hemorrhage or ramollissement. I have shown by repeated observations that as a general rule death is preceded in these cases, as in the preceding, by a sudden elevation of temperature, possibly reaching 40° or 41°. Thermometric observation here aids us in making a prognosis, for, as a rule, the temperature does not exceed, or only slightly exceeds, the normal level in apoplexy, which depends on hemorrhage or cerebral softening of recent date, when there is no inflammatory complication; hence sudden rise of temperature is in such a case an indication of most unfavourable augury.* So far, I have only met with very few exceptions to this rule.

As I have indicated, there is a thermic character by which apoplexy with or without convulsions, resulting from a recent lesion (hemorrhage or softening), may be distinguished from those apoplectiform or epileptiform attacks which sometimes supervene in long-standing cases of hemiplegia. In the latter case, in fact, the temperature always rises more or less from the beginning,† whilst in true apoplexy dependent on cerebral softening or hemorrhage of recent occurrence, there is at the commencement an almost constant fall of temperature below the normal.

What is the physiological explanation of the phenomena which I have just described ? Wunderlich and Erb, who were the first to direct attention to this subject, have admitted as an explanation that certain parts of the nervous system have

---

* *Mémoires de la Société de biologie*, vol. iv., 4th series, 1867, p. 92.

† The comatose state which brings to a close most cases of cerebral tumour is also accompanied by a sudden rise of the central temperature; I have seen this occur several times, and it is shown by a case reported by Ladame, *Symptomatologie und Diagnostik der Hirngeschwülste.* Wurzburg, 1865, p. 164.

normally an inhibitory [*modératrice*] influence on the sources of bodily heat. Now if these supposed inhibitory centres happen to be profoundly injured, the result will be that the chemical processes productive of heat will go on in a disorderly manner, and consequently a sudden and sometimes enormous elevation of temperature will occur.

But where are these inhibitory or regulative centres situated? The recent experiments of Tscheschichin appear to give an answer to this question.* They are as follows : If you cut through the cord at different levels, the limbs become warmer on account of the consequent vaso-motor paralysis ; but at the same time there is cooling of the central parts, depending partly on the loss of heat, partly on the weakness of the heart caused by the accumulation of blood at the surface. But if a carefully made section passes through the cord where it joins the medulla oblongata, the central temperature almost immediately rises, and reaches after two or three hours a very high level. At the same time the pulse and respiration grow more rapid. From these results the experimenter concluded that there are within the skull, above the spot indicated, inhibitory centres whose paralysis is the cause of an excessive and irregular production of heat.

It would be well if these experiments were repeated. If the results already published be confirmed they may usefully be brought into relation with clinical facts.

* *Deutsch. Archir*, 1866, p. 398.

LECTURE XXI.

SUMMARY.—Internal algidity.—Discrepancy that may exist between the temperature of external and of deep parts.—Lowering of the internal temperature in chronic diseases.—Cancer, anæmia, diabetes, phthisis.—Fall of temperature in acute diseases.—Effects of drugs and of poisons. — Physiological experiments. — Septicæmia, cholæmia, uræmia.—Affections of the heart.—Pleurisy, pneumonia, peritonitis.—Affections of the spinal cord.—Clinical meaning of collapse.—Algide pneumonia.—Pestilential diseases.

GENTLEMEN,—Hitherto I have only taken into consideration pathological states in which the temperature rises above the normal; but it is not uncommon, especially in the aged, to observe the inverse occurrence in the course of certain affections, that is, a real lowering of the temperature of the internal parts. It is to this point that I want to direct your attention to-day.

Though there are diseases of which the febrile state is a constant, necessary character, there are none which *necessarily* produce during their whole course a fall of temperature below the normal; so that *central algidity*—for so we call this condition—generally figures in the history of diseases as a mere incidental phenomenon, a symptom that is usually transitory. But its signification is often very serious.

Several of you will very likely be thinking of one of the most striking symptoms of Asiatic cholera, the cadaveric coldness of the limbs, and will regard the proposition I have just enunciated as rather too sweeping. But thermometry does not confine itself to external appearances, and what does it tell us in Indian cholera? In the algide stage, the temperature of the limbs no doubt falls markedly below the usual level, less, however, than the sensation experienced by the observer's hand would lead him to suppose. In hands and feet, even in the intensest cases, the thermometer indicates 35°, 31°, 29° (95°, 87·8°, 84·2° F.). But during all this time, contrary to all expectation and to the information furnished by a thermometer in the axilla, the internal temperature is not generally changed. This is a fact, the demonstration of which I began to make at the time of the epidemic in 1866,* and which has since been confirmed in the

* Note on the rectal temperature in Asiatic cholera, *Comptes rendus des séances et mémoires de la Soc. de biol.*, vol. xvii. Paris, 1866, p. 197.—On the fall of temperature in disease, by Cherbach, *Thèse de Strasbourg*, 1869.

most striking manner by researches on a larger scale undertaken
by Guterböck in Germany, and by my colleague M. Lorain in
France. Out of 74 cases collected by this latter author, the
rectal temperature sank to 35° four times, and to 34° only once.
It rose in five cases to 40° (104° F.), and in all the other cases
it varied between 37° and 38° (98·6° and 100·4° F.). Thus in
cholera itself, hitherto considered as the type of algide diseases,
the cooling is all external and does not reach the central parts
of the body.

There are, moreover, a considerable number of morbid conditions beside cholera in which various degrees of this difference
of temperature between the superficial and the deep parts are
met with. In certain forms of dying, for example, it is not uncommon to find the temperature rise in the rectum to the limits
of hyperpyrexia, although the extremities are cold. And observe
that the inverse event never occurs. The increase of temperature
in the external parts is never greater than that in the interior,
unless perhaps in one case, that of a local inflammation. John
Simon concluded from his experiments that an inflamed region
is a spot where the temperature may rise some tenths of a degree
above that of the arterial blood which comes to the part. The
recent experiments of Weber have confirmed this result.[*]

When it is no longer a case of inflammation but of a simple
neuroparalytic hyperæmia such as occurs in certain forms of
paralysis, or again in certain febrile states—pneumonia for
example [†]—the temperature of the hyperæmic parts always
remains below that of the deep parts.

I. But let us return to central algidity. I have already told
you that it rarely occurs persistently during the course of a
disease. The few examples of this condition that may be mentioned relate to chronic diseases. In the first rank must be
placed cancerous affections, but only when certain conditions are
present ; when, for example, there is loss of flesh and wasting,
reaching almost to marasmus. Thus it is especially in gastric
and hepatic cancer that central algidity is observed. When

---

[*] The recent observations of Jacobson and Bernhardt (*Berlin Centralblatt*, 1869,
No. 19), of Landieu (id.), and of Schneider (id., 1870, No. 34), seem to confirm Hunter's
opinion, and consequently to contradict the results obtained by Simon, Billroth, and
O. Weber.

[†] R. Lépine, *De l'hémiplégie pneumonique, Thèse de Paris*, 1870.

these circumstances do not exist, then, in the most diverse forms of the disease, the temperature remains normal, or there is even a slight rise of the thermometer. This year I have convinced myself of this fact from the observation of a pretty considerable number of women suffering from cancer—mammary, uterine, and facial. These same conditions of inanition and marasmus may also be met with in other diseases than cancer ; thus I may mention profound anæmia, diabetes, and some cases of phthisis   The temperature may often remain depressed for a long time—36° (96·8° F.) or less, for example—but this does not prevent the temporary occurrence, especially towards evening, of a relative rise of the temperature to the extent of a degree or more ; and this is sometimes indicated by a rigor.   Under these circumstances the weight of the body diminishes continuously and rapidly, although the temperature continues to sink to the last (Zehrfieber, O. Weber).

No doubt it is also on account of the inanition that a more or less persistent lowering of temperature has been pretty frequently observed (Wolff) in subacute or chronic forms of insanity, with symptoms of depression—chiefly in melancholia with stupor. But the explanation that I am putting forward is not applicable to all cases of this kind. Quite recently, in fact, Dr. Loewenhardt, of Sachsenberg, has reported two cases of insanity, in which the almost incredible rectal temperatures of 31°, 32°, 32·5° (87·8°, 89·6°, 90·5° F.) were observed, and lasted some weeks without nutrition appearing to be seriously interfered with.   One of these patients was excited, the other erotic, and both took sufficient food.*

II. It is especially as an incident in the course of acute diseases that the study of central algidity is interesting.

First of all let us find out what are the chief conditions which give rise to lowering of temperature in these cases.

A great many substances employed as *drugs* have the effect of inducing a more or less decided fall of the central temperature. It is especially when they are taken in almost toxic doses, and also when they are taken during the febrile state, that the action of these drugs is shown in its full energy.   In this way digitalis, sulphate of quinin, calomel, and even alcohol act.

* *Allgemeine Zeitschrift für Psychiatrie.* Berlin, 1868, vol. xxv., p. 685.

But when they are administered in a healthy state, they must be given in comparatively enormous doses in order to produce a fall of a few tenths of a degree. This, for example, occurs in the case of alcohol.*

When these substances are taken in toxic doses they usually occasion a considerable lowering of the temperature, which perhaps, as I have already pointed out, is one of the chief causes of death. Among the substances which give rise to this result, I may refer to chloroform, ether, alcohol, opium, belladonna, nicotin, phosphorus, and the majority of acids—sulphuric, oxalic, hydrocyanic, etc.†

It is interesting to note that although many drugs and poisons have the power of lowering the central temperature, a very limited number can raise it. We cannot mention more than three or four substances which have the power of raising the bodily temperature. These are: neat, strong coffee, tea (Lichtenfels and Frölich), but to a less degree, musk (Wunderlich), and lastly, curare, which, according to the researches of Voisin and Liouville, gives rise to a true febrile state, in which the central temperature may rise as high as 40° (104° F.).

We may here consider the variations of temperature caused by the action on the organism of morbid poisons, of animal or vegetable substances undergoing putrefaction.

The majority of putrid substances introduced into the blood in physiological experiments have the effect of raising the internal temperature, and of causing a feverish attack, with shivering, quickening of pulse, loss of body weight, etc. The numerous and oft repeated experiments recently conducted by Billroth, Weber, Fischer, Bergmann, and many others, have nearly always given the same results; and fever may be caused not merely by the injection of putrid substances, but also by that of the products of tissue-metamorphosis, obtained, for example, from an inflamed wound, even when there is no trace of putrefaction.‡

---

* Sydney Ringer, The Influence of Alcohol, etc. (*Lancet*, 1866, Oct. 25th).—H. C. Gell and Sydney Ringer, The Influence of Quinine on the Temperature of the Human Body in Health (*Lancet*, 31st Oct., 1868).

† Brown-Séquard, *Soc. de biologie*, vol. i., p. 102, 1849.—Wyss, Case of poisoning by sulphuric acid (*Archiv der Heilkunde*, 2 Heft, 1869).—Magnan, Case of poisoning by alcohol (*Gaz. des Hôpitaux*, 1869, No. 82).

‡ Venom appears to act in the same manner. Case of Snake (Cobra) Bite, successfully treated by Suction, Liq. Potassæ, and Brandy. By John Shortt, *Lancet*, April 16, 1870.

According to modern researches, you know, traumatic fever is produced in a similar manner. The liquids secreted on the surface of wounds and loaded with products formed by the destruction of tissue, penetrate by diffusion through the walls of lymphatics and veins and mingle with the blood. In this way they would set up a febrile condition by reason of their *pyrogenic* power, the existence of which experiments have recently demonstrated.

Experiment has likewise shown that blood taken from a febrile animal gives rise to fever when injected into the veins of a healthy animal. The same thing occurs after a considerable withdrawal of blood, which, in a healthy individual, after giving rise to a brief lowering of the temperature, then produces a real febrile state. On account of the decrease of tension which the loss of blood has caused in the vascular system, the products of the normal metamorphosis of tissue suddenly enter the circulation in great quantity, and there behave like pyrogenic substances. This, at least, is the interpretation given by Bergmann and Frese, the authors of these experiments.*

It seems established, therefore, that the majority of septic substances contained in morbid fluids have the property of giving rise to fever. But it is likewise true that a certain number of substances of this kind have an exactly opposite action on the organism. Thus, for example, in the experiments of Weber and Billroth, the injection of decomposed animal substances, such as putrid pus, occasioned a very notable fall of temperature, usually followed in a little while by a more or less intense febrile state, but in other cases persistent, and even growing steadily worse till death, which in such a case generally comes on rapidly.

It is difficult to foresee with certainty what putrid substance when injected into the blood will give rise to fever, and what other, on the contrary, will cause internal algidity, for under the head of putrid or septic bodies are included substances of the most varied chemical constitution. It is at any rate very probable that the same substance which, taken at a certain point in the putrid fermentation, will cause fever, will, if employed at a more advanced period of the process of decomposition give rise, on the contrary, to lowering of the temperature. The bodies, the presence of which in putrescent matter has been determined by Chemistry, vary according to the nature of the substances which

* *Centralblatt*, 1869, No. 2.

have given rise to them, and according to the different phases of the putrid fermentation. Now among these bodies are a certain number which when injected alone into the blood have the effect of lowering the temperature of the body. Such are, according to the harmonising experiments of Billroth, Weber, and Bergmann, carbonate of ammonium, butyric acid, hydrosulphuric acid, and sulphide of ammonium. So that if these bodies happen to predominate over the pyrogenic substances in a fluid, it is easy to understand what will be the effect produced on the system by the injection or absorption of such a liquid.

These facts, borrowed from experimental pathology, give us, I think, the key to a certain number of seemingly contradictory facts observed in human pathology.

There are, in fact, forms of septicæmia with fever, and others with internal algidity. Sometimes, indeed, these two states, apparently opposed in nature, may follow each other in the same individual without the original conditions having been apparently modified.

I may refer, in this connection, to what happens in cases of traumatic or spontaneous gangrene, extending over a considerable portion of a limb. You are aware of the well-known fact that even when the circulation of blood in a gangrenous limb is completely stopped, and when clots have already formed in both arteries and veins, the sphacelated part may act as a source of infection. This had been already recognised in practice, but Kussmaul's experiments have shown its full importance. He injected a certain quantity of iodide of potassium under the skin of a limb thus apparently separated from the rest of the body, and four hours later he found traces of the iodide in the urine. It cannot be doubted after this that putrid substances from sphacelated parts may themselves penetrate into the circulating current. The infective phenomena to which they give rise are manifested sometimes as intense fever, sometimes, on the other hand, as internal algidity. We frequently observe this succession of phenomena in the cases of spontaneous gangrene which occur in this hospital, and which are generally the result of atheromatous obliteration or thrombosis of the chief arterial trunks of a limb. If in such a case the patient withstands the infection for some days, and especially if the gangrene assumes the moist form, you may see the central temperature sink steadily to

36°, 35° (96·8°, 95°), and in one case which I saw to 34·5° (94·1° F.). In a case of this kind death comes on amid symptoms of profound collapse; icy skin, cold sweats, almost imperceptible pulse, &c.

How do the substances in question act in causing such a rapid and considerable lowering of the internal temperature? It is supposed that they have the effect of destroying a very large number of blood-corpuscles, or at least of suddenly annihilating their respiratory power. There would arise in such a case, to employ an expression used by Williams, a *necræmia*, or death of the blood. Although preserving their physical characters, the corpuscles thus changed would have lost their chemical properties. In cases where this change in the corpuscles became general, a rapid lowering of the temperature would be the consequence.

But it is very probable that, independently of this action, some substances affect the heart, paralysing its movements. This is what happens in the case of bile. Every time that a certain quantity of it enters the blood, it causes both a slowing of the heart and a lowering of the internal temperature (Leyden, Röhrig). Experiment, indeed, has lately told us which alone, among the numerous components of the biliary fluid, give rise to the retardation of the cardiac contractions and the internal algidity.

We now know, contrary to the opinion of the ancients, that the whole of the bile, or at least its essential constituents, pass into the blood in simple jaundice, such as is caused by occlusion of the bile duct. Now in spontaneous, just as in experimental jaundice, one finds these fundamental elements of bile in the blood and urine. In both cases, moreover, slowing of pulse and fall of temperature may be observed.

Röhrig* has shown that these effects are due to the presence of the biliary acids. Injected by themselves into the circulation they lead to the same result.

On the contrary, nothing of the kind is caused by the cholesterin, colouring matters, or fats. By the simple fact of their slowing and weakening the contractions of the heart, the presence of the biliary acids in the blood would cause a fall of temperature. But Van Dusch and Kühne have shown that they also have the

* *Archiv der Heilkunde*, 1863.

property of destroying the blood corpuscles, and this latter action
no doubt aids considerably in producing the lowered temperature.*

There also occurs in most cases a very remarkable lowering
of the internal temperature in uræmia.†

III. After what I have just told you with regard to the
mechanism of the fall of temperature caused by the introduction
of septic matters into the blood, you will not be surprised to
meet with this same occurrence in certain *organic or functional
affections of the heart.* It is a fact that the majority of diseases
which weaken the action of the heart tend to cause a lowering of
the internal temperature. It is easy to understand that enfeeblement of the circulation when carried to a marked degree may
be a circumstance very unfavourable to the performance of the
chemical processes which maintain the heat of the body. It is
known, besides, that when cardiac weakness is pushed to its
extreme limits, as in syncope, the blood traverses the capillaries
without undergoing any modification, and appears in the veins
with the bright colour of arterial blood. Now in cases of this
kind the internal temperature falls, and it falls too in a very
remarkable manner, where matters do not go so far.

Among the affections of the heart itself which are accompanied
by a diminution of the internal temperature, I may mention to
you, as an example, a case of rupture of the heart with effusion
of blood into the pericardium, which we observed together in this

---

* Virchow's *Archiv*, xiv.

† One of my pupils, Dr. Bourneville, has recently published a series of researches,
from which it appears that in *uræmia* from whatever cause (parenchymatous nephritis,
pyelitis, cystic degeneration of the kidneys, calculous obliteration of the ureters, etc.),
and whatever the symptomatic form which it assumes (comatose, apoplectic, or convulsive form), there is in all cases a fall of internal temperature. This lowering of temperature increases in proportion as the nervous symptoms get worse, and in certain cases
the temperature has sunk *below* 30° (86° F.). On the contrary in *puerperal eclampsia*,
which several authors still connect with uræmia, Bourneville has noticed a constant
elevation of temperature, an elevation which goes on increasing from the commencement up to the fatal termination. A temperature of 42° has been observed in some
cases of this kind (107·6° F.). Bourneville has also collected some observations
relating to the modifications which the internal temperature undergoes in cerebral
apoplexy (hemorrhage and softening of the brain), which confirm in all respects the
results which I have myself published. Moreover, having observed the temperature
hour by hour in some apoplectic cases, he has made evident the influence on the
thermometric tracing of the production of fresh foci of hemorrhage, or the bursting
of the effused blood into the ventricles (See Bourneville, *Etudes cliniques et thermo-
métriques sur les maladies du système nerveux.* Paris, 1873).

hospital. An old woman who fainted one morning in her dormitory was immediately taken to the infirmary, where we found her in a state of syncope, which lasted nearly the whole day. A second faint occurred towards evening, and death took place suddenly. During this long syncopal period, which came between the two fainting fits, the beats of the heart were feeble, frequent, and irregular, the pulse was almost imperceptible, and the rectal temperature was 36° (96·8° F.).

You are aware that in cases of asystole dependent on organic disease of the heart, from time to time attacks occur which are characterised by feebleness and irregularity of the cardiac impulse, cyanosis, and coldness of skin. During these attacks I have several times seen the internal temperature sink to 35° or 36°, and after the attack soon rise again to the normal. In *acute pericarditis* and *endocarditis*, as I stated during my early researches, sometimes a rise and sometimes a notable fall of temperature is observed. It is the same with *peritonitis*. The observations of Wunderlich have fully confirmed the results that I then obtained.

It will very likely appear singular at first sight to find inflammations which sometimes affect a very large surface, such as the whole extent of a large serous membrane, giving rise to a lowering of the central temperature. Nothing is more certain, however. For example, pericarditis supervenes in a case of lobar pneumonia ; you might fancy that from such a combination there ought to result a hyperpyretic rise of the curve; nothing of the kind occurs, however. Either the curve remains as it was, or more frequently, to judge from my often-repeated observations, it experiences an unusual fall. The production of such a depression in the course of a pneumonia hitherto regular in its course has several times induced me to examine the heart carefully, and to recognise the presence of a pericarditis, which would otherwise have escaped me. *Diaphragmatic pleurisy, pneumothorax from perforation, traumatic peritonitis, peritonitis from perforation, internal strangulation,* also generally occasion a fall of internal temperature at least for a time.

It is true this is not an invariable result, but still it is pretty common. In such a case the central algidity sometimes persists or goes on increasing till death, whilst at other times it is soon replaced by an excessive rise of temperature.

However it be, it will no longer astonish you to find more or less violent irritation of the serous membranes, and especially of the peritoneum, give rise to these effects, if you think of the results of experiment. You are aware that a blow on the epigastric region, the ingestion of a cold fluid * when the body is sweating, may cause sudden death, apparently by way of syncope. Now Brown-Séquard has shown that excitation of the semilunar ganglia has the effect of causing syncope. According to him excitation of these ganglia is transmitted by the cord to the medulla oblongata, and thence reflected to the pneumogastric nerves, irritation of which causes stoppage of the heart in diastole. When less intense, this excitation of the great sympathetic may cause a *permanent diminution in the power of the heart*, and thus give rise to a kind of syncopal state which is more or less persistent, and to a lasting depression of temperature.†

It is, no doubt, in a similar manner that most great disturbances of the nervous system first show themselves by a syncopal state, with internal algidity, which may or may not be followed by reaction.

Magendie proved by experiments, which have been confirmed by Cl. Bernard,‡ that any intense irritation of the peripheral nerves, such, for example, as that caused by the crushing of a limb, has the effect of lowering the blood pressure ; the researches of Mantegazza have shown us that in such a case a lowering of the central temperature occurs.§

After certain traumatic lesions of the cord, Brown-Séquard has observed profound collapse, complete suspension of reflex actions, and passage of bright blood into the veins. At the same time there was diminution of the internal temperature.

The same process may be relied on to explain the syncopal state, which, as a good many practitioners have observed (Abercrombie, Portal, Watson, Grisolle), marks the onset of an apoplectic attack from hemorrhage or softening, and which, according

---

* See on this subject the interesting memoir of M. A. Guérard, *Sur les accidents qui peuvent succéder à l'ingestion des boissons froides* (*Annales d'hygiène*, vol. xxxvii. Paris, 1842).

† See Brown-Séquard (*Archives de Médecine*, 1856, vol. ii., pp. 440, 484).—(*Lectures on Physiology and Pathology*, 159).—Bernstein, Herzstillstand durch Sympathicus-Reizung (*Centralblatt*, 1863, No. 52, and 1864, No. 16).—Eulenburg and Guttman, Pathologie des Sympathicus (in *Archiv für Psychiatrie*, 1869, Bd. ii., heft. 1.

‡ *Leçons*, etc , vol. i., p. 267.

§ Schmidt's *Jahrbuch*, 1867, i., 153.

to my observations, is accompanied by an actual lowering of the
temperature of the deep parts.

IV. We have thus discussed the chief circumstances in which
lowering of the internal temperature occurs. Now in most cases
in which this depression of temperature takes place suddenly, it
is indicated externally by coldness of the surface of the body,
and by a number of other alarming symptoms. This group of
symptoms has been called *collapse* by Thierfielder * and Wunderlich, to whom we owe a remarkable essay on this clinical
question, which is too much neglected among us.† But the condition of collapse may also arise in cases where the central
temperature remains normal, or even rises above the normal, and
according as one or other of these different cases occurs will the
prognosis and the therapeutic indications be remarkably different.
Thus collapse is sometimes the almost certain forerunner of a
fatal termination, sometimes it indicates what is no doubt an
alarming situation, but one which the resources of our art, when
well applied, may perhaps succeed in bringing to a favourable
issue. Sometimes, lastly, collapse is but the exaggeration of
phenomena, which almost always occur to a certain extent when
some febrile diseases end in rapid and favourable defervescence.

You see at once by this simple account how much a study of
collapse should interest the practitioner, since every time that
this collection of symptoms comes before him there is a problem
to solve, a prognosis to be made, a particular group of therapeutic measures to be brought into operation ; moreover, there is
no time to lose, for the symptoms of collapse may rapidly lead
to an unfortunate conclusion.

Symptoms of this kind are very commonly met with in very
various cases in the aged, and in individuals weakened with previous disease or alcoholism. But it is especially when it comes
on in the course of acute febrile diseases that collapse merits
your attention ; it is under these circumstances that I want to
study it with you, and to try to make out its chief characteristics.

Suppose, for example, we have a case of lobar pneumonia, and

* *Archiv für physiolog. Heilk.*, 14th year, No. 2.
† In the excellent article "Chaleur," in the *Nouveau dictionnaire de médecine et de
chirurgie pratiques* (vol. vi., p. 808, 1867) M. Hirtz has made very clear the interest
attaching to the study of collapse.

S

let us take a well-marked case. Up to the sixth or seventh day all has gone on as usual; the pneumonia is intense, but its progress has been regular; the temperature is 39° or 40° (102·2°, 104° F.), and the external signs of the febrile state are well-developed. Suddenly, in the course of a few hours, the scene changes, the physiognomy is altered, the eyes are sunken, the cheeks and nose pale and chill; the extremities are cold and cyanotic; the body is covered with cold sweat; there is great prostration of strength, sometimes even delirium; the impulse of the heart is weak and irregular, and its sounds are dull and distant; the pulse is thready, sometimes quicker, sometimes slower than before; the respiratory movements are rapid and deep.

What in such a case is the meaning of this group of alarming symptoms?

The observation of the internal temperature will supply you with precious indications: 1stly, If while the external symptoms of algidity arise, the central temperature remains elevated or rises to the level of hyperpyretic temperatures, death is certain. The process of dying is already begun. Doubt soon becomes no longer possible; the pulse still further quickens, and the laryngo-tracheal râle is not long in appearing. 2ndly, If, on the other hand, at the same time that the symptoms of collapse appear, the central temperature sinks decidedly, or descends to normal or less than normal, the doctor's position is more difficult, for in some cases a fatal termination is again before him, and will before long supervene, while in other cases convalescence will commence in a few hours, and a grave prognosis inconsiderately given might thus be belied in the most direct manner. Here you must take into very serious consideration the indications furnished by the other symptoms which accompany the lowering of the central temperature.

If the collapse is but the exaggeration of the ordinary symptoms of rapid and favourable defervescence, then, while the central temperature is falling, the respiratory movements and the arterial pulsations grow slower and more regular; the prognosis is favourable in such a case, even when some disquieting symptom like intense delirium has come on.*

If, on the contrary, while the internal temperature is falling

* Weber, *Med. Chir. Trans.*, vol. xlviii., 1865.

the frequency of the pulse and of the respiratory movements remains as before, or even increases, the situation is exceedingly grave. Soon, whatever you do, you see that death is at hand. And whilst just now we were led to give a favourable prognosis, in spite of the appearance of violent delirium, here we must still give a grave prognosis, even when the defervescence may have given the patient a feeling of relief.

This was the case in a woman of 54, weakened by uterine cancer and attacked with lobar pneumonia, whom you have observed in our wards. About the seventh day of the disease, at the time when rapid defervescence set in, this woman noticed a remarkable feeling of relief, which deceived several of you, but which soon gave place to death.

I have been talking to you of the collapse which occurs in lobar pneumonia when defervescence sets in; this is the most usual case. But the same group of symptoms may appear at all periods of the disease.

When the disease is at its height, the occurrence of collapse most frequently results from a complication, such as pericarditis, violent diarrhœa, or perhaps, especially in old people, it appears under the influence of the excessive action of a drug such as tartar emetic or digitalis. The prognosis you will make varies remarkably in such a case. It depends especially on the influence of the measures brought to bear on the complication, or to make up for the injury caused by the unsuitable use of drugs.

Collapse may also appear during the invasion of pneumonia; in this case it is usually transitory and soon gives place to more or less marked reaction; in other cases, however, it persists during the whole course of the disease, which then almost always ends in an unfortunate manner.

These *algide* forms of pneumonia are tolerably uncommon even in the profoundly debilitated individuals whom we meet with in such numbers in this hospital. Several of you, however, have had the opportunity of observing a remarkable example of this form in our wards. A woman called L——, 71 years of age, was attacked with lobar pneumonia, and presented from the onset and during the whole course of the disease a number of symptoms which made her resemble a cholera patient. The extremities were cold and deeply cyanosed, the face livid, the eyes sunk, the voice inaudible. There was no diarrhœa, the

s 2

alvine evacuations being few; the urine was pale and scanty, and contained a considerable proportion of albumen. The rectal temperature oscillated between 38° and 38·4°, never reaching 39° (100·4°, 101·1°, 102·2° F.). The feeble, almost imperceptible pulse varied from 100 to 108. At the autopsy the lower and middle lobes of the right lung, throughout, presented the most marked features of granular red and grey hepatisation. This lung weighed about a kilogram more than the left. The kidneys showed no appreciable change.

This variety of collapse is one of the characters of the malignant form of most pestilential diseases; thus it is observed in yellow fever, plague, typhus ;* and is also met with in malarial poisoning.† I have several times observed it in the variola of old people, which, as you know, frequently assumes the hemorrhagic character. In these cases, at the very time when dark pustules were appearing on various parts of the body, the extremities were cold and cyanotic, the prostration of strength was extreme, and the rectal temperature varied between 36° and 37° (96·8°, 93·6°).

I am far from having exhausted the subject I proposed to talk to you about, but I should be afraid of fatiguing your attention if I multiplied examples ; moreover, I have said enough, at least I hope so, to make you feel the great interest which attaches to thermometric investigations both in general clinical work and in that among the aged.

* Charcot, articles, "Typhus Fever," "Pest," "Yellow Fever," in the 4th vol. of the *Elémens de pathologie médicale* of A. Requin. Paris, 1868.

† Griesinger, *Treatise on Infectious Diseases.*

LECTURE XXII.

CEREBRAL HEMORRHAGE AND SOFTENING OF THE BRAIN.—MORBID ANATOMY OF CEREBRAL HEMORRHAGE.

SUMMARY.—Cerebral hemorrhage and softening of the brain.—Importance of studying them.—Their *rôle* as causes of death and infirmity.—Formerly designated under the name of apoplexy.—Apoplexy and paraplexy.—Apoplectic symptoms originate in the encephalon.—Discovery of cerebral hemorrhage as the cause of certain cases of apoplexy.—Cerebral hemorrhage came to be considered as the cause of every apoplexy.—New interpretation of the word apoplexy.—Discovery of cerebral softening as a cause of apoplexy.—Of some other affections which may give rise to apoplexy.—Analogies which may be drawn between hemorrhage and softening. —Of the supposed identity in nature of these two diseases.—They depend on lesions of the same vessels, but on lesions which differ in the two cases.

Of cerebral hemorrhage.—Its greater simplicity should give it the first place in the study of encephalic diseases.—Hemorrhages in the brain occurring as secondary lesions in certain diseases.—Encephalic hemorrhage dependent on diffuse arterio-sclerosis.—Its seat.—Spread of the foci.—Opening of the foci into the ventricles or on the surface of the encephalon.—Number of the foci.—Symmetrical disposition of the foci.

GENTLEMEN,—We commence to-day the study of diseases of the nervous centres. This series of lectures will be devoted to cerebral hemorrhage and softening, two diseases which, in many respects, are particularly deserving of our attention. Thus, they carry off by rapid death a large number of persons every year. According to the mortality statistics of London for a period of five years, which Dr. Mushet* has recorded in his treatise on apoplexy, there is one death from apoplexy in forty-four; and, as you know, that expression refers to a group of symptoms which is especially associated with cerebral softening and hemorrhage. Moreover, should the apoplectic attack, which usually characterises the onset of these two diseases, not be followed by speedily fatal symptoms, it is very rare for the patient to return completely to his previous state of health, or to recover the integrity of his momentarily suspended functions. In the immense majority of cases he only retains life at the expense of deplorable infirmities. He is left with more or less complete hemiplegia, most frequently rendering him incapable, and even condemning him to perpetual confinement in bed. The intelligence itself rarely escapes com-

* A Practical Treatise on Apoplexy (Cerebral Hemorrhage), p. 81. London, 1866.

pletely, and remains more or less profoundly clouded, a condition which may go on to complete dementia. I can enable you to judge of the heavy tribute which we pay to these diseases by giving you some statistics from the reports that Vulpian and I drew up at the hospital of the Salpêtrière. We have of course rejected from our calculation the patients who are placed in the wards devoted to mental diseases. Out of about 2,000 inmates there are at the Salpêtrière 1,000 healthy women, who have no other claim to assistance but age and poverty, and 1,000 others who have been admitted because they suffer from infirmities which are reckoned incurable. Now, of these thousand invalids, 400 are blind ; 200 are hemiplegic ; 100 have affections of the spinal cord, such as locomotor ataxy and paraplegia ; 100 more come on account of the different forms of chronic articular rheumatism, an affection which was the special object of our studies last year. So that hemiplegia seems to give rise to the fifth part of our infirmities ; and although every persistent hemiplegia does not necessarily depend on cerebral hemorrhage or softening, these two diseases are at any rate by far its most frequent cause. It was, you know, these two affections which ancient symptomatic Medicine specially designated by the common name of *apoplexy*.

You are aware that to the ancients, to Galen for example, apoplexy meant the sudden loss of sensation and motion all over the body, the respiratory movements being, however, exempted ;* and to this definition was afterwards added the exemption of the circulation.† Besides this apoplexy properly so called, Galen and most of the physicians who have followed him, down to Boerhaave,‡ have also described *paraplexy* or parapoplexy; it was

* *Commentary on Aphorism* 42, 2nd section, and *The Parts affected in Disease*, lib. iii., c. 10.

† The well-known definition of Boerhaave may be here recalled :—Quæ (apoplexia) dicitur adesse, quando repente actio quinque sensuum externorum, tum internorum, omnesque motus voluntarii abolentur, superstito pulsu plerumque fort‌i, et respiratione difficili, magna, stertente, una cum imagine profundi perpetuique somni.—*Aphor.*, § 1008.

‡ Paraplexia est levior apoplexia ad paralysin magis accedens, vel quando alterutro saltem in corporis latere, aut certo membro, immobilitas et sensus privatio animadvertitur.—Galen, c. 2 in prorrhet., t. 50.—B. Castelli, Lexicon *medicum.*

Locus vero affectus in apoplexia exquisita est totum sensorium ; in paraplexia vero ejus quædam pars præ cæteris, reliquis quodammodo, sed tamen minus pressis. —Boerhaave, *Aph.*, § 1013.

See also Gendrin, *Traité philosophique de médecine pratique*, vol. i., p. 381. Paris, 1838.

a sort of attenuated apoplexy, in which the loss of motion and sensation was less generalised, and might remain restricted to one side of the body or even to a single arm. Paraplexy in this latter sense is therefore nothing but hemiplegia of sudden onset, arising from any cause. But if it is true, as is now admitted, that in the majority of cases these two symptomatic groups depend either on softening of the brain or on cerebral hemorrhage, it is equally true that they may be found associated with entirely different affections. You see from this, that, according to its traditional meaning, this old word apoplexy should only be applied to a group of symptoms, to what used to be called a *syndrome*, and that it is only by an abuse of the term that it is now sometimes made to serve as the designation of a definite disease or even of an anatomical lesion.

Before the intervention of pathological anatomy it was admitted that the encephalon is the seat, the starting-point, of apoplectic phenomena, and hypotheses were not wanting with respect to the nature of the change which thus suddenly attacks the brain. Galen had supposed that the ventricles became suddenly distended by a cold and melancholic humour. Others suggested that bile and phlegm were blocking the vessels ; and Willis supposed that there was rather an arrest or suffocation of the animal spirits.

It seems to us as though it would have been more natural to seek in the brain, which was supposed to be attacked, for the lesion which might be found there ; as though it would have sufficed to look in order to find, and to substitute reality for hypothesis, the demonstration of hemorrhagic or softened foci not requiring great refinement of investigation. But these notions, which seem to us now-a-days so simple and so clear, are only the outcome of a long and difficult infancy ; and it has needed all the labour of Wepfers, Valsalvas, and Morgagnis to demonstrate that certain apoplexies are due to an effusion of blood into the substance of the brain and into the ventricles.

But the morbid anatomists of that period only saw the most apparent aspect of the matter ; having discovered scarcely more than recent hemorrhages, they were for the most part led to admit that effusion of blood into the brain is always fatal. It was only after some time that old foci were recognised, and that, seizing the connection between them and recent hemorrhages, we have been able to reach the notion of the relative curability and the possible transformations of these effusions.

In this respect the labours of Rochoux have been epochal, and rightly so, for they have powerfully aided to make our knowledge definite with regard to cerebral hemorrhage. But at the same time Rochoux was one of the first who had to alter the classical meaning of the word apoplexy. Thus his first researches, which date from 1814,[*] clearly betray the tendency which this author had to refer most, if not all, cases of apoplexy to intra-encephalic hemorrhage ; true, he describes congestion and serous effusion into the ventricles, but he hardly does more than refer to them as quite secondary, and as being able to simulate apoplexy. To him, in short, cerebral hemorrhage is *par excellence* apoplexy, it is actually apoplexy. Thus diverted from its primitive meaning, the term apoplexy was made to pass from the language of semeiology into that of nosography or pathological anatomy.[†] You know how this new meaning has itself been outdone in the application of the term apoplexy to internal hemorrhage in the liver, spleen, lung, and indeed in any parenchymatous tissue.[‡]

Still, about that period important progress was realised. Rostan in 1819, then Abercrombie, Bouillaud, Lallemand, Andral, made known a disease which had not then been described, and

---

[*] *Recherches sur l'apoplexie,* Paris, 1814 ; and *Recherches sur l'apoplexie et sur plusieurs autres maladies de l'appareil nerveux cérébro-spinal,* 2nd ed., Paris, 1833.

[†] " With all deference to those who arbitrarily change the meaning of the term apoplexy, to those who recognise apoplexy only in intra-cranial hemorrhage, to those who from this restricted view proceed still further to abuse its meaning by calling every internal hemorrhage in a parenchymatous tissue, apoplexy ; with all deference, I say, to these violators of etymology and tradition, let us oppose the mania so common in our days, of upsetting the meaning of old terms, a mania a hundred times worse in my opinion than that of coining new words ; and in accord with ancient and with the best of modern, physicians, and also with the French Academy, let us use the word apoplexy wherever there is a disease characterised by sudden and more or less complete loss of sensation and motion without respiration and circulation being interfered with. But, they will say, that is a purely symptomatic definition. No doubt, we reply ; to preserve the term apoplexy for the language of symptomatology is precisely what we want to do, for it was created for this language, and not for the language of pathological anatomy. And though it is true that in the great majority of cases, apoplexy, as we define it, is the symptom of hemorrhage within the encephalon, it is no less true that it may occur as the symptom of cerebral hyperæmia, or indeed of a rapid effusion of serosity."—Requin, *Elements de pathologie,* vol. i., p. 430, 1843.

See on the same subject, Schützenberger and Hecht, in *Dict. encyc.,* etc. vol. v., part 2, p. 682.

[‡] Cruveilhier, *Dict. de médecine et de chirurgie pratiques,* vol. iii., art. " Apoplexy," Paris, 1829.

which till then had hardly been recognised ; softening of the brain took its place along with hemorrhage, and it was found that, like the latter, softening is usually indicated at the onset by an apoplectic attack.

At the present day it is agreed that the majority of cases of apoplexy depend on cerebral hemorrhage or softening ; but all cases, as I said, do not originate in this way; such are, for example, those which depend on hyperæmia or anæmia of the brain ; those which depend on sudden serous effusions occurring in the course of certain cases of dropsy ; those which characterise some of the cerebral manifestations of gout, rheumatism, uræmia, or malarial poisoning. Lastly, shall I mention what is still called essential, functional, or nervous apoplexy ? These different affections may be indicated by symptoms which present a more or less marked analogy with those accompanying hemorrhage or softening ; we shall have to recall this point when we treat of diagnosis ; but for the present we must concentrate all our attention on these two latter diseases.

Between cerebral hemorrhage and softening of the brain, as we shall have many opportunities of perceiving, there are indisputable points of contact and resemblances which justify us in drawing some analogy between them—and this as much in regard to anatomical seat as to symptomatic manifestation. You will even see, when we commence the clinical study of these affections, that though it is needful to keep them radically distinct in nosography, it is, on the contrary, almost always difficult, sometimes indeed quite impossible, to distinguish them by their symptoms. But some people have gone farther than this, and denied that there was any real difference in nature between them. Cruveilhier, who expressed his opinion that from an anatomical point of view they pass into one another by insensible transitions, saw little in them but two manifestations, different but regulated by analogous pathogenic conditions, of the same pathological state. This view has lately been developed anew in the recent edition of Valleix's treatise ; * and I may observe that one would be logically led to such a conclusion, if one regarded cerebral hemorrhage as dependent on arterial atheroma, a vascular lesion which is certainly at the bottom of most cases of cerebral softening.

* *Guide du médecin praticien*, 1866, vol. ii., p. 86.

We shall have to inquire, gentlemen, what we ought to think of this way of looking at the subject, which, it must be admitted, seems just now to be the dominant one. But I will tell you at once that our descriptions will tend to show, contrary to the prevailing opinion, that there is a well-marked line of demarcation between these two diseases; that the mixed forms, the transitions and hybrids, must be rejected as having no real existence ; that the two affections depend no doubt on a previous alteration of the same cerebral vessels, but that this alteration differs in the two cases. Senile softening of the brain depends in fact upon atheromatous degeneration of the arteries, through the obliteration of vessels which this consequence of endarteritis may cause, either directly or by giving rise to thrombosis. Cerebral hemorrhage, on the contrary, depends on a vascular change which is quite different, to a diffuse arterio-sclerosis, or better, a peri-arteritis, which had not been well described until lately, and to which the recent researches which I have conducted together with M. Bouchard enable us to refer the formation of miliary aneurisms. Now it is to the rupture of these aneurisms, whose pathogenic *rôle* had not even been suspected, that I shall be able to refer the great majority of cases of cerebral hemorrhage. But we need insist no longer on this point, which will be amply developed in what I shall have to say.

We shall first take up cerebral hemorrhage ; it will form an introduction to the study of diseases of the encephalon, because it is characterised by a simplicity which is not found in the others ; for the sudden tearing of the tissue of the brain by the irruption of blood realises in some degree the conditions, simple and relatively easy to analyse, which are sought in experiments on animals. From this point of view cerebral hemorrhage may to some extent be regarded as a typical disease among the affections of the brain. But these considerations are far from applicable to all hemorrhages within the skull ; and in order that we may have before us only one well-marked disease, we shall have to eliminate for the time certain affections which are also accompanied by effusion of blood into the brain or on its surface. Such are the meningeal hemorrhages which occur in false membranes, or result from the rupture of aneurisms of the arteries at the base ; such are also certain hemorrhages which are in a sense accidental, where the effusion of blood is quite a secondary matter or a complication, and which, being subordinate to other affections, possess no independent existence in nosography. Though forming only a very limited number of the cases of cerebral hemorrhage which come before us, these cases do not the less depend on very different pathogenic processes. There are cases of hemorrhage within the brain, which are usually referred to a change in the condition of the blood ; such are those sometimes observed in scurvy, purpura, typhus, pyæmia, melanæmia, and leucocythæmia. Other purely accidental hemorrhages may occur in the course of cerebral softening caused by obliteration of vessels. There are some which have their origin in a tumour of the brain, and follow the hyperæmia caused by cancer or glioma. We must mention also· capillary apoplexy, or hemorrhage by infiltration, an accessory lesion, which is not a special kind of cerebral hemorrhage, has no independent existence, and accompanies softening as well as the actual hemorrhage in which the blood collects in foci.

Having eliminated all these cases, we find ourselves in presence of a homogeneous group corresponding to the most common form of cerebral hemorrhage. This is, *par excellence*, sanguineous apoplexy. It bears the same relation to the other forms of cerebral hemorrhage as true hereditary epilepsy, for example, bears to the various symptomatic epilepsies. As it attacks a great number of old people, I might call it senile hemorrhage, if it was not for the fact that it may be found with the same characters at the other periods of life. Now we shall proceed to consider cerebral hemorrhage dependent on diffuse arterio-sclerosis.

Intra-encephalic hemorrhage dependent on diffuse arterio-sclerosis and miliary aneurisms.

In the case of an affection in which the organic lesion plays so important a part, it will seem natural to you that we should begin by studying its anatomy. It would perhaps be the logical method to point out to you first of all the vascular lesions on which the effusion of blood depends ; but I prefer to commence by studying the most readily comprehensible characters which hemorrhagic foci present. We shall find also in this preliminary study more than one argument which will be of use hereafter.

A focus of hemorrhage in the brain may be considered as to its nature, and as to the changes it undergoes at the different periods of the disease ; it must also be studied in its relation to the parts in the midst of which it forms, and especially with reference to its locality. It is this last point which we shall begin with in our anatomical study of cerebral hemorrhage.

The seat of the hemorrhage is very variable, but the effusion does not take place indifferently in any part of the encephalon; there are certain laws on this subject, which are made clear by an examination of the numerous observations which have been published up to the present time. I show you a table, the details of which have been supplied me by the statistics of Andral and Durand-Fardel. It is based on 153 observations, and will enable you to grasp the relative frequence of hemorrhage in the different regions of the encephalon.

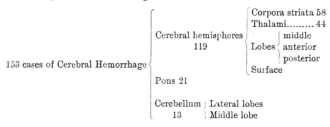

153 cases of Cerebral Hemorrhage	Cerebral hemispheres 119	Corpora striata 58
		Thalami......... 44
		Lobes { middle anterior posterior
		Surface
	Pons 21	
	Cerebellum 13	Lateral lobes / Middle lobe

There are some parts of the encephalon where hemorrhage is very exceptionally observed, or at least which are very rarely its primary seat ; such are the corpora quadrigemina, the cerebral peduncles, the medulla oblongata. Hemorrhage has scarcely ever been observed in the cornu ammonis or the corpus callosum.[*]

An attentive examination of the facts shows that it is especially in the grey substance that the hemorrhagic foci primarily form. The very small effusions are almost always limited to the grey parts ; the large collections of blood tear up the white matter, but it can generally be shown that they have their starting-point in a portion of grey matter.

I need not remind you of the distribution of the grey matter in the encephalon ; I will merely call your attention to an anatomical point which seems to me to have been rather neglected. What I want to point out to you is the existence of

* Rok.tansky, *Lehrbuch der pathologischen Anatomie*, vol. ii., p. 444.

that thin layer of grey matter which you see in this section beyond the corpus striatum, between the extra-ventricular nucleus and the surrounding convolutions of the insula ; it is what the German anatomists call the outer-wall, *Vormauer*, *Claustrum* (Burdach), or tæniform nucleus (Arnold, C. B. Reichert).* You will soon see the interest attaching to this little nucleus of grey matter from our present point of view.

The corpus striatum is the most frequent seat of effusion of blood ; hemorrhage occurs both in the lenticular and in the caudate nucleus ; it may be confined to the substance of the nucleus, but it may also extend farther and involve that white band which passes from the cerebral peduncle between the two nuclei, and which forms what is called in German nomenclature the internal white capsule of the corpus striatum. The anatomical arrangement that I am speaking of is of great importance in regard to the consequences of cerebral hemorrhage ; for, if the fibres of this capsule are torn through by the effusion, the result will be that they will undergo degeneration in their whole extent, through peduncle, pons, and medulla, extending even into the cord. This is a fact to which we shall have to return when we treat of secondary degenerations ; you will then see that if the hemorrhage is limited to the two grey nuclei of the corpus striatum, without involving the intermediate band, these secondary changes of the basal tracts and of the cord do not occur.

The thalami, together with the corpora striata, are the most common seat of hemorrhage ; and yet certain authors, especially M. Gendrin,† have announced the opinion that in the majority of cases the hemorrhage takes place outside the corpus striatum. This, gentlemen, is an exaggeration rather than an error, for next to the opto-striate bodies the spot most frequently attacked by hemorrhage is the claustrum or tæniform nucleus, which, as I showed you just now, is in fact situated outside the corpus striatum.

In the cerebellum the hemorrhage may occupy the convolutions, but more frequently is found in the rhomboidal body.

* Consult C. F. Burdach, *Von Baue und Leben des Gehirns,* 2nd ed., Leipzig, 1822, Plate iii.—C. B. Re'chert, *Der Bau des menschlichen Gehirns durch Abbildungen mit erlaüternden Texte dargestellt,* Leipzig, 1861, Plates iv., v., vi., vii., viii.

† Loc. cit., p. 449, 446.

The grey matter of the convolutions forms no exception to the rule; it, too, is often the seat of hemorrhagic accidents, only the foci rarely assume a great extent there, and are disposed in a way which I shall take care to mention farther on.

It is rare for the hemorrhagic focus to remain limited to the part where it originated; most frequently the effusion gradually increases in extent; it may then tear up the cerebral substance for considerable distances, or even burst out beyond it. In the latter case it may open into the ventricles or on the surface of the brain.

Usually the rupture takes place into the ventricles; the starting-point of the hemorrhage is then generally in the thalami or the corpora striata, sometimes in the cerebellum, in this latter case the rupture being into the fourth ventricle.

The orifice of communication is often small, and then the clot may extend no farther than one lateral ventricle; but if the tear be more considerable all the ventricles may be invaded by blood.

When the blood breaks through at the surface of the brain the starting-point of the effusion is generally in the pons, or in the cerebellum, or in the middle lobe of one of the cerebral hemispheres. A remarkable thing is that the hemorrhages which occur primarily in the convolutions rarely open externally. When the blood does reach the surface it is stopped under the meninges, or, bursting through, it spreads out in the great cavity of the arachnoid.

When the blood bursts through the surface of the brain or into the ventricles, the compressed or distended organ is generally pale; but it is congested when the effusion is slight, as Hasse pointed out.

The results of these ruptures are serious—death in the majority of cases, and sometimes speedy death. Apoplexy, which may be called fulminating [*foudroyante*], occurs in cases where the extravasation spreads beyond the cerebral substance. Death, however, is not an invariable consequence of this event; Rokitansky has observed recovery from hemorrhages which had penetrated into the ventricles, and I have had the opportunity of making several observations fully confirmatory of this fact.

We shall soon see the importance of these remarks; for when the effused blood tears up the cerebral substance and spreads beyond it, it gives rise to certain special events which modify the symptomatology of the disease ; thus, whilst hemiplegia is accompanied by flaccidity of the paralysed limbs, so long as the blood is confined to the interior of the nervous substance, it is accompanied by permanent contracture when the blood penetrates into the ventricles ; and, as Morgagni had already noted, you may observe epileptiform convulsions come on when the blood is effused into the arachnoid.

There is another point which I must mention to you, and which we shall have to make use of in forming our theory of cerebral hemorrhage ; this is the multiplicity and symmetry of the hemorrhagic foci.

It is quite rare to meet in the same brain with several recent foci of any considerable size ; but it is common enough to see, together with an immense hemorrhage in the corpus striatum, several small effusions scattered through the pons, the cerebellum, or the convolutions ; it is especially common to see beside a recent focus ochreous cysts, which are the evident traces of previous hemorrhage.*

In those cases where the foci are multiple you will often find that both hemispheres are involved, and that the effusions have occurred with some amount of symmetry. Thus, you will see in the specimen I show you both a recent focus just outside the corpus striatum and an ochreous cicatrix occupying the tæniform nucleus of the opposite side. You may often enough also see a recent effusion of considerable size in one thalamus, and another of more limited extent in the opposite thalamus. And nothing is more common than to meet with symmetrically placed foci in the two striate bodies.

* Consult Hughlings Jackson, *On Apoplexy and Cerebral Hemorrhage*, in Reynolds's "System," vol. ii., p. 508. London, 1868.—W. Ogle, *Path. Soc. Trans.*, vol. xv., p. 8.

LECTURE XXIII.

MORBID ANATOMY OF CEREBRAL HEMORRHAGE.

SUMMARY.—Demonstration of a case of hemorrhage with perforation into the ventricle not leading to death.

Continuation of the pathological anatomy of hemorrhagic foci in the brain.— Their shape.—Distinction between recent and ancient foci.

Condition of the contents of recent foci.—Transformation of the effused blood.—Condition of the limiting wall.—Softening by imbibition.—Capillary apoplexy around recent foci.

The formation of the limiting membrane marks the commencement of the second period.—Its growth.—Its structure.—Condition of the contents of ancient foci.—Last changes in ancient foci.

Secondary lesions of the nervous system.—Visceral lesions.—Nutritive lesions of paralysed parts.

GENTLEMEN,—Before continuing the study of hemorrhagic foci, which we commenced at our last meeting, I want to show you a rare pathological specimen, which will confirm an assertion which I based on the authority of Rokitansky, and on some analogous observations which I had previously collected. I allude to the possible curability of cerebral hemorrhage which has broken into the ventricles. The specimen I show you is most convincing.

It was the case of a woman of 60 who was attacked with hemiplegia about six months ago. She was admitted to the Salpêtrière as hemiplegic and incapable. After a sojourn of several months in this hospital she succumbed to a disease other than the cerebral one.

The autopsy showed us a hemorrhagic focus of considerable size, occupying the thalamus and corpus striatum of the right side. About its anterior third this focus communicates by a largish orifice with the lateral ventricle. You can see the yellow ochreous membrane which lines this focus, and in its centre a granular mass, also ochreous, and resembling fibrin, representing the vestiges of the clot, and formerly surrounded by a limpid fluid. I may add that in this case miliary aneurisms have been discovered in the grey matter of several parts of the encephalon. Having considered this case, which the chances of practice have

thrown in our way at the right moment, let us return to the study
of hemorrhagic foci.

We have already spoken of the number and site of these foci;
we must now study the focus itself. I shall describe it as it
appears directly after its formation ; then we will follow the
modifications which it undergoes with time, and which end at
last, when the patient survives, in the formation of a cyst or
even of a regular cicatrix. We shall, then, first study fresh, and
afterwards old foci.

I. *Recent Foci.*

What is of most importance and the greatest cause of varia-
tion in the other characters of recent foci is their size. Those
which are small are generally tolerably regular in shape ; their
walls are smooth and unbroken. If they are located in the substance of the convolutions they are usually round. Elsewhere,
in the claustrum for example, they are oval or almond-shaped ;
you might compare them to a button hole, and it looks as though
there had been simple separation of the nerve fibres rather than
rupture. The external appearance of the brain in these cases of
small hemorrhage is not perceptibly modified ; one sees no
difference in shape or volume between the two hemispheres ; and
were there not in some cases considerable injection of the pia-
mater, nothing in the aspect of the organ would lead to the supposition that any lesion existed. More frequently one finds
extensive effusions, perhaps of from two to eight or ten ounces
of blood (Rokitansky). The cavity is then anfractuous and
irregular, its walls are rough and broken. It is in such a case
that one often sees the tear involve the ventricular wall, and
thus establish a communication between the focus and the
ventricles. In such a case the brain is large and swollen, and
seems to fluctuate ; its consistence seems to be diminished, and
it flattens out when deposited upon the table. It often also in
these cases shows some degree of anæmia, and the convolutions
are pale and flattened.

We shall successively pass in review the characters presented
by the contents of the focus and its limiting walls. It is especially in this respect that the distinction which I pointed out to
you between recent and ancient foci is of importance. The

T

appearance and nature of the walls and of the contents of the focus vary in proportion to the progress of the reparative process, which in the most favourable cases is to end in the formation of a cicatrix. It is true these modifications take place gradually and imperceptibly, so that by restricting the name of recent foci to those which are examined during the first month, and calling those which have already passed the beginning of the second month, ancient foci, we are establishing a rather arbitrary distinction, for the earliest reparative events begin before the second month; but in the continued series of these modifications we must for descriptive purposes make some sort of division. Now in assigning the commencement of the second month as the period when the focus may first be regarded as ancient, we date very nearly from the moment when the limiting membrane is first formed.

In the recent focus the effused blood is coagulated, but it does not separate into serum and cruor like that of a blood-letting; the clot is directly in contact with the wall. In small foci this blood, pure from all admixture, is fairly comparable to the clotted masses which are found at an autopsy in the cavities of the heart. In foci of considerable size it pretty frequently happens that the blood is mixed more or less intimately with a detritus of nervous matter and separate fragments of cerebral tissue. After eight or ten days important modifications have already taken place both in the blood itself and in the remains of cerebral pulp with which it may be mingled.

As to the blood, with the exception of a few details you will only find the usual modifications which this fluid undergoes when effused in almost any organ. The white corpuscles swell and undergo granular degeneration; the fatty granules with which they become crammed give them the appearance of granular corpuscles, but they are sharply distinguished from the other granular corpuscles, which we shall have to study later on, by preserving the essential characters of the normal elements from which they were formed; they are granular corpuscles in which the granules are bounded externally by an enveloping membrane, and in the interior of which one or several nuclei may be distinguished. The fibrin itself undergoes fatty degeneration, loses its striation, becomes granulated, and breaks down more or less completely into a granular detritus.

The changes which the red corpuscles undergo are of especial interest; for it is to the products of their metamorphosis that old hemorrhagic foci owe one of their most readily recognisable characters, their ochreous colouring. Little by little these corpuscles lose their colour by losing their hematin, but they retain their shape, remaining for some time as flattened or spherical bodies, but consisting entirely of globulin. At last, however, they shrivel up, become granular, and disappear by molecular disintegration. Meanwhile the hematin which has left the corpuscles has given a red tint to the serum in which it becomes dissolved, and impregnating the neighbouring parts, has communicated its colour to them; but after a certain time it becomes chemically changed, and is precipitated as a new substance called hematoidin. This product of the spontaneous decomposition of hematin, which latter only differs from it in chemical composition by having a molecule of iron in place of a molecule of water (Robin), appears in the foci of cerebral hemorrhage, as elsewhere, in two different states, the granular and the crystalline. In the former case, hematoidin appears in the form of irregular, amorphous granules, of various sizes and of a dark yellow colour; in the latter, it forms crystalline needles or lozenges of a beautiful blood-red colour. These crystals, which are oblique rhombohedra, are not only found when the hemorrhage is an ancient one; Virchow has seen them from the seventeenth day after the onset of the hemorrhage, and Lebert has met with them after three weeks.*

* In a note contributed to the *Société micrographique* (*Arch. de phys. norm. et path.*, May, 1868), M. Bouchard has studied the conditions which facilitate the absorption of the products of disintegration of blood in most organs, but cause these materials to remain indefinitely in the cerebral tissue, and give to old foci their lasting ochreous tint. In all organs where the connective tissue is characterised by fusiform or stellate cells with anastomosing processes, that is, in the immense majority of tissues, the products of disintegration of blood, granules of fat and hematoidin, infiltrate these cellular elements and spread through the networks formed by them, injecting, as it were, both the cells and the lymphatic channels. In this way there forms around the focus a zone of considerable extent and ochreous colour, the intensity of which goes on gradually diminishing in proportion as you advance towards the periphery, and in which you may see also that the granules of pigment, very numerous in the cells in the neighbourhood of the hemorrhage, become less and less numerous in proportion to their distance from the centre. There occurs, then, a migration of the coloured granules, which leave the seat of hemorrhage and allow the tissues gradually to resume their normal colour; and the ultimate disappearance of this blood pigment is due, no doubt, to its being at last carried off by the lymphatics, the radicles of which, as is well known, are in direct communication with the corpuscles of the connective tissue. This absorption of blood pigment by the lymphatic spaces and channels has its

While the changes which we have just mentioned are going forward, the clot as a whole becomes altered ; it condenses and loses its quivering consistence, its serous portion diminishing. The modifications which it undergoes are first observable at the periphery, so that the superficial layers become greyish and then ochreous, whilst the centre is still of a black-red, like lees of wine. At length the change involves the whole of the clot, which after a while presents the characters which I shall mention as belonging to ancient foci.

But before proceeding to this subject I must tell you what becomes of the fragments of nervous substance, which, as I have already observed, are pretty frequently mingled with the blood in foci of considerable size. These remnants may to a certain extent be compared with the fragments of divided nerves, for numerous experiments in which nerves have been cut have shown that nerve tubes thus parted from centres undergo a granular degeneration in the portion which has then lost its connection with its nucleus of origin. The myelin of each tube is converted into fatty granules. A similar necrobiosis seizes on the fragments of cerebral tissue which the hemorrhage has torn from the rest of the brain ; the nerve tubes which form these fragments having lost their connection with the cells from which they originate, and no longer receiving blood to maintain their nutrition, are rapidly transformed into drops of myelin, then into droplets and granules of fat. These granules, which unite into more or less regular masses, may form one variety of

---

analogy in the migration of coloured granules in a tatooed skin, and Follin and Virchow have shown that the latter penetrate into the lymphatic circulation.

In the encephalon matters happen otherwise, and the difference is in relation with peculiarities of structure, which would render such a migration impossible. The connective tissue of the nervous centres, the neuroglia, is formed of elements which do not anastomose, or at least, if the fibrillæ of the reticulum anastomose, it has never been shown that they form channels and bring the cellular elements into real relationship. Those cells which are in contact with the effused blood absorb plenty of pigment and fatty granules, but these granules remain enclosed in them. Again, the cavity of the perivascular sheath also becomes full of the granular *débris* of decomposing blood. But this sheath, which bears the name of lymphatic sheath, cannot be regarded as a true lymphatic canal, in spite of the conclusions at which Robin and His have arrived. You can inject these sheaths, but the injection never gets as far as a true lymphatic vessel or gland. The blood pigment from a cerebral hemorrhage, then, meets with none of the conditions which in other tissues facilitate its migration and disappearance. So that we must attribute the remarkable persistence of hematoidin in the foci of cerebral hemorrhage and the almost indelible ochreous tint of these foci to the absence of lymphatics and of a connective tissue with anastomosing cells.

granular corpuscles, which you will distinguish from those originating in leucocytes by their having neither enveloping membrane nor nuclei.

Thus, gentlemen, the blood pure or mingled with fragments of nerve tissue gradually becomes freed from its serous portion ; its solid elements undergo a granular and fatty metamorphosis which facilitates their absorption ; one element only, hematoidin, persists, because it is susceptible neither of solution nor of a sufficiently fine molecular division ; thus you will not be surprised to find that it gives to old foci their most striking characteristic.

But let us leave that subject for a moment and return to the study of the wall in recent foci. When you are examining a hemorrhage of recent date, and by extensively incising the focus have allowed the clot which it contained to escape, and when by means of a gentle stream of water you have more completely cleansed the wall from the remains of clot which have stuck there, you perceive, as I have said, that this wall, which is generally smooth when the hemorrhage has been scanty, is more frequently irregular and broken when the focus has attained a certain size. In this latter case, which alone need detain us, the surface is of a brownish red, infiltrated with blood, villous and flocky in appearance. A more minute examination shows that the inequalities which give it this aspect are formed of rags of brain substance or of broken vessels.

These small vessels, which extend into the focus, and the existence of which has already been announced by several authors, are sometimes blocked by little clots which surround and cap, as it were, the ruptured extremity. Hence results an appearance against which I must forewarn you, because it might easily lead you into error. These little masses of clot, suspended by filamentous vessels, simulate miliary aneurisms, and often microscopic examination is necessary in order that their true nature may be made out. (Plate VI., fig. 1.) We shall see that real miliary aneurisms may be found attached to the broken vessels which lie in the walls of large foci.

If you examine a section of the nervous tissue which surrounds the focus, you will find that it presents certain changes through a zone of three or four millimetres' thickness. In this zone the cerebral substance is softened, and is distinguished by its canary

yellow colour from the white-coloured surrounding tissue. These
lesions have been considered by some authors as the result of
softening precedent to the hemorrhage ; this is the *ramollissement hémorrhagipare* of Rochoux, and Todd has tried to rejuve-
nate it without bringing any very convincing reasons in support
of his opinion. I cannot enter now into a discussion to which
we shall have to return ; it is a subject which will ultimately be
treated with all the completeness that it allows of ; but I may
mention to you even now the reasons which show that this
softening is simply the result of infiltration by the serum of the
effused blood, that it is consequently secondary to the hemorrhage, and by no means a lesion preparatory to hemorrhage.
This œdematous infiltration by blood serum is in the brain the
analogue of the ecchymotic zone which surrounds the collections
of blood formed in external parts. A case reported by M. Bouchard in his thesis proves distinctly that it is the serum of the
effused blood which soaks the cerebral tissue in the neighbourhood of the hemorrhage. In the case to which I allude the
blood serum was strongly coloured by biliary pigment, and the
softened zone which surrounded the clot had a very marked
icteric tint, very different from the yellow colour of ecchymosis.
And then microscopic examination supplies data which suffice to
decide the question. If we were dealing with previous softening
we should find fatty granules after twenty-four hours, and granular
corpuscles after two days in the softened tissue, as is observed in
man and animals in real softening. Now there is none of this,
and the much more tardy appearance in cases of cerebral
hemorrhage of elements, which reveal a necrobiotic action,
indicates a process different from that of ordinary softening.
But the parts which become softened by imbibition at length
undergo fatty degeneration ; the nervous elements which formed
the softened zone disappear in great measure and give place to
new elements which result from a proliferating process in the
cerebral connective tissue. But this process, which is to end in
the formation of a limiting membrane, belongs already to the
second period.

This softened zone, which surrounds the blood from the
earliest period, is not always uniformly coloured. Most frequently you see, drawn on the yellow ground which it presents,
dots or red streaks of *capillary apoplexy*. This condition, which

is observed especially in foci with irregular walls, will be the object of our future studies, and we shall meet with it again elsewhere than in cerebral hemorrhage. I shall show you that this capillary apoplexy is not a real effusion of blood, that it is only an accumulation of blood, outside the vessels it is true, but confined to the interior of the lymphatic sheath, which is distended, not ruptured by it. We can then inquire what degree of credence is to be given to the opinion that these spots of capillary apoplexy form the starting-point of the hemorrhagic focus, and I hope to prove to you that this condition is, on the contrary, secondary.

II. *Old Foci.*

We will now commence the study of old foci. The reparative process which had already begun to take place in the wall during the former period becomes more and more evident. The focus is diminished in size ; the clot, as I said, is more solid and less bulky ; the surrounding œdema has disappeared ; the disintegration of the softened parts has caused the villous processes of the wall to disappear, and thus the wall looks cleaner ; it has at the same time acquired greater consistence owing to the formation of a limiting membrane, which henceforth separates the still healthy tissue from the hemorrhagic cavity.

This limiting membrane is already recognisable at the end of the first month. Cruveilhier has seen it on the twenty-fifth day* after the occurrence of the hemorrhage ; Lebert has discovered it only on the thirty-fifth ; and Rokitansky still later, at the end of the second month ; Förster thinks that it requires at least a month to form. Thus the period of its first appearance must be somewhat variable. The original extent of the hemorrhage, the quantity of effused blood, the grey or white character of the lacerated parts which form the wall, and doubtless many other conditions still unknown to us, probably hasten or retard the appearance of this limiting membrane.

However this may be, we can follow the process step by step which leads to the formation of this membrane. The connective elements, which took very little part in the formation of the torn cerebral tissue, have multiplied and given birth to a considerable number of nuclei in the substance of the tissue which is softened

* *Anat. path.*, book v., pl. 5.

by imbibition. The new tissue resulting from this hyperplasia does not form a separate membrane superposed on the nervous tissue ; it is not, as Cruveilhier pointed out,* a distinct new layer ; it is rather a proliferation accompanied by induration of the normal tissues in the neighbourhood of the focus. This tissue, which on its free surface has the appearance of a felted membrane, gradually loses this character as you proceed from the hemorrhagic cavity towards the normal nervous tissue. Its histological structure, which is not unlike that of ordinary membraneous tissue, presents a certain number of irregularly arranged wavy fibrils, and especially some ovoid or spherical nuclei, which are made very clear by colouring with carmine. These anatomical elements are imbedded in an amorphous substance, transparent but slightly granular. Numerous vessels penetrate this tissue, and the vascular walls are themselves thronged with nuclei. Other substances must also be mentioned as occurring in the substance of this tissue ; their presence is easily explained by the way in which the membrane is developed. At the time when proliferation commenced among the connective elements of the part softened by imbibition, the nervous elements of this part underwent fatty degeneration, and gave rise to granular corpuscles and isolated granules ; the blood which permeated the tissue in the spots of capillary hemorrhage became transformed into hematoidin. These various elements, the products of disintegration, have been enclosed in the newly-formed tissue, and are found in the substance of the limiting membrane. It is thus that you find, mingled with the essential structure previously described, nervous elements, granular corpuscles, granules of fat and pigment, and, lastly, crystals of hematoidin. It is especially to this last circumstance that the cicatrix of an old hemorrhagic focus owes that peculiar ochreous colouring (Pl. IV., fig. 3 b), which Cruveilhier considered to be indelible ; † some authors think that it becomes effaced in the end. All that I can tell you on the subject is that it persists for a very long time at any rate, and that I have found it very distinct in foci of ten or even fifteen years standing.

I shall be more brief in dealing with the contents of old foci. The clot, after contracting, persists a considerable time as a

---

* *Dict. de méd. et de chir. prat.,* art. "Apoplexy," p. 210.

† *Dict. de méd. et de chir. prat.,* art. "Apoplexy," p. 210.

solid mass, but at length it becomes reduced, in part at least, to an ochreous mud, which may still be found after five or six months, and even in some cases after several years, surrounded by a little limpid serum.

The modifications which we have just been studying in the walls and contents of old foci tend to bring about a state of things which is final and lasting, and which may be considered as the last term of the reparative process. This final condition, which is but a vestige of the original lesion, appears in two different forms : the cavity either remains as such, or it is replaced by a linear cicatrix. In the former case the cavity may be rounded and gaping, with indurated walls ; generally, however, this is only the case when the hemorrhage has been the cause of much destruction ; more frequently it is elongated like an almond, and here and there the walls come into contact with each other and contract adhesions. The linear cicatrices, which are not met with so frequently, are only an exaggeration of this latter condition ; the union of the walls has become complete, and every trace of a cavity has disappeared.

We have now completed our anatomical study of hemorrhagic foci ; but, omitting the lesions on which the production of the hemorrhage depends, a subject which we shall commence at our next meeting, there would still be many points which I should have to study with you if I intended to give you a complete account of the anatomical lesions which are associated with cerebral hemorrhage. A study of them will find a more fitting occasion elsewhere, and to-day I merely want to mention them to you summarily.

These lesions of secondary development may be met with in the nervous system itself, in the viscera, and in the paralysed limbs.

The different portions of the nervous system are not independent of one another ; there is a sort of solidarity between them, and a lesion of one portion may influence the rest in various ways. It is in this way that, as a consequence of old cerebral hemorrhages, nutrition may be affected either in the injured hemisphere or throughout the brain ; thence results a kind of atrophy, which is evidenced by the diminution in weight of the affected lobe or of the whole encephalon. In this latter case you find the convolutions small and of a yellowish colour, while the ventricles are enlarged; the condition is very like that of senile atrophy of the brain.

Other alterations in the nervous system depend on a process that is quite peculiar. The fibres which have been separated from their nuclei of origin in the grey matter by the tearing of the cerebral tissue undergo fatty degeneration in their whole extent. As a consequence, you can, starting from the focus, trace out bands of secondary degeneration, which follow the normal distribution of the nervous bundles, not only in the brain itself but through the basal tracts, and even in the cord. This important study of the secondary degenerations of the spinal cord deserves a place to itself.

As to the visceral lesions, such as pulmonary consolidation and hemorrhage from the gastric mucosa, they are more particularly connected with morbid physiology and clinical medicine, and we shall have an opportunity of returning to them.

I shall also postpone, till we are considering the symptomatology of cerebral hemorrhage, the study of those nutritive lesions which come on early or late in the paralysed parts.

LECTURE XXIV.

DIFFUSE PERIARTERITIS AND MILIARY ANEURISMS.

SUMMARY.—Arterial lesions which give rise to cerebral hemorrhage.

Diffuse periarteritis with miliary aneurisms.—The rupture of these aneurisms is the most frequent cause of hemorrhage in the brain.—Description of diffuse periarteritis.—Structure of the arteries and arterioles of the brain.—Modifications which the various coats of these vessels undergo in diffuse periarteritis.—There is no atheromatous degeneration in this case.—Mode of formation of miliary aneurisms.—Chief characteristics distinguishing diffuse periarteritis from nodular endarteritis.—These two affections may occur separately or appear together in the same patient.

Description of miliary aneurisms.—They are usually visible to the naked eye.—Varieties in their aspect.—Their favourite sites.—Their number.—Their texture and its modifications.—Various ways in which these aneurisms undergo spontaneous cure.

Rupture of miliary aneurisms.—Formation of hemorrhagic foci.—Persistence of the lymphatic sheath in some cases.

Statistics relating to the habitual presence of miliary aneurisms in cerebral hemorrhage, whether old or recent.—Cases in which cerebral hemorrhage does not depend on rupture of miliary aneurisms.

Relation between miliary aneurisms, aneurisms of the arteries at the base, and aneurisms in other parts of the body.

A few words of history.

Comparison of miliary aneurisms with the other intra-cranial aneurisms.—Hemorrhages resulting from the rupture of these aneurisms.—Anatomical and clinical differences between these hemorrhages and those occurring within the brain.—Frequency of aneurisms of the arteries at the base.—Slight importance of atheroma in the production of these aneurisms.—Their relation to aneurisms of the viscera and limbs.

GENTLEMEN,—The arrangement which I intend to follow in this anatomical account leads me to talk to you to-day about the changes in the cerebral vessels, on which cerebral hemorrhage depends, as a more or less direct consequence.

I showed you before that, according to the researches which Bouchard and I have undertaken, the rupture of certain small aneurisms is the immediate cause of the extravasation of blood in the very great majority of cases of hemorrhage within the brain ; these aneurisms, which we propose to call *miliary aneurisms,* will soon be the subject of a detailed description ; but they are themselves only one of the results, and indeed the last term, of a peculiar morbid process in the arterial walls, the study of which must first occupy us.

Later on we shall discuss other vascular changes to which authors are in the habit of referring most cerebral hemorrhages. Fair criticism of the opinions expressed on this subject will then, I don't doubt, convince you that it is only the variety of arterial induration ending in the production of miliary aneurisms, that plays any really peculiar part in the pathogenesis of hemorrhage within the brain.

I. *Diffuse Periarteritis.*

I am not in a position to decide whether the lesion in question may affect all parts of the vascular system of the encephalon, but I can state that it mainly attacks the small arteries. The true capillary vessels, the biggest of which do not exceed ·1 mm. in diameter (Robin's *capillaires de la première variété*), are, it is true, rarely quite free ; but they never appear so profoundly changed as the vessels of more complex structure, already visible to the naked eye, and called arterioles or veinlets by most anatomists (Robin's *capillaires de deuxième et de troisième ordre*). The arteries at the base, and their larger or smaller branches which ramify in the meninges, are frequently affected by this morbid process.

A. Before beginning to study the details of this arterial lesion, I think it well to recall a few peculiarities in the normal structure of the capillaries and arteries of the encephalon. We shall thus be enabled to follow more readily the modifications to which the disease gives rise in the histological structure of these vessels.

It has long been noticed that the arteries at the base of the brain have very thin walls in proportion to their calibre, and it is here the adventitious or connective-tissue coat which is remarkable for its extreme tenuity. Some have been inclined to see in this anatomical condition a kind of normal predisposition to rupture of arteries. I do not believe that this opinion is based on very solid foundations. According to Dr. Gimbert's very important work * on the comparative structure of the arteries in the different parts of the body, it is especially the elastic fibres, that is, the agents of passive resistance, which are specially scanty in the arteries at the base of the brain ; but the active elements,

* Mémoire sur la structure et sur la texture des artères, *Journ. de l'anat. et de la phys.*, etc., 1865, p. 565 ; and *Dissertation inaugurale*, Paris, 1865.

the muscular fibres, are abundant, the basilar artery, for example, presenting in an equal space more unstriated fibres than the thyroid does ; in this way no doubt sufficient compensation is effected. I shall do no more than point out this peculiarity of structure, which, however, does not exclusively affect the comparatively large arteries at the base, but is also found to some extent in the very fine arterioles distributed through the interior of the cerebral pulp. We must examine these arterioles with care, for they are the vessels which bear miliary aneurisms, and which consequently supply the blood in ordinary cerebral hemorrhage.

The walls of these vessels, as you know, consist of three coats one within another : —

(1) The most internal is lined on the inside with a layer of epithelioid cells, which are inseparable from one another, and in this way differ from those occurring in the larger arteries. It consists itself of a homogeneous membrane, which is inlaid with ovoid nuclei, whose long axis lies in the direction of the vessel.

(2) The middle coat is formed of involuntary muscular fibres, arranged in rings encircling the internal tunic. These muscular elements become more numerous and closer packed the further you proceed from the capillaries towards the actual arteries. You thus find one, two, then three layers one over another ; their arrangement is very regular, and they are not found mingled with elastic fibres. One peculiarity deserves special mention, namely, that the plain fibres are more abundant in the cerebral arteries than they are in any other part of the body in arterioles of corresponding calibre.

(3) The external coat is the one which is called adventitious ; its structure is somewhat different from that of the arterioles in other parts of the body. It is to be observed, in the first place, that it ceases to be evident some time before the vessel grows free of its muscular coat and becomes a true capillary ; again, elastic elements seem entirely absent, and it is composed almost exclusively of connective tissue, very fine on the small vessels, thicker and more fibrous on the larger trunks. This tissue has a regular longitudinal striation. The cellular elements which are imbedded in it are scanty ; there are a few narrow fusiform corpuscles, which lie in the direction of the vessel. Where the adventitia becomes very thin, these corpuscles become no more

than mere nuclei outside the muscular coat; they are comparable in their arrangement to the oval nuclei of the internal layer, but they are always smaller in size.

So you see we find, as I said, that the arterioles of the encephalon present the same characters as those which I mentioned to you as belonging to the large arteries at the base; namely, the abundance of muscular elements, the relative paucity of elastic structures, and the remarkable tenuity of the adventitia. I have still to describe to you an anatomical arrangement which seems to belong exclusively to the small arteries of the encephalon and cord.

I refer to that additional tunic the existence of which has been demonstrated by Robin in the vessels of the encephalon and cord, which His has of late studied afresh, and which is now commonly spoken of as the lymphatic sheath. This membrane really forms a sheath, enveloping the small blood-vessels, especially the arterioles, and accompanying them from the point where they emerge from the arteries of the pia-mater as far as the point where they split into true capillaries; the capillaries are quite free of this sheath. It is not applied directly to the actual wall of the vessel, but the vessel floats freely in its cavity, bathed by the liquid with which it is filled. It is important to notice that in the normal state the lymphatic coat or sheath is fine and transparent, structureless, and merely dotted here and there with a few nuclei, which resemble to some extent the nuclei of the neuroglia (myelocytes).* The external surface of the sheath is bordered by the nervous tissue with which it is in close contact; its internal surface, according to His, is covered in the larger arterioles by an epithelium, which Bastian thinks he has traced as far as the minutest branches. I shall not attempt to decide this question, which is still under discussion, and in order to conclude with what it is important you should know concerning the anatomy of lymphatic sheaths, I will merely remind you that the liquid which they enclose seems to be normally almost transparent, and that it is only in a state of disease that it is found to contain a large number of

---

* The sheath which surrounds the larger trunks (arteries of the corpus striatum, for example) does not consist solely of a structureless membrane; it has besides a layer of connective tissue in which are found a number of cellular elements, assuming the most varied forms. In the aged these elements frequently become vesicular (Lépine, *Soc. Biol.*, 1867).

the elements which are figured in the plate accompanying Robin's memoir.*

B. The lesion which I am going to describe may act upon all the layers, the normal arrangement of which I have just recalled to you; but it does not occur simultaneously, or with equal intensity, in all these structures; it may be said as a general rule to progress from without inwards; when the change is slight the outer coats are alone affected, and when it has attacked the whole thickness of the vessel, it is still the outer coats in which the morbid process appears most advanced. It is therefore, you see, a case of *periarteritis*, and the lesion in question is thus sharply distinguished by its first characteristic from that which leads to atheromatous degeneration of the arteries, and which is rightly called *endarteritis*.

Another characteristic of this lesion is that it is essentially *diffuse*, in the sense that it is not limited to a particular arteriole, or even to a separate portion of the intra-cranial circulation; it tends to extend beyond the arterioles, which are, however, its principal seat, and to spread to the whole arterial system of the brain. On the one hand we must admit that the true capillaries frequently participate in the morbid process, and, on the other, that the larger arteries of the base and meninges are often the seat of a morbid change like that which more particularly affects the small vessels of the cerebral substance. I must now point out the histological modifications which take place during the progress of this disease in the different vascular tunics, beginning with the most external. My description will apply especially to the arterioles.

In the lymphatic sheath we have first to note a multiplication of those nuclei, which, as I told you, are somewhat like those of the neuroglia; this is nearly constant, and usually considerable; the membrane becomes loaded with nuclear bodies, spherical or ovoid, but rather irregular in outline, and contracting and becoming clearer under the action of acetic acid. Carmine and fuchsia stain these nuclei. They may develop in numbers so prodigious as to interfere with the study of the subjacent parts. The degree to which this multiplication of the nuclei of the sheath goes is always in relation with the actual intensity of the vascular lesion. You may notice that a good many of these

* *Journal de la Physiologie*, vol. ii., pl. 6, fig. 3, 1859.

numerous nuclei appear constricted, thus assuming a bilobed
aspect, or the appearance of a bean ; this is, no doubt, to be
regarded as the commencement of a process of segmentation,
and there is every reason to believe that the proliferation of
these bodies takes place, at least partially, in this manner.
(Pl. IV., fig. 1.)

There are cases where, instead of this multiplication of its
nuclei, the only lesion presented by the lymphatic sheath is a
striated wavy condition, scarcely modified by acetic acid ; in such
a case the membrane is considerably thickened.

In either case the cavity of the sheath may appear nowise
abnormal. Sometimes, however, you may see some vesicular
cells floating in the fluid which it contains ; you may also discover in it fatty granules and granules of hematoidin, but this
fact is not peculiar to the affection before us, and is observed
tolerably often in the most varied circumstances of old age.

In the adventitia the lesion may also be met with in two
different forms. Sometimes, and this is the usual case, the only
lesion is an often enormous multiplication of the nuclei, which
collect in confused masses and become quite irregular in their
arrangement ; this form of lesion may extend as far as the finest
arterioles. At other times you find merely a more or less
marked thickening of the membrane. Its thickness may sometimes be such as to equal the calibre of the vessel. In such a
case the tissue of the adventitia appears longitudinally striated
and dotted over with pretty frequent fusiform nuclei, lying in
the same direction as the vessel. Thence results a fasciculated
appearance, in consequence of which the arteriole assumes the
semblance of a band of fibrous tissue. (Pl. IV., fig. 1, D.)

It is at least very probable that, in the case of the adventitia
as well as in that of the lymphatic sheath, this fibroid state corresponds to the extreme stage of the morbid change, the first
phases of which are characterised by the multiplication of nuclei.
It is, moreover, occasionally possible to recognise the various
transitional states between these two extremes of an identical
morbid process.

The muscular coat may in its turn become affected, and the
lesion which you find in such a case consists in the atrophy and
disappearance of the muscular elements, this occurring without
fatty metamorphosis. This lesion is first shown by the diminu-

tion and separation of the transverse striæ of the artery, which here and there disappear completely. It is usually less extensive than the change in the lymphatic sheath and the adventitia; it is never observed except in the spots where these latter are already markedly involved in the irritative process; it is often absent in vessels in which the superficial coats are already beginning to be changed, and it is always most marked in spots where these latter are most profoundly diseased.

After all this, it will be clear to you that the change of the muscular coat is a secondary and consecutive lesion, dependent on the indurating inflammation of the more superficial layers.

I can now point out to you, before entering into the details of a complete description, the modifications of shape and size which the arterioles may present, when they have become the seat of these morbid changes in the muscular coat. Wherever the unstriated fibres are decidedly diminished, and especially where they have completely disappeared, the vascular wall, deprived of its means of resistance, yields to the lateral pressure of the blood; thus are produced dilatations of various forms, sometimes cylindrical, sometimes fusiform, moniliform, or saccular. (Pl. V., fig. 3; Pl. VI., figs. 3, 4.) These last, of which I shall treat directly under the name of miliary aneurisms, are the most important of all. A noteworthy thing is that the various forms of vascular dilatation, and especially miliary aneurisms, scarcely ever appear when the external coat has reached a certain degree of fibrous metamorphosis and has become notably thickened, even when the atrophy of the muscular fibres is very pronounced. On the other hand, multiplication of the nuclei of the adventitia is almost always very decided at spots where the vessel has been distended into an aneurism.

Of the arterial coats the internal is the one which is most slightly and tardily affected in the disease which we are considering. There may be no lesion here at all when the other coats are already deeply involved. The morbid change is evidenced here, as in the adventitia, by a varying amount of multiplication of the nuclei, which lose their ovoid shape and regular arrangement. This lesion may be traced as far as the vessels in which the internal coat frees itself of the external and muscular layers and begins to constitute the sole wall of the true capillaries.

U

The capillary vessels are thus sometimes affected in the same way as the arterioles ; the same may be said of the very small vessels of the pia-mater, which in such cases often bear globular dilatations, which Virchow has already observed, and which he referred to *saccular ectasis*. As to the larger branches of the circle and the meninges, I have often seen them with fusiform dilatations, or with true saccular aneurisms, at the same time that the arterioles presented the most manifest signs of diffuse periarteritis with or without miliary aneurisms, and this cannot be regarded as a chance coincidence.*

After the description which you have just heard, it will, I think, be superfluous to enter into much detail in order to satisfy you as to the name of *diffuse periarteritis*, which I have selected to designate the arterial lesion which we are considering. That there is at the commencement an irritative process is sufficiently evidenced by the multiplication of nuclei in the lymphatic sheath and adventitia ; and we know that these two layers, the most external of the arterial coats, are always the first affected and the most seriously involved. The atrophy of the muscular fibres of the middle coat is a consecutive and secondary phenomenon. We know also that in this form of arteritis the lesion mainly affects the very small arterioles of the cerebral substance, but that the change may spread on the one hand to the true capillaries, on the other to the large arteries at the base. Lastly, without mentioning the usual accompaniment of miliary aneurisms, there is one trait peculiar to this affection which it is important to make conspicuous in a summary description, namely, that the morbid process may pass through all the phases of its development without ever leading to fatty degeneration of the structural elements.

We have now summed up the most essential characteristics of diffuse periarteritis. They will appear still more striking to you, when at another meeting we compare them with those distinctive of nodular endarteritis, a change so frequently observed in advanced age affecting the cerebral arteries, leading almost inevitably to atheromatous degeneration of these vessels, and

---

* Several cases showing this coincidence have been collected in the inaugural thesis of a student of the Salpêtrière, M. Durand (*Des anévrismes du cerveau*, Paris, 1868). An analogous case, a very remarkable one, has been published lately by Dr. Paulicki of Hamburg, in the *Deutsche Klinik*, vol. xix., p. 449, 1867, with the title, *Mehrfache kleinere Aneurysmata an den Basilararterien des Gehirns und in Gehirnsubstanz.*

commonly assumed, though quite mistakenly, in my opinion, as the usual starting-point of hemorrhages within the brain. The commencement of the disease in the internal coat, its preference for the arteries of the base and their chief branches, the almost constant presence of the products of fatty degeneration in the midst of the diseased structures, the absence of vascular enlargements of the nature of miliary aneurisms, these are the characters of endarteritis which I shall have to bring into prominence. But it is easy for you to perceive already how radical are the differences which separate these two chief forms of chronic arteritis from one another.

I do not mean to say that these two forms of chronic inflammation of the arteries may not coexist in the same individual and at the same spots in the vascular system. On the contrary, this coincidence is really pretty frequent. Thus, in reviewing all the cases of cerebral hemorrhage ending in death, which have been collected for nearly two years at the hospital of the Salpêtrière, I find that atheroma of the arteries of the base and arteritis with miliary aneurisms occurred simultaneously, and to almost the same extent, in about one-third of the cases; in a second third the coincidence was still present, though the atheroma was but slight. But in the last third of these cases, the lesions of endarteritis were completely absent; the periarteritis was free from all complication, and could alone be regarded as the starting-point of the extravasation of blood; from which we may make the legitimate induction that in ordinary cerebral hemorrhage diffuse periarteritis is the only really peculiar lesion to which we can refer. But this is a point to which we shall have to return presently.*

II. *Miliary Aneurisms.*

A. It is on the convexity of the cerebral hemispheres at the surface of the convolutions that miliary aneurisms may be most readily observed and studied. After the removal of the pia-mater they may be seen at the summit or on the sides of the gyri, or again at the bottom of the sulci which separate them, in the form of little spherical grains of shining aspect, and which

* This result is confirmed by the analysis of 69 cases in the *Archives de physiologie,* p. 733, 1868.

seem to be to some extent imbedded in the grey matter. If the
search for these little bodies is sometimes a long and delicate
process in the deeper regions of the encephalon, this is by no
means the case with those which are placed superficially. The
slightest attention is required in order to discover them at once,
for there is no need to arm oneself with a microscope, or even
with a lens; all miliary aneurisms indeed are visible to the
naked eye; their diameter varies from ·2 mm. to 1 mm. But it
is well to have recourse to a lens to grasp details better. You then
perceive, by raising the aneurism, or displacing it with needles,
that these enlargements have formed upon vascular threads, and
you can generally distinguish pretty easily the afferent and
efferent vessel. It is also generally possible to recognise these
small vessels even with the naked eye, for their diameter, which
I have never noticed less than $\frac{1}{30}$ mm., may be as much as a
quarter of a millimetre.

Whether miliary aneurisms are observed at the surface of the
convolutions or in the substance of the cerebral tissue, they
present some variations in external appearance of which I must
speak to you. Modifications in the condition of the walls or
contents of the aneurism account for these differences. If the
wall is formed of the dilated internal coat simply covered by the
adventitia, it is often very thin. At other times, on the contrary, it is notably thickened on account of the proliferation of
the connective tissue of the adventitia, which is united to the
internal coat, and also pretty frequently contracts intimate adhesions with the lymphatic sheath. The wall becomes more or
less opaque on account of the thickening which it has undergone.
From these peculiarities it happens that, when the walls of the
aneurism are thin, and when the blood which it contains circu-
lates freely, owing to the permeability of the afferent vessels, the
aneurism has the appearance of a bright or dark red glomerulus ;
but when, on the contrary, the blood has become stagnant
because of the growth of concretions in the vessel leading to the
aneurism, or when it has coagulated primarily in the aneurismal
cavity, it will there have undergone the disintegrative changes
with which you are already acquainted, and then the aneurism
acquires from the hematoidin, which it contains, a brown
ochreous colour, which is sometimes very marked. You will
often notice in such cases that the hematoidin stains of a yellow

or brown tint the surrounding cerebral tissue to some distance from the aneurism.

In cases where the fibrous overgrowth has thickened the aneurismal wall, and this occurs especially with aneurisms situated deeply in the cerebral substance, the little swellings have a slightly bluish colour if the blood has remained fluid, greyish if the stagnation of the blood has allowed the white corpuscles to collect together, brownish if the blood has already undergone some amount of disintegration, and yellowish if the coagulation took place long enough ago to allow fatty or even calcareous granules to predominate over the deposits of hematoidin.

It is well to point out that, in relation with these differences in appearance, and influenced by the causes which determine them, aneurisms present very marked differences in consistence.

Thus some are soft and fragile, and are ruptured by the least pressure, allowing the blood to escape in a liquid condition and of normal appearance ; others are denser and firmer, and somewhat elastic, and hence resist better when one squeezes them, allowing their contents to escape by the orifices of the vessels which lead to the dilated parts ; others still are hard, and sometimes even acquire the consistence of a grain of sand.

B. Miliary aneurisms may be met with in almost every part of the encephalon ; there are, however, certain regions which they more especially frequent. In the convolutions, as you are aware, they are very commonly observed ; this is not because they are really more frequent there than in some other parts, but, owing to their more superficial position, they seem to offer themselves to the attention of the observer. All aneurisms in the convolutions are not, however, apparent without preparation and by the mere removal of the pia-mater ; there are some which dip so far into the grey matter as to be enveloped on all sides ; there are others which are buried more deeply still, and are situated in the zone which connects the cortex with the white substance. It is clear that such aneurisms can only be discovered by numerous and very close incisions made perpendicularly to the surface of the brain. (Pl. IV., fig. 2.)

Whenever you meet with miliary aneurisms in the convolutions you may be sure that there are others deeply buried in the cerebral tissue. The convolutions, as I said, are not the sole or even the favourite seat of aneurisms. The result of the observations which I have collected leads me to arrange the regions of the encephalon, where aneurisms occur, in the following order of diminishing frequency. The thalami and the corpora striata must be mentioned first, then come the pons, the grey matter of the convolutions, the claustrum, the cerebellum (especially the parts in the neighbourhood of the rhomboidal body), the cerebellar peduncles, and lastly, the centrum ovale. In the medulla miliary aneurisms are, I believe, infinitely rare. I could not affirm that this arrangement is in absolute conformity with reality; but I do not think it can be far otherwise. I may observe, however, that the high place occupied in this table by certain regions, such as the pons or the convolutions, is probably partly due to the fact that in these parts the discovery of aneurisms is relatively easy.

C. It is almost impossible, as you will readily understand, to estimate accurately the number of miliary aneurisms which, in a given case, the encephalon may contain. Incisions made into the organ cannot be sufficiently delicate or sufficiently numerous for us to be sure that not one of the little enlargements has escaped our search. In some cases of cerebral hemorrhage I have not been able to find more than two or three miliary aneurisms, in spite of the most careful search; but at other times, on the contrary, more than a hundred can be counted on the surface of the convolutions, whilst in most of the sections through the central nuclei of grey matter a large number may also be counted.

D. We know how, in consequence of the atrophy of the plain fibres of the muscular coat, the internal and external tunics become distended by the pressure of the blood and produce miliary aneurismal dilatations. In their subsequent course these little aneurisms undergo modifications of texture, so that what we may call their normal structure becomes changed. Numerous anatomical researches enable us to understand all the phases and degrees of these various modifications. It may be said, without falling into the error of teleology, that these changes sometimes consist of a kind of reparative process, giving rise to spontaneous cure of the aneurism, or, at least, making it harmless; but that at other times they have the effect of diminishing the thickness or strength of the vascular walls and thus favour their rupture.

When blood passes from a narrow vessel and suddenly enters an aneurismal cavity, the diameter of which may be ten times as great as that of the vessel, and the sectional area therefore a hundred times as great, it necessarily experiences there a marked retardation of flow; now these conditions are present in the case of miliary aneurisms. Consequently it is not uncommon for the white corpuscles to accumulate in these aneurisms where the current is least perceptible. A layer of granular semi-liquid material sticks these corpuscles together, and in this way little masses are formed which may be the starting-point of concretions sufficiently large to fill up and completely obliterate the cavity of the aneurism. At other times the blood coagulates first in the afferent or efferent vessel, and the clot gradually spreads into the cavity of the sac. In either case the coagulated blood undergoes the usual transformations, and after a time the aneurism, having become impermeable, is filled with a mixture of fatty granules and of grains or crystals of hematoidin. In such a case rupture is not to be apprehended.

The same result may be brought about in quite a different way; the walls of the sac exhibit occasionally a kind of induration with considerable thickening, dependent on the mutual adhesion and even fusion of the internal coat, the adventitia, and the lymphatic sheath. The three tunics now form but a single membrane, which is formed of connective tissue with fusiform corpuscles, and the thickness of which is sufficiently great to resist the extremest pressure of the blood current.

Aneurisms whose walls have undergone this sclerotic thickening generally contract abnormal adhesions to the neighbouring nervous tissue, the connective elements of which have also proliferated. It is not uncommon in such a case to see numerous capillaries spreading over the surface of the enlargement in the same way as vasa vasorum.

The conditions favourable to the rupture of miliary aneurisms are less easily perceptible. It is at least very probable that the chief thing is an excessive atrophy of the walls and a consequent diminution of their strength. However it be, this rupture may occur, as I have many times ascertained, either at the neck of the aneurism or at that part of the enlargement which is farthest from the orifice of the sac. I have often discovered it in the aneurisms removed from the walls of a large hemorrhagic focus.

But it is easier to recognise it in the case of certain small foci whose diameter scarcely exceeds that of a hempseed, and the interior of which is generally occupied by a single aneurism.

E. One word on these small hemorrhagic foci, the study of which is, as you will see, very interesting in reference to the pathogenesis of cerebral hemorrhage. They may occur in almost all parts of the encephalon, but they are met with especially in the grey matter of the convolutions; their number is variable; as many as three, four, or even more, may be counted in the same brain, and it is not uncommon to find them accompanying a large hemorrhagic focus in patients who have succumbed to an apoplectic attack. They look like little bloody clots of globular form, and may be easily isolated from the neighbouring parts. It might be supposed at first that one of these foci was a very large miliary aneurism; but a careful dissection discloses the fact that, though the blood clot is not in immediate contact with the cerebral tissue, and is separated from it on all sides by a transparent and very fine membrane, yet this latter is nothing else than the lymphatic sheath considerably distended, and in the centre of the clot you find the miliary aneurism of the usual size, and maintaining its connection with the vessel on which it has grown. In the wall of the aneurism it is often possible to recognise the fissure which has given passage to the blood.

So you see these little hemorrhagic foci represent the first stage of sanguineous apoplexy, but it is doubtless rare for things to remain thus; excessively distended by the pressure of the blood the lymphatic sheath usually ends by bursting. The blood then spreads into the nervous tissue and tears it, thus forming an apoplectic focus of considerable size.

F. This, gentlemen, in my opinion is the mode of production of intra-encephalic hemorrhage in the very large majority of cases. This conclusion I have already presented to you many times during this lecture, and I have endeavoured to base it upon the most varied evidence. It is now time to introduce numbers: now, in a total of 26 cases of cerebral hemorrhage collected at the Salpêtrière in my wards during eighteen months (11 cases of old and 15 of recent hemorrhage), miliary aneurisms were not once absent, and when we have examined them carefully in the walls of a recent focus, we have on several occasions found them ruptured, and have been able to determine that the clotted contents of the aneurism was continuous with the clot of the effusion. To these 26 cases I might add 6 others in which Vulpian has also perceived the coincidence of miliary aneurisms and hemorrhage, and 8 more which have been collected in various hospital wards by several observers. Two of these cases were observed by my teacher Béhier and formed the subject of one of his clinical lectures. This makes a total of 40 cases of hemorrhage within the brain in which the presence of miliary aneurisms has been well and duly determined. I might multiply still further the number of cases to be cited in support of my assertion. Thus, Gull found a ruptured aneurism in the midst of a hemorrhagic focus in the pons. Out of a total of 16 cases in which Heschl found miliary aneurisms in this organ, though he did not recognise their pathological *rôle*, death occurred in two owing to cerebral hemorrhage. There is, moreover, no doubt that Cruveilhier in one case,* and Calmeil in another,† saw these same aneurisms accompanying cerebral hemorrhage, but without suspecting their nature. Any one may easily convince himself of this by reading the observations made by these authors.‡

At the commencement of our studies on this subject, and before cases were multiplied as they have been since, we were led to suppose that it is only *senile* hemorrhage which depends on the presence of miliary aneurisms. Making our observations in a hospital for old people, we did not for some time meet with miliary aneurisms except in apoplectics of advanced age. But since the first communications in which we asserted the pathological function of these aneurisms, I have had the opportunity of finding them in a woman of 51, who died of cerebral hemorrhage ; again, one of the cases reported by Béhier related to an adult ; and quite recently Bouchard has found numerous miliary aneurisms in the brain of a man of 20, who had succumbed to sanguineous apoplexy.§

* *Anat. pathol.*, bk. xxxiii., pl. 2, fig. 3, Obs. p. 5.

† *Traité des maladies inflammatoires du cerveau*, vol. ii., p. 522. Paris, 1859.

‡ Since the period when this lecture was given, the number of my observations has been considerably increased ; at the present time (Nov., 1868) it exceeds 80. See Charcot and Bouchard, Nouvelles recherches sur la Pathogénie de l'hemorrhagie cérébrale, *Archives de physiologie*, Nos. 1, 5, 6, 1868.

§ Out of 80 cases of cerebral hemorrhage with coincidence of miliary aneurisms, the history of which is given in the last mentioned publication, and in which the age is noted, there are 13 cases of patients not more than 55 years old ; these cases are thus distributed : 55 years, 2 ; 54 years, 1 ; 52 years, 1 ; 51 years, 1 ; 50 years, 2 ; 47 years 2 ; 45 years, 1 ; 43 years, 1 ; 40 years, 1 ; 20 years, 1.

You see, gentlemen, the rôle of diffuse periarteritis and miliary aneurisms tends to grow more and more prominent in the pathogenic history of cerebral apoplexy. I have no doubt that we shall be led some day to refer to this same organic cause a certain number of cases of cerebral hemorrhage, which have hitherto been referred to the influence of a blood change, or to still other causes. In support of this opinion I will only mention the two following cases. It is well known that Beau and Duchassaing were obliged to regard anæmia as the cause of some cases of cerebral hemorrhage, and adduced some examples which seemed at first sight to confirm their view of the matter.* Now there was a woman admitted into the Salpêtrière, 51 years of age, whom repeated hemorrhages, caused by a uterine polypus, had for many years thrown into a state of profound anæmia ; she rapidly sank under an apoplectic attack with hemiplegia. At the autopsy I found in the brain a large hemorrhagic focus with miliary aneurisms perfectly developed and in large numbers. The arteries at the base and their chief branches showed no trace of atheromatous lesion.

In a case of severe jaundice consequent on complete obliteration of the bile duct, which was observed in Vulpian's practice, death ensued as a consequence of cerebral hemorrhage. On this occasion also miliary aneurisms were found distributed in large numbers through different portions of the encephalon. If the search for aneurisms had not been made, one might perhaps have been led to consider the cerebral effusion in the first case as the result of profound anæmia, and it is almost certain that the second would have been regarded as a direct consequence of the hemorrhagic diathesis which so frequently accompanies grave icterus.

But although in my opinion the majority of cases of cerebral hemorrhage have their starting-point in the rupture of miliary aneurisms, I by no means go so far as to maintain that every case has such an origin. Without doubt there are cases—and their number is considerable—in which the effusion depends on causes quite different. But cases of this kind must on all accounts form a group to themselves, and in due time we shall devote to them a special notice.

G. There is one question which must often have presented

* Duchassaing, Mémoire sur certaines affections cérébrales qui dépendent de la chloro-anémie, *Journal de médecine*, Dec., 1844, p. 354.

itself to your minds during the course of this description, and I cannot avoid mentioning it by the way—have miliary aneurisms any relation to the aneurisms of other parts of the body? If it were strictly true that these latter are necessarily dependent on arterial atheroma, as is usually supposed, the question would at once be decided in the negative, since miliary aneurisms depend on a vascular lesion which has nothing in common with endarteritis. In that case they would depend on morbid changes quite distinct in nature from each other. Several authors, and especially Bizot,* Virchow,† Broca,‡ and Richet,§ have already protested against the common opinion, and have pointed out that aneurisms of the visceral cavities and of the limbs are not by any means always the result of atheromatous alteration in the arteries. As for aneurisms of the arteries at the base of the encephalon, I can assert, both from the observations of Gouguenheim and Lebert, and from my own, that they have usually no essential connection with atheroma, a character which associates them with miliary aneurisms, with which, moreover, they pretty frequently coexist. From what precedes it appears probable that these intra-cerebral aneurisms, and those of the other visceral cavities, as well as of the limbs, may develop simultaneously in the same person, under the influence of the same cause acting upon the whole arterial system; neither is it improbable that in the interior of other viscera than the brain, saccular dilatations will be found growing on the finest arterioles, altogether resembling miliary aneurisms. Hitherto no case can be cited in support of these views; they are, however, worthy, in my opinion, of further investigation.‖

H. I desire to give you now a few words on the history of this subject.

* Bizot, quoted by Lebert, *Virchow's Handbuch*, vol. v., § 2, p. 11.
† Virchow, *Cellular Pathology*.
‡ Broca, *Traité des tumeurs*, vol. i., p. 147.
§ Richet, quoted by Lefort, article " Aneurism," in the *Dictionnaire encyclopédique*, p. 529.
‖ While these pages were in the press, M. Liouville communicated to the Société de Biologie three cases, taken from Vulpian's practice at the Salpêtrière, in which the coincidence of miliary aneurisms in the brain with aneurisms of small size on the arterioles of various viscera was observed. In the first case there were on the two branches of the splenic artery two aneurisms of the size of a pea, rounded and with thick walls, but still permeable. In another patient there were real miliary aneurisms met with under the visceral layer of pericardium and under the mucous coat of the œsophagus. (Liouville, Reports of the *Société de Biologie*, 1868.)

There is no doubt that miliary aneurisms were noticed and described, at least in certain portions of the encephalon or its membranes, previously to the publication of the researches which Bouchard and I made together; but it is equally certain that no one before us had comprehended or even suspected the important part which these aneurisms, and the arteritis which causes them, are called on to play in the pathogeny of cerebral hemorrhage.

Cruveilhier* was no doubt the first to see, and figure in his atlas, these little bodies which we speak of as miliary aneurisms. But he thought that they were little apoplectic foci, "globules of blood," as he called them, in immediate contact with the nervous substance, and not aneurisms at all.

Virchow † has long described those little saccular aneurisms which develop on the arterioles of the meninges ; he has carefully indicated the most important peculiarities of their structure, and made known the chief phases of their growth ; he has even expressed the opinion that the rupture of these aneurisms is the cause of intra-cranial hemorrhages in more cases than is commonly supposed. But I do not think it is possible to extract from the works of this great observer a single passage in which he makes mention of similar aneurisms situated in the interior of the cerebral substance, in the striate body for example, or the thalamus, which can be regarded as the cause of hemorrhage in the encephalon.

The case in which Gull‡ found a ruptured aneurism in the centre of a hemorrhagic focus, occupying the pons, seems to have been considered by that author as quite exceptional.

Meynert § and Heschl ‖ have observed and described miliary aneurisms in the interior of the pons and in other parts of the encephalon, but I do not think they dreamt of establishing any connection whatever between the existence of these aneurisms and the production of sanguineous apoplexy. Their principal object seems to have been to criticise a hypothesis of Schröder van der Kolk, and to inquire whether these vascular dilatations exert any influence on the development of epilepsy.

* *Anatomie Pathologique*, part xxxiii., pl. II., fig. 3. See the case reported at page 5 of the same part.

† *Archiv für path. Anat.*, vol. iii., p. 442.—*Handbuch*, vol. i., p. 241.

‡ *Guy's Hospital Reports*, 1859, p. 281. § *Centralblatt*, 1864, p. 528.

‖ *Wiener medicinische Wochenschrift*, 1865, 6 and 9 Sep.

After this retrospective examination you will allow us to consider the opinion which we entertain concerning the *rôle* of aneurisms in the production of cerebral hemorrhage as quite our own, and we shall be permitted to assume the whole responsibility of it.

I do not wish to leave the subject of miliary aneurisms without dwelling a few moments on the analogies which they offer to the larger aneurisms of the arteries at the base of the brain. I told you just now of the coincidence, which does not seem to be very uncommon, of these latter with miliary aneurisms ; I relied on this coincidence when I said that they were no doubt dependent on the same arterial change. But the coincidence of these two varieties of aneurism, pretty frequent as it is, is not the sole argument that may be made use of in favour of their identity in nature ; for I think there are striking resemblances to be observed between them. Thus, as Lebert has remarked, the walls of aneurisms which occur on the arteries of the circle are rarely atheromatous, even in persons of advanced age.* Although beyond the limits of the enlargement the vessel may sometimes be atheromatous, this is the case much less frequently than you might be inclined to suppose.† These analogies, though negative, deserved to be mentioned ; neither miliary aneurisms nor other intra-cranial aneurisms are dependent on arterial atheroma, and this circumstance is alone sufficient to suggest the supposition that these two forms of aneurism differ only in the calibre of the diseased arteries, and not in the nature of the primary lesion.

But there are other traits of resemblance. Aneurisms of the arteries at the base of the brain—this observation is also Lebert's —have generally thin walls ; and if they are in the form of a pouch, the orifice of communication between the cavity of the sac and the lumen of the vessel is usually large ; both these conditions peculiarly predispose to rupture. Thus, out of

* H. Lebert, On Aneurisms of the Cerebral Arteries, in *Berliner klinische Wochenschrift*, No. 20, 14th May, 1866.

† In a case of intra-cranial aneurism of the right internal carotid, recently published by W. Ebstein of Breslau, the walls of the dilatation were thin like those of the normal artery, and showed no trace of atheromatous change. The other arteries at the base of the brain offered all the characters of health in this patient, with the exception of some opaque spots of little importance. (*Wiener med. Presse*, 10th Jan., 1869).

86 cases which that author has collected, rupture occurred 48 times, that is to say, in nearly three-fifths of the cases.

The immediate effect of the rupture is the formation of a more or less circumscribed effusion of blood within the skull. Sometimes this effusion occupies the arachnoid cavity, sometimes it is sub-meningeal, and in this latter case it has sometimes been noticed to be restricted within tolerably narrow limits, and to lacerate the nervous substance in its neighbourhood. In this way is produced a softening *by attrition*, resembling the zone of soften-ing, which frequently exists around intra-cerebral effusions con-sequent on the rupture of miliary aneurisms. This fact, I may say in passing, is of importance for us, because it will help to show how slight a foundation has the theory of *ramollissement hémorrhagipare*.

From the clinical point of view these two kinds of aneurism will likewise deserve to be associated. We shall see, in fact, that rupture of aneurisms on the circle of Willis gives rise to a form of fulminating apoplexy, which we must liken to that resulting from hemorrhage within the brain. There is still another clinical analogy which I must mention to you: in the same way as miliary aneurisms produce in their neighbourhood an irritation of the cerebral tissue, which is manifested by more or less definite symptoms, so the larger aneurisms at the base may also give rise to a form of encephalitis in the superficial portions of the encephalon near them; but the symptomatic manifestations of this are more serious.

Aneurisms of the arteries at the base of the brain do not con-stitute a very rare lesion. During the last ten years the number of observations concerning them has much increased, and I am disposed to think that they will continue to be regarded as more common in proportion as they are looked for more attentively.*

---

* I borrow from the thesis of M. Durand, a pupil of the Salpêtrière, the following table, which corrects and completes that of Lebert:—

LOCALITY OF ANEURISMS ON THE ARTERIES AT THE BASE OF THE BRAIN IN 128 CASES.

Internal carotid	21	Basilar trunk	36
Anterior cerebral	13	Vertebrals	5
Anterior communicating	2	Superior cerebellar	1
Middle cerebral	34	Cerebellar, locality not stated	1
Posterior communicating	8	Inferior cerebellar	3
Posterior cerebral	3	Middle meningeal	1

Durand, *Des anévrismes du cerveau*, Thèse de Paris, 1868.

Most of the published cases relate to enlargements of some size, and there are not many in which the aneurisms are very small (size of a pea, for example). Everything, however, tends to the opinion that in reality these small aneurisms are not really less common than the larger dilatations, and that hitherto they have generally been overlooked. We must therefore expect to see aneurisms of the circle assuming greater importance in practice from day to day.

May the analogy be pushed still further, and, having shown the affinity between miliary aneurisms and the other intra-cranial aneurisms, may we also establish some relationship between miliary aneurisms and those of the viscera or limbs? I have already touched on this subject, and I have told you that the common opinion, which attributed these latter to arterial atheroma, has been forcibly shaken. Atheroma is no doubt a cause of aneurisms, but these may not be the most numerous ; atheroma, again, may be observed in the walls of an aneurismal pouch, but very frequently this is only a consecutive change, a mere complication, and is far from being the primary and funda-mental event. What is of most importance is the weakening of the arterial walls, which seems to be due to the atrophy of the middle coat. There are, therefore, no essential differences to point out between the aneurisms of the intra-cerebral vessels and those of the other parts of the system. But will clinical or anatomical observation, besides showing the coincidence of these two forms of aneurism, succeed in proving that they are the result of the same general affection of the arterial system? This is probable, but it is a point which can only be demon-strated by further investigations.

[*The three preceding chapters form part of a second series of lectures, the rest of which have never been published.*—TRANSL.]

FINIS.

INDEX.

LONDON:
PRINTED BY JAS. TRUSCOTT AND SON,
Suffolk Lane, City.

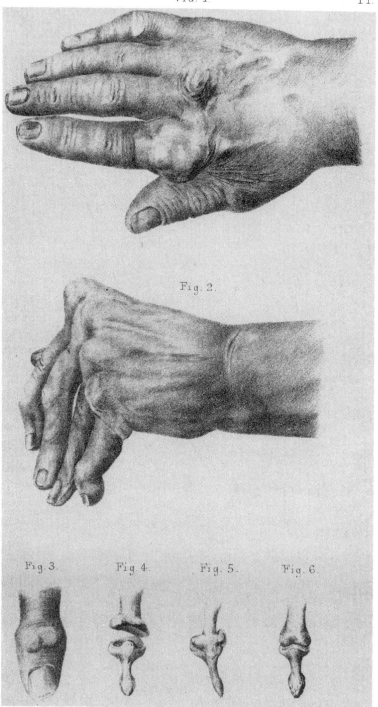

Fig. 1.   Pl. 1.

Fig. 2.

Fig. 3.   Fig. 4.   Fig. 5.   Fig. 6.

P. Linckerbauer ad nat. del.

Pl. II.

Fig. 1.

Fig. 2.

Fig. 3.

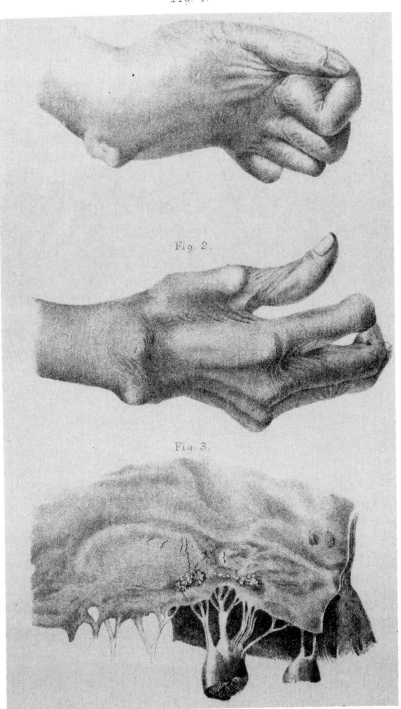

P. Lackerbauer et Charcot ad nat. del.

West Newman & Cº lith.

Pl. III.

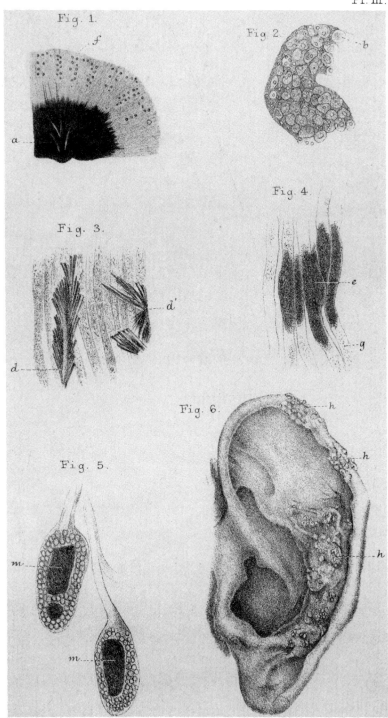

Fig. 1.

f

a

Fig 2.

b

Fig. 3.

d'

d

Fig. 4.

e

g

Fig. 5.

m

m

Fig. 6.

h

h

h

Cornil et Charcot del

West Newman & Cᵒ litᵗ

Pl. IV

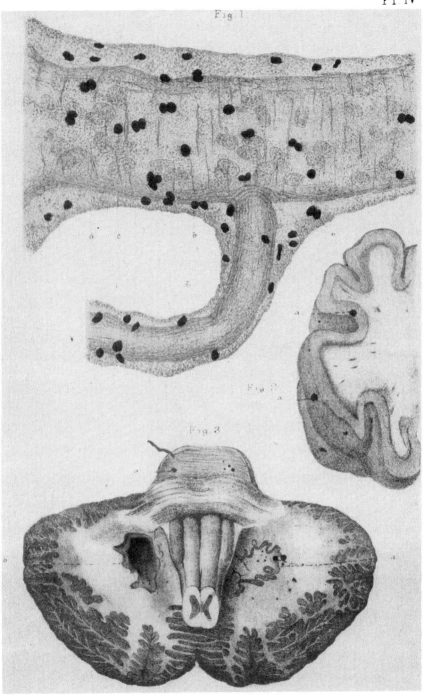

Fig 1

Fig 2

Fig 3

Charcot ad nat del.   West Newman & Co. lith.

Pl. V.

Fig. 1.

Fig. 2.

c

b

a

Fig. 3.

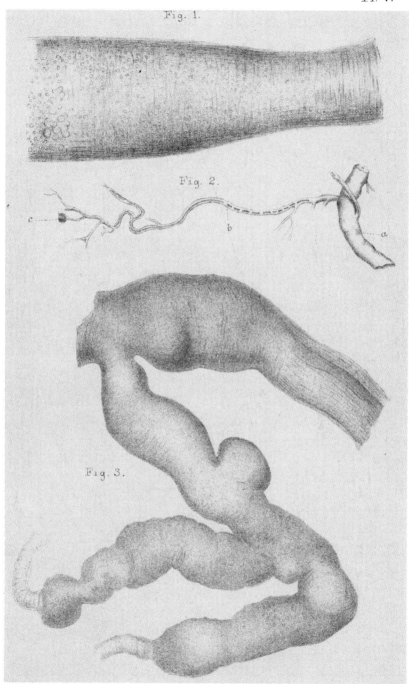

Charcot ad nat. del.

West Newman & Cº lith.

Pl. VI

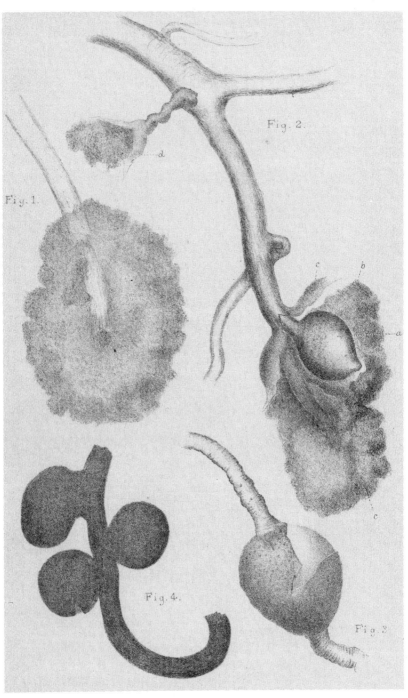

Charcot ad nat del.

West Newman & Co. lith

AGING AND OLD AGE

An Arno Press Collection

(Armstrong, John). **The Art of Preserving Health.** 1744

Canstatt, Carl. **Die Krankheiten des Hoheren Alters Und Ihre Heilung.** 1839

Carlisle, Anthony. **An Essay on the Disorders of Old Age, and on the Means for Prolonging Human Life.** 1818

Cavan, Ruth Shonle, et al. **Personal Adjustment in Old Age.** 1949

Charcot, J(ean) M(artin). **Clinical Lectures on Senile and Chronic Diseases.** 1881

Cheyne, George. **An Essay of Health and Long Life.** 1724

Child, Charles. **Sensecence and Rejuvenescence.** 1915

Cicero, M(arcus) T(ullius). **Cato Major.** 1744

(Cohausen, Johann Heinrich). **Hermippus Redivivus.** 1771

Cornaro, Luigi. **The Art of Living Long.** 1917

Cowdry, E. V., ed. **Problems of Ageing.** 1939

Cumming, Elaine and William E. Henry. **Growing Old.** 1961

Day, George E. **A Practical Treatise on the Domestic Management and Most Important Diseases of Advanced Life.** 1849

Department for the Aging, City of New York. **Older Women in the City.** 1979

Floyer, John. **Medicina Gerocomica.** 1724

Gruman, Gerald J., ed. **The "Fixed Period" Controversy.** 1979

Gruman, Gerald J., ed. **Roots of Modern Gerontology and Geriatrics.** 1979

(Hufeland, Christoph Wilhelm). **Art of Prolonging Life.** 1854

Jameson, Thomas. **Essays on the Changes of the Human Body at Its Different Ages.** 1811

Kirk, Hyland Clare. **When Age Grows Young.** 1888

Kleemeier, Robert W., ed. **Aging and Leisure.** 1961

Lessius, Leonard and Lewis Cornaro. **A Treatise of Health and Long Life With the Future Means of Attaining It.** 1743

MacKenzie, James. **The History of Health, and the Art of Preserving It.** 1760

Martin, Lillien J(ane) and Clare de Gruchy. **Sweeping the Cobwebs.** 1933

Minot, Charles S. *The Problem of Age, Growth, and Death.* 1908

Nascher, I(gnatz) L(eo). **Geriatrics.** 1914

Pearl, Raymond and Ruth DeWitt Pearl. **The Ancestry of the Long-Lived.** 1934

Ramon y Cajal, S(antiago). **El Mundo Visto a Los Ochenta Anos.** 1934

de Ropp, Robert S. **Man Against Aging.** 1960

Stieglitz, Edward J. **The Second Forty Years.** 1946

Sweetser, William. **Human Life.** 1867

Thoms, William J. **Human Longevity.** 1873

Tibbitts, Clark, ed. **Living Through the Older Years.** 1949

Tolstoy, Leo. **Last Diaries.** 1960

Vercors (pseud. Jean Bruller). **The Insurgents.** 1956

Warthin, Aldred Scott. **Old Age.** 1929